ORGANIC VOICE DISORDERS

Assessment and Treatment

ORGANIC VOICE DISORDERS

Assessment and Treatment

Edited by

Wm. S. Brown, Jr., Ph.D.

Professor and Chair

Betsy Partin Vinson, M.M.Sc.

Director of Clinical Education
Department of Communication Processes and Disorders
University of Florida

Michael A. Crary, Ph.D.

Professor and Chair
Department of Communicative Disorders
College of Health Professions
University of Florida Health Science Center

SINGULAR PUBLISHING GROUP, INC.
SAN DIEGO · LONDON

MW

11/21/02

Contents

Contributors

Diane Bless, Ph.D.
Professor
Waisman Center Voice Lab
Otolaryngology, Head and Neck Surgery
University of Wisconsin
Madison, Wisconsin

Wm. S. Brown, Jr., Ph.D.
Professor and Chair
Department of Communication Processes
    and Disorders
University of Florida
Gainesville, Florida

Nicholas J. Cassisi, M.D.
Professor and Chair
Department of Otolaryngology
University of Florida
College of Medicine
Gainesville, Florida

Françoise Chagnon, M.D.
Department of Otolaryngology
Montreal General Hospital
Montreal, Quebec
Canada

Raymond S. Colton, Ph.D.
Professor
Department of Otolaryngology
SUNY Health Science Center
Syracuse, New York

Donald S. Cooper, Ph.D.
Professor
ENT Research
USC Medical School
Los Angeles, California

Mark S. Courey, M.D.
Medical Director
Vanderbilt Voice Center
Assistant Professor
Department of Otolaryngology
Vanderbilt University Medical Center
Nashville, Tennessee

Michael A. Crary, Ph.D.
Professor and Chair
Department of Communicative Disorders
College of Health Professions
University of Florida Health Sciences
    Center
Gainesville, Florida

Charles N. Ford, M.D., F.A.C.S.
Professor, Otolaryngology, Head and Neck
    Surgery
Center for Health Sciences
University of Wisconsin Hospital and
    Clinics
Madison, Wisconsin

Ann Glowaski, M.D.
North Central Florida ENT Associates
Gainesville, Florida

Douglas M. Hicks, Ph.D.
Director, The Voice Center
Head, Speech-Language Pathology
Department of Otolaryngology and
    Communicative Disorders (A71)
The Cleveland Clinic Foundation
Cleveland, Ohio

Joel C. Kahane, Ph.D.
Professor
Director of the Anatomical Sciences
    Laboratory
School of Audiology and Speech-Language
    Pathology
The University of Memphis
Memphis, Tennessee

G. Paul Moore, Ph.D.
Distinguished Service Professor, Emeritus
Department of Communication Processes
    and Disorders
University of Florida
Gainesville, Florida

Thomas Murry, Ph.D.
Professor
University of Pittsburgh
Eye and Ear Institute
Pittsburgh, Pennsylvania

Robert H. Ossoff, D.M.D., M.D.
Guy M. Maness Professor and Chair
Department of Otolaryngology
Vanderbilt University Medical Center
Nashville, Tennessee

Thomas R. Pasic, M.D.
Assistant Professor, Otolaryngology, Head
    and Neck Surgery
Center for Health Sciences
University of Wisconsin Hospital and
    Clinics
Madison, Wisconsin

Lorraine Olson Ramig, Ph.D.
Professor
Department of Communication Disorders
    and Speech Science
University of Colorado
Boulder, Colorado

Christine Sapienza, Ph.D.
Assistant Professor
Department of Communication Processes
    and Disorders
University of Florida
Gainesville, Florida

R. E. (Ed) Stone, Jr., Ph.D.
Associate Professor
Vanderbilt Voice Center
Vanderbilt University Medical Center
Nashville, Tennessee

Betsy Partin Vinson, M.M.Sc.
Director of Clinical Education
Department of Communication Processes
    and Disorders
University of Florida
Gainesville, Florida

Hans von Leden, M.D.
Professor
Los Angeles, California

Peak Woo, M.D.
Department of Otolaryngology
Mt. Snow Medical Center
New York, New York

Gayle E. Woodson, M.D., F.R.C.S.
Professor
University of Tennessee
College of Medicine
Department of Otolaryngology
Memphis, Tennessee

Foreword

When I returned from the Naval Service at the completion of World War II and settled in Chicago, my practice included a high percentage of patients with vocal problems. Somewhat to my surprise, for I had been trained at a highly respected institution, I discovered that I knew very little about the physiology of phonation. Even worse, I felt that the standard medical therapy for the care of the professional voice users was inadequate and sometimes even deleterious.

At this crucial period in my professional development, I attended a meeting of the Chicago Society of Otolaryngology, during which G. Paul Moore, Ph.D. showed one of his high-speed motion pictures on laryngeal vibrations. I was fascinated! Could these mysterious "traveling waves" assist me in providing better care for my patients? I was determined to find out, and a few days later I was on my way to the Evanston campus of Northwestern University where Dr. Moore served as an Associate Professor of Speech. There and then started a professional association which affected the development of our two specialties, and a friendship which has lasted for more than 40 years and which eventually spanned a continent.

Regrettably, the Department of Speech at Northwestern University did not have the resources for our utopian program. However, Dr. George Shambaugh, the renowned otologic surgeon and Chairman of the Department of Otolaryngology at Northwestern University Medical Center, agreed to give up two rooms of his own meager allotment for the first interdisciplinary voice research laboratory on the North American continent. We began our studies of the larynx with an expansion of the photographic analyses which Paul Moore had pioneered. At the same time, we set up the first multidisciplinary voice clinic which included representatives from the fields of laryngology, speech pathology, pediatrics, neurology, and psychiatry to assure a more comprehensive approach to the clinical diagnosis and treatment of patients with complex vocal problems.

Two or three years later when the facilities at the Medical Center proved inadequate for our expanding program, two grateful patients, Mr. William E. Gould of Chicago and his wife Harriet, provided the necessary resources in a commercial building near the Medical Center. Paul Moore became the Director of the new "Institute of Laryngology and Voice Disorders." In this capacity, Paul conducted and supervised research on normal and pathologic human subjects and animals, gross and microscopic anatomic studies, stroboscopic tests, photographic analyses at normal and ultra-high speeds (up to 5,000 pictures per second), acoustic evaluations of the voice involving normal and artificial larynges, and a series of other physiologic and patho-physiologic examinations.

On the basis of these studies, we were able to refute Husson's neuro-chronaxic theory of phonation, which was then in vogue in France and some other European countries, and to reaffirm the myo-elastic theory which had been elaborated by the

German physiologist, Johannes Muller, in the first half of the 19th century. Our experiments also led to the recommended term "aero-dynamic" theory of phonation as more appropriate for this phenomenon. A series of educational motion pictures was the by-product of this research. For their outstanding work, Paul and his associates were honored with several national and international awards which brought honor to our Institute and to our country. About this time, Paul Moore also developed the first portable apparatus for television via indirect laryngoscopy, an impressive accomplishment given the state of technology almost 40 years ago!

Throughout this period, Paul stressed the need for a team approach for better care of phoniatric disabilities. We traveled together to colleges and universities all over the Midwest, and we lectured together at major medical and speech conventions to broadcast this new concept of collaboration for both research and clinical care. At first, not all of our colleagues were inspired by this deviation from their standard program, but gradually the message took hold as our results became apparent.

Undoubtedly, the highlight of Paul's affiliation with Northwestern University and the Institute of Laryngology and Voice Disorders was his role in the First International Voice Conference which brought clinicians and scientists from 23 countries together in Chicago during the spring of 1957. The participants included leading educators and clinicians from the fields of speech pathology, laryngology, and music (singing), and the presentations covered every then known facet of phonation. For many of the visitors, this conference presented the first opportunity to watch Paul Moore's team spirit in action.

A few years after this great demonstration of voice as a multidisciplinary science, Paul Moore accepted the chairmanship of the Department of Speech at the University of Florida, and shortly thereafter, I moved the Institute of Laryngology and Voice Disorders to Southern California. In his new position, Paul climbed from success to success. With his ingenious pupil, Harry Hollien, Paul developed the renowned Institute for the Advanced Study of Communication Processes (IASCP) which attracted scholars and scientists from the North American continent as well as Europe. Numerous contributions to the literature document the spirit of exploration and discovery at this center of experimentation and learning.

For Paul Moore, honor followed honor and award followed award: In 1961, the Presidency of the American Speech and Hearing Association (ASHA), in 1962 the Merit Award of the American Academy of Ophthalmology and Otolaryngology and the Gould Award (of the William and Harriet Gould Foundation in Chicago). In the same year, Paul was elected to the Editorial Board of the *Archives of Otolaryngology*, and a few years later to the Editorial Board of the *Folia Phoniatrica*. In 1964, he received the international Barraquet Award, and in 1974, the University of West Virginia presented him with the honorary degree of Doctor of Science. In 1976, he was given the Teacher/Scholar Award of the University of Florida, and in the following year, the Honor Award of the Florida Language, Speech and Hearing Association. Also, in 1977, Paul was elected President of the American Speech and Hearing Foundation (ASHF), and in 1979, he delivered the Chevalier Jackson Lecture of the American Broncho-Esophagologic Association. A special lecture at the Voice Foundation's Annual Symposium on the Care of the Professional Voice was named the G. Paul Moore Lecture.

In addition to all his other responsibilities, Paul found the time to serve on important consulting assignments at the National Institute of Health, at the Vocational Rehabilitation Administration, and on various advisory boards of the Division of Chronic Diseases, the National Institute for Neurologic Diseases and Blindness and the National Institute for Neurologic Diseases and Stroke. He also served with distinction on the American Board of Examiners of Speech Pathology and Audiology.

Last but not least, Paul has traveled all over the North American continent as a Visiting Professor and as a popular lecturer. His professional engagements have taken him as far as the Union of South Africa. In 1977, Paul was promoted to the position of Distinguished Service Professor at the University of Florida and in 1980 received the exalted status of a Distinguished Service Professor Emeritus. Yet today, 18 years later, Paul Moore is still active in his beloved Communication Sciences Laboratory (presently called the Institute for Advanced Studies of the Communication Processes), and is in demand as a valued lecturer.

Paul has collaborated in the preparation of 15 textbooks, authored more than 60 articles, and produced numerous films, videotapes, and exhibits in his chosen field of voice production. He has seen his dream of elevating the field of phonation to a respected science come to fruition, and he has been one of the acknowledged leaders in this new specialty. So it seems only just that this book, *Organic Voice Disorders: Assessment and Treatment*, be dedicated to this distinguished educator, scientist, academician, and clinician in recognition and appreciation of his pioneering approach to voice as a multidisciplinary art and science.

Hans von Leden, M.D.

Preface

Organic Voice Disorders: Assessment and Treatment is an edited textbook for individuals who have an interest in studying human voice production. It is intended to be a definitive text that reflects the current trends in prevention, assessment, diagnosis, and treatment of voice disorders. The authors of the chapters represent a cross section of active individuals in medicine, speech-language pathology, and professional voice use who have been influenced by Professor G. Paul Moore's teachings, writings, and/or collaborative efforts.

In 1950, Dr. Moore published what, at the time, was also a definitive text to guide those who were studying and researching the human voice. Entitled *Organic Voice Disorders*, it has served as the inspiration for the development of this book. In his original text, Dr. Moore stressed the need for interdisciplinary teamwork in researching, diagnosing, and treating voice disorders. Through his own interactions with professionals in medicine, music, engineering, and speech-language pathology, Dr. Moore developed an empirical database for understanding phonatory dysfunction and formed the foundations for modern voice examination and treatment.

The book is divided into four sections. Section I (Chapters 1–4) is a study of the anatomical and physiological aspects of the voice. In Chapter 1, Donald Cooper, Ph.D., presents an historical perspective of the study of voice and its disorders from its inception to present day practices.

Spanning a period of over 2,000 years, Dr. Cooper has written an unparalleled history of the study of vocal production.

Chapter 2 is an updated version of the anatomy chapter written by Dr. Moore in *Organic Voice Disorders* (Moore, 1950). In a companion chapter, Raymond Colton, Ph.D. describes the physiology of normal vocal fold function. The major emphasis of Chapter 3 is discussion of the acoustic and perceptual dimensions of normal voice. Dr. Colton offers a review of the work of Dr. Moore and his colleagues with high speed films and discusses how it relates to the work of other investigators of vocal physiology. Information from stroboscopic analysis of vocal fold vibration is also presented.

In Chapter 4, Joel Kahane, Ph.D., expands the anatomical and physiological chapters a step further, looking at lifespan changes in the larynx. Dr. Kahane presents information on the structure and function of the larynx in infancy, childhood, adolescence, and adulthood.

Section II of the book, chapters 5–7 provide an overview of the assessment and treatment of voice disorders. In Chapter 5, Gayle Woodson, M.D., discusses the need for interdisciplinary approaches in research, assessment, diagnosis, and treatment of voice disorders. Dr. Woodson specifically addresses the contributions and interactions of otolaryngologists, speech-language pathologists, internists, neurologists, psychiatrists, psychologists, gastroenterologists, pulmonary specialists, voice teachers, and speech scientists in research and clinical roles.

Chapter 6 is authored by Diane Bless, Ph.D. and Douglas Hicks, Ph.D.. Drs. Bless and Hicks provide an overview of strategies, instrumentation, and procedures available to assess and diagnose normal and abnormal voice production. A variety of approaches to treatment are discussed in Chapter 7, also by Hicks and Bless. This chapter offers an explanation of procedures, strategies, and instruments that can be used to treat a wide range of organic voice disorders.

In Sections III (Chapters 8–13) and IV (Chapters 14–16), specific voice disorders are presented. In each of these chapters, the authors provide a definition of the disorder and discuss etiological, demographic, medical, and social factors and considerations. They describe the onset and course of the disorder, as well as information related specifically to diagnosis and treatment of the disorder. Finally, the importance of interdisciplinary interaction in handling patients with voice disorders is stressed in each chapter.

Section III is dedicated to discussion of voice disorders related to inflammation, edema, and lesions. In Chapter 8, Peak Woo, M.D., offers an in-depth discussion of a variety of factors that can irritate the larynx and result in vocal change. Dr. Woo also presents the etiological and symptomatic features of acute and chronic laryngitis, and their implications for assessment, differential diagnosis, and treatment.

In Chapter 9, Francoise Chagnon, M.D., and Ed Stone, Ph.D. discuss benign focal lesions of the vocal folds (polyps and nodules). Guidelines for the decision-making process involved in differential diagnosis and appropriate courses of treatment are provided.

Intracordal lesions, that is, lesions of Reinke's space, are discussed by Mark Courey, M.D. and Robert H. Ossoff, D.M.D., M.D. in Chapter 10. Several disorders, including sulcus vocalis, scar tissue, true cysts, mucosal retention, and polypoid corditis, are discussed.

Charles N. Ford, M.D., presents information related to the relatively rare, but potentially life-threatening, problem of laryngeal papilloma in Chapter 11. The temporary and prolonged effects of papilloma in both childhood and adulthood are presented. In Chapter 12, Thomas Pasic, M.D. follows a similar format as he discusses information related to laryngeal ulcers. Differential diagnosis and treatment of contact ulcers due to voice abuse, prolonged endotracheal intubation, and gastroesophageal reflux are discussed. Voice disorders associated with malignant lesions of the larynx are the topic of Chapter 13 by Nicholas J. Cassisi, M.D., Christine Sapienza, Ph.D., and Betsy Partin Vinson, M.M.Sc. Discussion of the role of a variety of specialists in the care of the patient and his or her family provides the health-care professional with insight into the multidimensional problems associated with malignancies.

The final section of the book, Section IV, is dedicated to the study of voice problems due to movement disorders. In Chapter 14, Michael Crary, Ph.D. and Ann Glowaski, M.D. address the pervasive problem of vocal fold immobility. Drs. Crary and Glowaski present an in-depth explanation of the causes, evaluation, and treatment of voice disorders due to vocal fold immobility. Specific neurological disorders that can result in voice disorders is the topic discussed by Lorraine Ramig, Ph.D., in Chapter 15. Dr. Ramig addresses a variety of disorders including myasthenia gravis, myotonic muscular dystrophy, Parkinson disease, Huntington's disease, and essential tremor. The last chapter of the book, *Spasmodic Dysphonia*, by Thomas

Murry, Ph.D. and Gayle E. Woodson, M.D., answers many of the questions frequently asked about this chronic and often disabling voice disorder. A comprehensive discussion of the pathophysiology of this disorder, as well as guidelines for definitive diagnosis and treatment, is offered.

Organic Voice Disorders: Assessment and Treatment offers a unique opportunity for students and professionals intersted in studying the voice and its disorders to do so from the perspective of the otolaryngologist and the speech-language pathologist, both of whom are key members of a voice care team. The historical and current perspectives on voice care are presented in keeping with the philosopies of Dr. Moore, whose influence in this realm of study spans almost 60 years.

It has been an honor and a privilege to work on this book in honor of G. Paul Moore, and we sincerely thank all of those who so willingly contributed to this project. We consider ourselves to be very fortunate to work with Dr. Moore on a daily basis and to have the continuing opportunity to benefit from his knowledge and dedication as he teaches professionals and students from many disciplines about the mystery and magic of the human voice.

DEDICATION

Organic Voice Disorders: Assessment and Treatment
is dedicated to G. Paul Moore, Ph.D., whose
teachings, research, and writings have influenced
literally thousands of professionals in the field of voice
for nearly six decades.

CHAPTER 1

THE DISCIPLINE OF VOICE: AN HISTORICAL PERSPECTIVE

DONALD S. COOPER, PH.D.
HANS VON LEDEN, M.D.

The multifaceted discipline of voice has called on contributions from many specialties for its creation, just as does its clinical practice. In this chapter, we will start from the development of varying conceptions of the human voice and vocal production, descriptions of the structures that underlie it, and their pathology. These factors have been prerequisites for the gradual recognition of voice-related disorders of the larynx and the creation of the corresponding professional specialties.

The pulmonary system, which provides the power source for the voice, has been the subject of a rich harvest of monographs and reviews during recent decades. Consequently, this chapter will emphasize the physiological role of the larynx in voice production, which is more often the focus of clinical concerns for voice. Not all aspects of this work have been the subject of the careful preliminary study that Moore (1937, 1991) gave to the history of the optical examination of the larynx and phona-

tion; thus, only further special investigations will make it possible to see the contributions of many researchers in a just perspective.

EARLY CONCEPTS OF VOICE AND ITS PRODUCTION

Some artifacts and traditions of peoples outside the Western written tradition suggest a primitive effort to conceptualize breath, voice, and speech. For example, ancient Egyptian artifactual representations of the lungs and trachea are interpreted as representing the connection between continuity of breath on the one hand and life or the soul on the other (Panconcelli-Calzia, 1957b). However, the interpretation of such images may be unclear when it is not supported by a verbal tradition, as in the Biblical references to speech problems. In the East, the seminal tradition stemmed from China. The ancient Chinese textual tradition makes it clear that laryngeal function and voice production were the subject of Chinese medical thought at least two millennia ago and perhaps much earlier (Hübotter, 1929). In the early Chinese view, exhaled air from the lungs caused motion of the hyoid bone, the thyroid cartilage, and the tongue in speaking (Huard & Wong, 1959). However, as in the West, religious prohibition of dissection obstructed the development of anatomical and physiological knowledge during the early period (Kleiweg de Zwaan, 1917).

The earliest civilizations to make lasting contributions to the understanding of voice production were those of ancient India and Greece. The languages of their texts, Sanskrit and Greek, like many languages of Europe and Western Asia, stem from an earlier unwritten common language known as Indo-European, which was spoken about seven millennia ago in some area of prehistoric Eurasia. The Latin word *vox*, from which the English term "voice" is ultimately borrowed, descends from an Indo-European term indicating the acoustic emission of voice, particularly in religious and legal aspects (Ernout & Meillet, 1967).

The Voice of the Indian Tradition

Early Indian scholars turned to the analysis of grammar and phonetics, which they essentially invented to preserve a correct interpretation and pronunciation in the oral tradition of their sacred religious texts. The phonetic sources for our knowledge stem broadly from the first millenium B.C. Although the anatomical knowledge of the larynx shown by Indian medical treatises of roughly the same age is very slight (Kutumbiah, 1962), the ancient Indian phonetic and musical treatises show a considerable understanding of voice production. The phonetic treatises recognized air as the vehicle of the voice, the need for

the development of subglottal pressure, the glottis and the opening and closing of the larynx for voice, perhaps the oscillatory character of voice production, and the relation of pitch control to vocal fold tissue mechanics (Allen, 1953). A variety of sources such as manuals for actors and medical treatises describe voice characteristics, disorders, and their medical treatment (Savithri, 1988).

Voice in the Age of Philosophers

The first hints of early Greek concepts of voice come from the fragments of the pre-Socratic philosophers. Certain prerequisite concepts for the study of voice are found among the followers of the early Greek philosopher Pythagoras who lived from approximately 580–500 B.C. At least the later followers of this school gradually developed a qualitative understanding of such preliminary concepts as the relations between frequency of vibration, auditory pitch, and the length of strings. Certain basic concepts of the transmission of sound through air also were recognized (Hunt, 1978).

We are on firmer ground when we reach an age from which more extensive continuous texts are available. Hippocrates (who lived approximately from 460–370 B.C.) had to refute primitive beliefs such as the notion that the lungs were filled with fluid. He was aware of the role of air as a carrier of sound and the need for participation of the lungs and the integrity of the airway, and he recognized the significance of the articulators for speech, but it is not clear that the Hippocratic school recognized the role of the larynx in voice production (O'Neill, 1980). In his treatise on epidemics, Hippocrates invoked the loss of speech or voice as a symptom of diseases such as wasting, fever, and delirium (Panconcelli-Calzia, 1942).

Although Aristotle, who was born around 384 B.C. and died in 322 B.C., is best known as a philosopher, he was trained as a physician, and biology was a basic sphere of his activity. However, he gives few details on the anatomy and physiology of the larynx. He describes the mechanism of voice production as "the impact of the air that is exhaled by the soul which is in these regions, against the artery (as it is termed) is voice." The term "artery," as used by Aristotle, refers to the trachea. Thus, Aristotle defined the essential character of voice production as a mechanical interaction between the air-stream and the structures enclosing the airstream.

Aristotle was also a careful observer of pubertal voice changes and of the effects of aging, sex differences, and castration on voice. He discussed voice disorders that accompany deafness and nasality. Arisotle also studied the effects of intoxication and desiccation on speech, the effects of eating on professional performance, and the effects of illness, fever, and exercise on voice production (Pan-concelli-Calzia, 1942).

Descriptions of the healing of psychogenic loss of voice in the temple of Asklepios are echoed by similar treatments attributed to Christian clerics (e.g., Gregory of Tours, 538–594 A.D.) during the Middle Ages. A different group, voice professionals and their teachers, must also be recognized from the fifth century B.C.: singers, actors, orators, and statesmen such as Antiphon, Pericles, Demosthenes, and Aristides used daily vocal exercises, prescribed by a special profession of voice teachers (in Greek, *phonaskós*), to strengthen their voices (Reich, 1950; Habermann, 1987).

Voice in the Hellenistic World: Galen

The next historical figure in the study of voice is the Greek physician Galen of Pergamon, who lived about 131–201 A.D. Galen practiced in Rome for much of his life. In his treatise, "On the Usefulness of the Parts of the Body" (quoted after May, 1968) and in his anatomical writings, Galen provided the first genuine portrayal of the structure and function of the larynx. Fragments of a separate treatise on the voice survive. Galen provided anatomical details primarily based on animals. The major cartilages are described, although the two arytenoids are considered as a unit. The vocal folds are termed "membranous lips." He describes the muscles of the larynx, and his own discovery of the recurrent laryngeal nerve. The epiglottis and the closure of the larynx in swallowing are also described in detail. Galen notes that voice cannot be produced without narrowing of the glottal passage. He is clear that "voice is first formed in the larynx" (I, 402). "The larynx is the principal and most important instrument of the voice" he says (II, 385). Although one can point out significant errors in Galen's treatment, they appear against a recognizable anatomy and physiology of the larynx which makes him by far the greatest contributor to the study of the larynx in the whole of antiquity.

Galen also provides examples of various types of clinical disorders of voice and the throat (Habermann, 1987). He distinguishes inflammations of the external neck from those within the larynx that endangered the airway, and warns against vocal abuse. Baths, change of air, blood-letting, bland food, and a variety of lozenges were recommended for treatment. O'Neill (1980) has traced the continuity of ancient views of voice and speech and their disorders through the middle ages.

The Voice of the Practical Romans

The Romans added little to the understanding of voice. Roman medical writings are either compilations of paraphrases from Greek medical writings, or uncritical collections inferior to existing

Greek knowledge (Singer, 1959). However, practicing physicians made use of the understanding of the structures underlying voice for new treatments. For instance, a functional recognition of the role of the windpipe and airflow in voice is implied by the description of the operation of tracheotomy by Antyllus, a Greek physician who practiced in Rome during the second century A.D. The successful penetration of the airway was indicated by the outrush of air from the trachea and the cessation of voice (Weir, 1990).

Much of the practice of Greek and Roman teachers of voice professionals is summarized in the lengthy treatise on the training of orators by the Spanish-born Quintilian (about 35–95 A.D.), whose professional activity took place mainly in Rome. He is clearly aware of the connection between health of the larynx and that of the voice, although with little specificity regarding particular disorders. A variety of vocal exercises in reading and crying aloud, speaking, singing, laughing, and declamation were recommended. Beyond general bodily health and exercise, special procedures such as defecation and massage before exercises in public speaking were advocated (Habermann, 1987).

Greek learning was lost to most of Western Europe after the fall of Rome in 476 A.D. During this period, the language of learning in Western Europe was Latin. Most of the medieval Latin texts of Galen, as well as of a number of other important Greek authors, reflect translation from Arabic (Sarton, 1955). We shall see why.

ISLAMIC MEDICINE AND THE VOICE

With the spread of Islam in the seventh century, Arabic conquests began to extend as far as Spain in the West and Central Asia in the East. Many works of Greek learning and science were translated into Arabic in the Middle Eastern area, and other important translations into Arabic came from Chinese and Indian sources. Scholars within the Islamic cultural sphere also built on the information they received; particularly in the Iberian peninsula, translations from Arabic to Latin often brought this wealth of learning to Europe, especially after the partial reconquest of Spain by the Christians which was marked by the fall of Toledo in 1085. The treatment of voice disorders by important early Islamic medical figures who wrote in Arabic has been described by Daoud (1965), and, in a broader context of speech, O'Neill (1980).

Although all noted here were Persians by birth, they are known by their Arabic names; the Latinized names under which their works circulated in Latin translation are in parentheses: Al-Razi (Rhazes) of Baghdad (865–925); 'Ali ibn el Abbas (Haly Abbas), born near Shiraz, who died in 994; and Ibn Sina (Avicenna) of Bokhara (980–1037).

Other Arabic works were eclipsed in the European view by Avicenna's encyclopedic treatise on medicine, the Medical Canon, based on Greek and early Arabic writers. His many other works include a short treatise on the physiology and acoustics of speech, written in 1024. Like Galen, he describes only the major cartilages of the larynx. He also specifies the laryngeal muscles and their functions in opening, closing, and narrowing the glottis. The effect of the change of angle between the cricoid and thyroid cartilages on voice fundamental frequency change is specified, but is attributed to resulting changes in laryngeal width. In Avicenna's view, a high fundamental frequency is produced when the glottis is narrowed, and a lower one when it is widened. Acoustic subtypes of voice disorders and the physiological and behavioral bases of voice disturbances are considered in the Canon, and recommendations are included for voice rest and breathing exercises.

Not only medicine, but also the fields of musical acoustics and phonetics bear witness to a considerable knowledge of the larynx and voice within the medieval Islamic cultural sphere (Hunt, 1978).

THE REVIVAL OF LEARNING IN EUROPE

After the initial wave of Greek learning in Latinized Arabic dress reached Europe, with the waning of the Dark Ages the next priority of European learning was the recovery, editing, and interpretation of the Greek and Latin texts in which classical knowledge survived. The fall of Constantinople to the Turks in 1453 brought learned Greeks to Western Europe to teach Western scholars and personally collaborate in publication of recovered classical texts by means of the new moveable type (Sarton, 1955).

However, the influence of classical learning was not always beneficial. For centuries it was blindly followed not only by scholars and humanists, but also by physicians, even when the development of knowledge made reference to it for biological and physical information quite anachronisitic. Not only in many medieval illustrations, but in early printed books, the larynx was often ignored and omitted in anatomical figures (Panconcelli-Calzia, 1940, 1942, 1957a). In reaction against this scholastic tradition, the appeal to dissection and the testimony of one's own observations to settle scientific issues marked the revival of critical and scientific learning in a substantial sense, rather than simply the ability to copy out of a book (Sarton, 1955).

THE RENAISSANCE AND EARLY BAROQUE PERIODS IN ITALY

The Medical School of Bologna

Rare exceptions aside, dissection was prohibited in both the Moslem and Christ-ian worlds; the first university whose professors turned systematically to dissection of man as the basis for anatomy was that of Bologna at the beginning of the fourteenth century. The first new anatomical treatise based on examination of the cadaver came in *Anatomy* by Mondino dei Luzzi (1270–1326), professor of anatomy in Bologna. Although barely more than a manual for dissection, Mondino's treatise was the first anatomy of the larynx to be unmistakably based on human material (Panconcelli-Calzia, 1943).

Jacopo Berengario da Carpi, who lived about 1460–1530, was professor of surgery at the University of Bologna in the early sixteenth century. His commentary on the anatomy of Mondino and an original treatise entitled *Brief Introduction* (1522 A.D.), with excellent woodcuts, mark his claim in the history of anatomy. While Galen and Avicenna had treated the two arytenoid cartilages as a single structure, Berengario noted their dual nature. This observation was also made by Leonardo da Vinci and Vesalius.

Leonardo and the Larynx

The contributions of Leonardo da Vinci (1452–1519) to the study of speech and voice have been the topic of a monograph worthy of its subject by Panconcelli-Calzia (1943). Because Leonardo's findings and conclusions were unknown until the investigations of his notebooks at the end of the nineteenth century (O'Malley & Saunders, 1952), it is difficult to relate them to subsequent history. Sometimes Leonardo's information was drawn from animal larynges. He was the first experimenter of record to study voice production with the excised larynx preparation (Cooper, 1993), and his practical experiences in hydraulics doubtless underlie the insight with which he discussed aerodynamic aspects of voice production. He clearly understood the mutually exclusive three functions of the larynx, noting on a notebook page with figures of the larynx that, "One cannot swallow and breathe or emit sound at the same time."

Aesthetic and Performance Aspects of Voice

We can note only samples of developments relating to the professional voice (Reich, 1950). Much of the medieval development of Western formal music had been for religious service. The rules of medieval choral liturgical musical performance were first codified in print by Conrad von Zabern in his treatise on choral performance in 1474. The scholarly physician Girolamo Mercurialis (1531–1616), who was active in Padua and Pisa, revived the classical vocal exercises described above under Quintilian in his 1569 book on the art of gymnastics and discussed disorders of speech and voice in his 1583 treatise on pediatrics (O'Neill, 1980). A creative extension of antiquity came in the establishment of Italian opera at the end of the sixteenth century, and in early Baroque theories of music and singing, with the participation of figures such as Camillo Maffei, singer, physician, and author of a discourse on the voice in 1562 (Habermann, 1987).

The Larynx and the Padua Anatomists

The importance of the University of Padua in anatomical studies is partly explained by the circumstance that it began as an offshoot of the University of Bologna. It produced distinguished medical graduates such as William Harvey (circa 1602) who studied with Fabricius and Casserius. Here we find a gradually more specialized series of contributions to laryngeal anatomy.

The Flemish physician and anatomist Andreas Vesalius (born Andreas van Wesele in 1514) of Brussels was the effective creator of modern anatomy (O'Malley, 1964). His main professorial period was in Padua between 1537 and 1542, although he also lectured in Bologna in 1540. His great treatise, *On the Structure of the Human Body*, was published in Basel when he was only 28 years old; a second edition appeared in 1555. Vesalius spearheaded a thorough turn to the reconstruction of human anatomy based on the witness of the anatomist's own studies of human specimens. He recognized differences between the human larynx and those of animals commonly used for demonstration. Garrison and Hast (1993) have made available an English translation of Vesalius's treatment of the larynx based on both editions of his treatise.

An eyewitness account of Vesalius' lectures in Bologna in 1540 makes clear that Vesalius was generally aware of the role of the vocal folds in voice production, regarding them as "the proper instrument of voice." Considering terminological divergences in the denomination of the vocal folds, which still persist today, Vesalius provides a memorable comment: "When we have understood the operations of the vocal cords, we may call them Petrus, Paulus, Johannes, or whatever we want, for I will not fight about words" (Heseler, 1959).

We turn briefly away from Padua to note Bartolomeus Eustachius (about 1500–10 to 1574), who practiced as a physician in Rome. His *Anatomical Figures* included fine copperplate anatomical illustrations of the larynx, more naturalistic than the figures of Vesalius. However, they were not published until 1714 (Panconcelli-Calzia, 1940, 1957a, 1961; Weir, 1990).

Returning to the Padua anatomists, the modern name "cricoid" (Greek: "ring-like") used by Galen to describe the only circular cartilage of the larynx was reinstated by Gabriele Falloppius (1523–1562). Falloppius' *Anatomical Observations* (1561) include extensive material on the muscles of the head and neck, including the larynx. Hieronymus Fabricius ab Aquapendente (1537–1619) provides an extensive treatment of the larynx on the basis of comparative anatomy in his work *On Vision, Voice And Hearing* (Venice, 1600). Julius Casserius (1552–1616) was the author of the book *Anatomical Treatise on the Organs of Voice and Hearing*, published in 1600–1601, which includes valuable information on laryngeal anatomy and function, and phonation (Hast & Holtsmark, 1969). Giovanni Battista Morgagni (1682–1771) of Padua is famous as a founder of pathological anatomy (including that of the larynx). He also greatly expanded knowledge of the histology of the larynx. Investigating the ventricular folds and laryngeal ventricles, he gave due credit for their discovery to Galen (Panconcelli-Calzia, 1940; Weir, 1990).

THE VOICE OF REASON IN THE ENLIGHTENMENT

Although it is clear from the above discussion that the gross structure of the larynx was well known by the early seventeenth century, the exploration of details continued in the work of such eighteenth century anatomists as G. D. Santorini (1681–1737) and Peter Camper (1767). Fink (1975) narrates the discovery of the smaller laryngeal cartilages.

With some injustice to intervening figures, to some of whom we will return, we must shift our attention to the many contributions of the Enlightenment which set the stage for the modern study of voice (Panconcelli-Calzia, 1941). The French physician C. Perrault (1613–1688) compared the mechanism of voice to wind instruments. The mathematical physicist J. Sauveur (1653–1716) clarified the concept of the harmonics of a periodic sound and the analysis of the vibration of strings. The underlying mathematics of the vibra-

tion of strings was the subject of profound discussion, on which was based the analysis by Joseph Fourier (1768–1830) of arbitrary functions which underlies modern spectral analysis.

At the beginning of the 18th century, the prevailing concept of voice relied on the antique view that voice was produced in the trachea much as sound is produced in a flute. Galen, still influential, had recognized the importance of the larynx in voice production, but still attributed a considerable phonatory role to the trachea. The French physicist D. Dodart (1634–1707) shifted emphasis from the trachea to the larynx itself as the generator of voice; in his view, vocal intensity and pitch were controlled by variations in glottal width and airflow.

The French anatomist A. Ferrein, whose life spanned the period between 1693–1796 (Cooper, 1989a), changed the rules of the game by his publication in 1741 of an extensive empirical study of voice production in human and animal excised larynges. In these preparations, the function of all laryngeal muscles except the vocal fold muscles can be simulated in order to adjust the larynx for phonation, while an airflow supplied by human lungs or a machine excites the larynx to produce voice. The approximation of the vocal folds was found to be necessary for phonation, whatever the airflow. Emphasizing the concept of the vibrating string which was under vigorous discussion by contemporary mathematicians, Ferrein concluded that the vocal cords, as he called them, were both a string and a wind instrument. He incorrectly maintained that voice was generated by the vocal folds like a vibrating string, and described experiments, some quite impossible and others misinterpreted, which he claimed to support this view. Thus, despite Ferrein's enormous contribution in opening the door to the empirical study of phonatory physiology, crucial discoveries in the understanding of voice production had to wait for scientists of following centuries.

A remarkable summary of what had been attained in the physiology of voice by the mid-eighteenth century can be found in the eight-volume treatise *Elements of the Physiology of the Human Body* (1757–1766) by A. von Haller (1708–1777), a testy Swiss-German of wide and profound learning. His chapter on voice and speech in the third volume includes an impressive qualitative summary of the physiology of phonation, with clinical applications; the deficiency of the physical conceptualization is indicated by the fact that quantification is essentially absent, as in the work of Ferrein.

DIRECTIONS TOWARD THE MODERN STUDY OF VOICE PHYSIOLOGY

The Larynx Under the Microscope

After Galen, the centuries had seen the gradual clarification of the gross anatomy of the larynx. Beginning with the improvement of microscopy in the early nineteenth century, and extending through the middle of the present century, there starts the age of histology, including the establishment of the theory of cells, especially as the unit of the nervous system. From about 1960 onwards this horizon has been extended toward the biochemistry and ultrastructure of laryngeal structures, although the attentive observer can note isolated related studies from the beginning of this century. An early landmark in this development is the work of the Strasbourg anatomist and physiologist E. A. Lauth (1803–1837) on the yellow elastic fibers of the larynx (1835), already noted by J. Müller (1837) and soon followed by the study of the subtypes of the laryngeal epithelium (1838) by J.

Henle (1809–1895) in Zürich. The nineteenth century also built on the foundations laid during the Enlightenment for understanding the acoustic aspect of voice production.

The Origins of Source-Filter Concepts

Johannes Müller (1801–1858), professor of physiology at the University of Berlin, one of the most distinguished physiologists of his time and teacher of many of the greatest succeeding figures of German physiology, inserted a 123-page section "On Voice and Speech" in the second volume of his great *Handbook of Human Physiology* (1837). Müller carried out experiments on voice production in excised larynx preparations, published in this work and in a separate short monograph *On the Compensation of Physical Forces in the Human Larynx* (1839). Whereas Ferrein's critics, including von Haller, had complained that the quality of the voice produced by the excised larynx did not match that of the usual speech sound, in some of his experiments Müller (1839) studied voice production in a preparation with both a human larynx and head to demonstrate that the missing link for perceptually natural quality of the resulting sound was the vocal tract. By appropriate manipulations he was able to produce the vowels [u, a] and the consonants [m, w].

It is easy to underestimate the significance of this work from a modern perspective. Although some statements of Aristotle invited confusion as to the source of vowel distinctions, even in antiquity there was sporadic recognition of the separability of the role of supraglottal articulators from that of the larynx, as in Seneca's question, "What is the voice, save tension of the air moulded by a stroke of the tongue so as to become audible?" (Naturalium Quaestionum Bk 2.6, 3–4: Hunt, 1978). However, we come to a clear distinction of the functions of the vocal tract and the larynx in the generation of vowels first in the work of J. Matthiae (1586), who appears as an explicit critic of Aristotle's statement that vowels are produced by the voice and the larynx. He emphasizes that vowels are distinguished by the changing shapes of the mouth (Panconcelli-Calzia, 1940). The role of supraglottal articulators was also clearly recognized by the English mathematician John Wallis (1653). Stumpf (1926) relates how the Kiel scholar Samuel Reyher (1679) subtracted out the harmonic contribution of the larynx to vowel production by analyzing the resonant frequencies of German whispered vowels; he published the approximate pitches of the second formants in musical notation. Musically gifted specialists such as the composer J. P. Rameau (1726) placed these resonances in an acoustic framework by analyzing by ear the upper harmonics of vowels.

This separability of the acoustic characteristics of the vocal tract from those of the laryngeal voice source was implemented on a practical level by ingenious physically minded inventors such as W. von Kempelen (1734–1804) and C. G. Kratzenstein (1725–1795), who constructed artificial speaking devices in which an improvised voice source fed a signal to an acoustic resonator serving as an artificial vocal tract. From the other end, Dodart (1703) had clarified that the trachea's role in voice production was limited to providing an air supply from the lungs (Ungeheuer, 1962), and Ferrein (1741) had provided the experimental proof that voice, in fact, emanated from the larynx, with a crucial and even exaggerated role attributed to the vocal folds. However, in view of the severe criticism of the sound produced by Ferrein's preparation in terms of its difference from usual voice, what remained was the demonstration that the specific laryngeal source used by Ferrein

could be combined with an appropriate supraglottal resonator to produce a realistic sound. The irregularity of the shape of the larynx makes it a nontrivial task to join an artificial resonator on an excised larynx; this has been achieved only by a few investigators in the present century (first by W. Trendelenburg and O. Wullstein, 1935). The experiment of J. Müller (1839), which simply left the larynx together with a natural resonator, was thus the best alternative, but was deceptively complex in its implications.

Although Müller could not surmount his own limited preparation in physics and chemistry, or the limited development of acoustic theory and measurement in his day, others succeeded in clarifying the question. Aware of the eighteenth century findings which had succeeded in isolating vowel resonances, R. Willis (1829) concluded on the basis of experiments with vowel-like sounds from organ pipes that, although the fundamental frequency might vary, the quality of the sound depended only on the length of the pipe. Reviewing the work of Kempelen, Kratzenstein, and Willis in a journal article, the physicist and instrument maker C. Wheatstone (1802–1875) pointed out in 1838 that, in fact, the sound emitted by the glottal source excited the multiple resonances of the vocal tract. The treatise *On the Sensations of Tone* (First edition, 1863) of the great German physicist and physiologist H. Helmholtz (1821–1894) gives Wheatstone fundamental credit for this discovery. It is worthwhile to cite Helmholtz's summary: "For the vowels of speech are in reality tones produced by membranous tongues (the vocal cords), with a resonance chamber (the mouth) capable of altering in length, width, and pitch of resonance, and hence capable also of reinforcing at different times different partials of the compound tone to which it is applied" (1877, p. 103). Helmholtz recognized two formants (resonances of the vocal tract) in front vowels, but only one in back vowels. Underlying his statements is the assumption that, according to Fourier's analysis, the intensity and phase of the harmonic components of the sound emitted by the larynx were altered by the vocal tract; that is, it acted as an acoustic filter (Ungeheuer, 1962). This explanation was accepted in the authoritative treatise on acoustics by Lord Rayleigh (J. W. Strutt, 1877, 1894) and is fundamental to subsequent work on the acoustic theory of speech production, under the label of source-filter theory. The preceding development provides only a partial solution for the nature of sound generation in the larynx, but it does grant the right to consider this question separately from the filter properties of the vocal tract. Although voice and speech shared in the progress of technical acoustics during the late nineteenth and early twentieth centuries, more detailed solutions to both questions have been discovered during the second half of the present century. The study of the acoustics and mechanics of the voice source has shifted from the territory of physiologists to that of engineers, physicists, and specialists in acoustics, among whom the names (in alphabetical order) of J. W. van den Berg, G. Fant, J. L. Flanagan, O. Fujimura, K. Ishizaka, K. N. Stevens, J. Sundberg, and I. R. Titze are eminent. Apart from technical works, an overview of the implications of such research is provided by Sundberg (1987) and Titze (1994).

The Control of the Larynx by the Nervous System

Other developments made it possible to refine knowledge of many aspects of laryngeal function. Crucial was the advancement of knowledge concerning electricity. Once this foundation was laid in the first half of the nineteenth century,

the mid-nineteenth century work of the German physiologist E. Du Bois-Reymond (1818–1896) rapidly and definitively established not only the electrical character of nerve conduction, but also the techniques for the application of electricity for the physiological investigation of excitable tissues, primarily nerve and muscle. This discovery forms the background for the many detailed studies of laryngeal nerves during this period (Weir, 1990), which in an anatomical sense continued the work of eighteenth century scientists, such as that of C. S. Andersch (1791) and J. Swan (1830). After the description of the superior laryngeal nerve by the physician Thomas Willis (1621–1675; distinguished for his studies of the anatomy of the brain), the sensory function of the internal branch of the superior laryngeal nerve and motor function of the recurrent laryngeal nerve were studied by a rapid succession of British physicians, by J. Hilton and E. Cock in 1837, by J. Reid in 1838, and by M. Hall in 1841 (Weir, 1990). The French physiologist F. Magendie (1783–1855) included among his studies of nerve physiology observations of the effects of laryngeal nerve activation.

However, the fundamental conceptual armamentarium for the investigation of laryngeal neurophysiology was not available until the demonstration first of the cell as the basic unit of the animal, especially in the work of T. Schwann (1810–1882) and R. Virchow (1821–1902) in the decades around 1850, and then the demonstration of the neuron as the particular type of cell which is the building block of the nervous system (S. Ramón y Cajal, 1852–1934). The maturation of histological techniques at that time makes Cajal's work the approximate landmark at which detailed information on laryngeal neuroanatomy and neurophysiology became usable.

This epoch was also a productive period for studies of the central neuroanatomy and neurophysiology underlying basic motor control of the larynx, especially in Germany and Austro-Hungary, in the work of researchers such as the neurophysiologist S. Exner (1846–1926); the laryngologists F. Semon (1849–1921), H. Grabower (1849–1914), and L. Réthi (1857–1924); the otolaryngologists A. Onodi (1857–1920) and J. Katzenstein (1864–1922); and the physiologist R. Du Bois-Reymond (1863–1938). Details of these developments are too technical to be presented in this chapter. The significance of many of these studies for voice production is well put in context by Lullies' (1953) treatise on the physiology of voice and speech, and the rich bibliography of Wyke and Kirchner's survey (1976) of the neurology of the larynx makes a point of giving credit to older, but still valid, research.

Another important topic for motor control broached at this time was the presence of muscle receptors in the larynx. A number of early studies at the turn of the century did not find muscle spindles in some muscles in the cranial nerve territory, but H. Nakayama observed muscle spindles in the human laryngeal muscles in 1911, followed by N. Nakamura in 1915. Other studies during this period made clear the presence of a sensory component in the recurrent laryngeal nerve (C. Sherrington, 1894; J. Katzenstein, 1900), as has been repeatedly confirmed in subsequent research. Laryngeal sensory studies have expanded in recent years and found a new context and stimulus as part of respiratory neurophysiology.

During the period following World War I, another subject opened for study was the specialized character of laryngeal muscles. P. Grützner (1902) had already commented on the rapid character of their contraction on the basis of optical observations. At first the topic belonged exclusively to the French. A study of the chronaxie of thyroarytenoid muscle in which its rapidity of response was shown

(F. Moura Campos, A. Chaucard, & B. Chauchard, 1927) was followed in turn by a general study of the chronaxie of the larynx by P. Dumont (1933). Aside from the careful study of canine thyroarytenoid muscle by Y. Laporte and P. Bessou (1956), the study of dynamic aspects of laryngeal muscles was neglected until A. Mårtensson (1964), M. H. Hast (1966 et seq.), and H. Hirose and T. Ushijima et al. (1969) clarified on the basis of animal studies the contrast between the relatively fast contractile properties of the thyroarytenoid, lateral cricoarytenoid, and interarytenoid muscles compared to the slower posterior cricoarytenoid and cricothyroid muscles. Related studies in man have been tentative.

Although some initial biochemical findings in regard to laryngeal muscles were available early, as in F. Imhofer's (1914) observation of the increase of lipofuscin around the nuclei in aging thyroarytenoid muscle, only about 1960 did studies of histochemistry, ultrastructure, and more recently immunohistochemistry begin to appear which illuminate the physiological and metabolic properties of laryngeal muscles. In 1974, L. Edström, C. Lindquist, and A. Mårtensson demonstrated the fatigue-resistance of laryngeal muscles and made important contributions to its metabolic explanation, illustrating the power of combined physiological and biochemical studies. The relevant chapters in Kirchner (1986); Ford and Bless (1991); Blitzer, Brin, Sasaki, Fahn, and Harris (1992); and Titze (1993) orient to recent progress in the neurology of the larynx.

The Power-Source for Speech

The power for voice production is the product of airflow and subglottal air pressure. We shall begin by sketching the development of the measurement of the respiratory quantities which provide the driving force for voice production; this area has been surveyed by Panconcelli-Calzia (1940, 1961).

In 1681, the Italian physician and physicist G. Borelli (1608–1679) described a device for the measurement of inspired quantities of air. The refinement of the spirometer by the English physician J. Hutchinson (1811–1861), made public in 1844, led to the quantitative analysis of the compartments of the lung volume. After a hundred years of development of the kymograph, a rotating drum on which movements were recorded on paper as a function of time, dynamic registration of speech respiratory movement was achieved by K. Vierordt and K. Ludwig (1816–1895) in 1855. The adoption of this technique by French investigators such as E. J. Marey (1865) and A. Piltan (1887) led to its application by the French experimental phonetician P. Rousselot in his dissertation (1891), with succeeding expansion of its application in the study of speech, especially by the pioneer phoniatrist H. Gutzmann, Sr., of Berlin and various collaborators (1894, 1895, 1909). After approximate indications of the air expended on various speech tasks by J. Guillet (1857), J. Gad (1887), and P. Rousselot (1891), the first quantitative indications of time-averaged volume velocities in phonation were published by L. Roudet (1900). More recently, procedures have been developed to estimate the time-varying glottal volume velocity waveform by physical or computer techniques to eliminate the effects of the vocal tract on the glottal flow signal (Rothenberg, 1981; Scherer, 1991).

The determination of time-averaged subglottal pressure during phonation was achieved by the French physicist C. Cagniard de la Tour (1777–1859) in studies of tracheotomized men and women published starting in 1837. More systematic measurements of subglottal pressure during phonation in the excised larynx, including its interaction with vocal fold

tension in the control of fundamental frequency, were achieved by the German physiologist Johannes Müller (1839), by means of a manometer connected to the trachea, a procedure that was refined by E. Harless (1852). At the beginning of this century, Rousselot (1902) and E. A. Meyer (1913) published kymograms of subglottal pressures from tracheotomized subjects during phonation.

The German physician Harless (1853) had expressed the insight that subglottal pressures must vary dynamically during phonation, and the Belgian Jesuit Ch. Lootens had noted in the 1870s that, in a vibrating excised larynx, there were regions both of strong positive pressure and strong negative pressure; thus, subglottal pressures must vary in both space and time. Recordings of dynamically varying subglottal pressure were published first by O. Weiss (1914) based on the excised larynx.

After World War I, such measures became the domain of laryngologists: H. Gutzmann, Sr., and A. Loewy (1920) studied subglottal pressure in a subject with a tracheotomy, and R. Schilling (1925) did so in another patient with a tracheal fistula. More recently, J. van den Berg (1956) substituted measures of intra-esophageal pressure in normal subjects, in which he was followed by M. H. Draper, P. Ladefoged, and D. Whitteridge (1957) in a study of speech respiration. The correctness of this substitution has been challenged (L. H. Kunze, 1964) and defended (H. Schutte, 1980). Subsequently tracheal puncture (N. Isshiki, 1961) made direct subglottal pressure measures on normal subjects possible, but the frequency response was poor, and newer miniature pressure transducers have made possible measurements of time-varying subglottal pressures during speech, such as Harless longed for in 1853. The substitution of intraoral pressure measures for subglottal pressures in some maneuvers has expanded in recent use. Surveys of aerodynamic results, techniques, and basic concepts are provided respectively by Hirano (1981), Baken (1987), and Scherer (1991), with more general implications put in context by Sundberg (1987).

Optical Techniques for Observation of the Larynx and the Trajectory of Vocal Fold Vibration in Voice

The earlier history of the optical observation of the larynx and voice production has been described by Moore (1937, 1991). Schönhärl's classic monograph (1960) on stroboscopy in practical laryngology and Luchsinger (1970) provide a partial continuation of this account. The present discussion will narrow progressively from general optical observations to the analysis of the trajectory of vocal fold vibration.

Ferrein (1741) was the first to observe phonatory vibration of the larynx and publish a scientific account of his findings. Still, neither Ferrein nor other scholars who carried out similar experimentation, such as H. Dutrochet (1806), K. Liskovius (1814, 1846), or K. Lehfeldt (1835), could observe vocal fold motion in detail. The first to do so was probably Harless (1853), whose astuteness in matters of mechanics led him to the first application of stroboscopy in observation of the vibrating excised larynx. He found that the extent of glottal separation increased with subglottal pressure, although an increase of external tension of the fold decreased this effect.

After some less well-known applications listed by Moore (1937, 1991) and Weir (1990), the application of a simple dental mirror for the observation of laryngeal movement by the Spanish singing teacher Manuel Garcia (1805–1906) in 1855, and soon thereafter by the physicians L. Türck (1810–1868) and J. N. Czermák (1828–1873) (as narrated by Brodnitz in 1954 and Lesky in 1965), made

possible the observation of gross movements within the living human larynx. Although Türck made use of the laryngeal mirror before Czermák, undoubted priority is given to Czermák for the publication of stereoscopic photographs of the larynx (1861). The treatise on speech anatomy and physiology by the Leipzig otolaryngologist K. L. Merkel (1856, 1863) contains a rather convincing description of the mucosal wave. Between the publication of his first and second editions, Merkel had published a treatise on the larynx and pharynx (1862) in which he incorporated his own laryngoscopic observations.

French physiologists experimenting with excised larynx preparations and in living animals provided further evidence that the larynx would no longer phonate if the mucous membrane were removed (E. Fournié, 1866), and that the oscillation of the thyroarytenoid muscle during voice production was quite limited (E. Martel, 1885; M. Lermoyez, 1886). Lermoyez (1886), the author of a rich monograph on phonatory physiology, anticipated T. Baer (1975) in the finding that damage or removal of the vocal ligament led to loss of voice. The importance of these early findings has been underlined by the development of modern phonosurgery, which has emphasized the role of the subglottal mucosal membrane in voice production, and the risk of iatrogenic damage to the voice by uninformed or inept mucosal surgery.

Expanded application of stroboscopy (Moore, 1937, 1991) by T. Oertel of Munich (1878, 1895) in living subjects, and by D. Koschlakoff (1866) and L. Réthi (1896) in the excised larynx, led to Réthi's observation of the propagation of a wave upwards and laterally on the vocal fold during each vibratory cycle. Observations including remarkable stroboscopic photographs of glottal vibration by A. Musehold of Berlin (1897–1897; 1913) convinced him that there was a vertical as well as a horizontal component to vocal fold vibration. During the same period, the roentgenographic examination of the larynx was initiated by M. Scheier (1896). Scherer (1981) provides a detailed overview of the research on the geometry of the laryngeal airway in phonation found in related studies by subsequent researchers such as G. P. Moore, J. F. Curtis, and H. Hollien.

One year after the description of the first motion pictures of the laynx by L. Chevroton and F. Vlès (1913), soon followed by stroboscopic motion pictures by J. Hegener and G. Panconcelli-Calzia (1913), a pioneer study by O. Weiss (1914) of Königsberg published the first dynamic records of the medial-lateral vibration of the vocal folds of an excised larynx, recorded by shining a beam of light through the glottis onto a moving photographic film, as well as the first records of time-varying subglottal pressure. During the period between the two World Wars, the great Berlin physiologist Wilhelm Trendelenburg and his assistant O. Wullstein used a capacitive technique (1935) which made possible the recording of a second dimension of movement, primarily vertical. Another collaborator of W. Trendelenburg (W. Hartmann, 1938) substituted a second beam of light directed across the vibrating excised larynx to measure the vertical movement of the vocal folds quantitatively, suggesting a resolution of the motion of the vocal fold in a coronal section into X-Y coordinates. E. Müller (1938, 1939) attempted to combine the two records into a trajectory of the path of a tissue point on a coronal section of the vocal fold during vibration. Although details of his results were incorrect, they include much of extraordinary interest.

Schönhärl (1960) and Luchsinger (1970) describe postwar development in stroboscopy. In a landmark MIT dissertation, T. Baer (1975) essentially returned tó the technique of L. Réthi (1896), who

had stroboscopically observed the trajectories during phonation of brass particles on the vocal folds of excised larynges. Using carbon particles instead of brass, and reconstruction of their trajectories, Baer provided important information on the trajectories of laryngeal vibration in a coronal section of canine vocal folds.

S. Saito and colleagues successfully carried out E. Müller's program of resolving vocal fold motion into simple period variations of values of X-Y coordinates in the coronal plane. In a series of studies in excised larynges and animals, they tracked the motion of lead pellets inserted into the superficial layer of the vocal fold by means of X-ray stroboscopy (1981, 1983, 1985). Others such a T. Kaneko (1983) and J. Zagzebski (1983) used less invasive techniques such as ultrasonography to track the motion of vocal folds.

A more precise technique offered by high-speed photography, was initiated by research at Bell laboratories (1937) and continued during the postwar period by a number of investigators (Hirano, 1981), such as G. P. Moore and H. von Leden (1960, 1961, 1962), who with R. Timcke also contributed to the refinement of stroboscopic techniques. Such techniques are especially valuable for the analysis of events that depart from periodicity, such as a cough or clearing of the throat, so that their representation by stroboscopy becomes problematic.

VOICE AND THE LARYNX ENTER THE CLINIC

The Establishment of Prelaryngoscopic Medical Treatment of the Larynx

Laryngology and phoniatry, like speech and voice pathology, are recent developments in comparison to the basic anatomy and physiology of the larynx and voice. The early history of treatment of diseases of the throat concerns details of pathology, laryngeal trauma, syphilis, tuberculosis, and smallpox, diphtheria and laryngeal malignancies, scarlet fever, angina, and croup, which through the end of the eighteenth century were largely treated by general physicians. Following a progression initiated by Morgagni, the late eighteenth and early nineteenth centuries saw the detailed development of laryngeal pathology, resulting in the publication in 1829 of a detailed treatise of laryngeal disease by J. F. H. Albers (1805–1867) of Bonn and in 1836 of an English treatise of laryngeal disease by F. Ryland of Birmingham (1806–1857); (Weir, 1990). This recognition of laryngeal pathological anatomy legitimized the development of laryngeal surgical technique during the first half of the nineteenth century. However, the practitioners were largely flying blind during the prelaryngoscopic period.

Early Laryngoscopy and the Development of Voice-Related Laryngology

A development closely related to the contribution of Central European lands to laryngeal neurophysiology noted above was the institutional focus for the study of phonation and laryngology provided by the establishment of clinics for laryngology in Central Europe. The significance for this foundation of the clinical application of the laryngeal mirror and other optical refinements described above cannot be exaggerated. The competition between Türck and Czermák over priority in the clinical application of the laryngeal mirror generated an extensive clinical literature, such as Türck's classic treatise *Clinic of Disease of the Larynx and of the Airways* (1866), which contributed to establishing laryngology as a medical specialty.

Among the foreigners drawn to study in Austro-Hungary was the young English physician Morell Mackenzie (1837–1892), who learned laryngoscopy from Czermák in Budapest in 1859 and returned to establish himself in London as one of the most distinguished laryngologists of the world, leaving great treatises on laryngology and the foundation of the British school of laryngology as his legacy. A more recent giant of British laryngology, Victor Negus (188–1974) contributed both clinical publications and two editions (1929, 1949) of a classic monograph on the comparative anatomy and physiology of the larynx, complemented by the more recent work on the evolution and embryology of the larynx by the Dutchman J. Wind (1970) and subsequent research of M. H. Hast, J. A. Tucker, F. Müller, and R. O'Rahilly.

The development around the founding of the world's first laryngological clinic at Vienna General Hospital in 1870 by L. Schrötter von Kristelli has been described (Lesky, 1965; Höfer & Majer, 1980; Cooper, 1991). The Vienna School in the treatment of voice and speech disorders, headed by E. Froeschels (1884–1972) with a psychological and psychotherapeutic emphasis, contrasted with the organic emphasis of the Berlin school. Nineteenth century pioneers in the specialty of speech disorders such as K. L. Merkel of Leipzig (1812–1876) and A. Kussmaul of Berlin (1822–1902) prepared the way for the opening by Hermann Gutzmann Sr. (1865–1922) of a clinic for speech disorders in Berlin in 1891. B. Fränkel (1836–1911), an internist, founded Prussia's first laryngological clinic in Berlin in 1901, and Gutzmann, Sr. made phoniatrics a recognized academic specialty with his inaugural lecture at the University of Berlin in 1905. The research and clinical, organizational, and professorial activities of the senior Gutzmann, whose activities after 1905 increasingly turned toward voice, underlie the rich development of the medical treatment of speech and voice in Central Europe (Zehmisch, Siegert, & Wendler, 1980).

Max Nadoleczny (1874–1940), a student of Gutzmann, Sr., and Lermoyez, among others, made Munich a center for phoniatry and worked with equal distinction as researcher, clinician, professor, and founder of the German Society for Speech and Voice Medicine. After substantial contributions to the study of voice by such specialists as the physiologist J. E. Purkyně (1787–1869), J. N. Czermák, and the phonetician J. Chlumsky (1871–1939), an outpatient clinic for phoniatry was established in Prague in 1922 and entrusted to M. Seeman (1892–1975), a student of Gutzmann, Sr., who played a similar nuclear role. The Zürich phoniatrist R. Luchsinger (1900–1993) specialized in phoniatrics under the influence of Nadoleczny and, in collaboration with G. E. Arnold, produced a succession of editions which grew into a great handbook containing scientific and scholarly riches aimed at stengthening the scientific foundations of voice care (Luchsinger, 1970). The overseas movement of phoniatry may be exemplified by the Italian R. Segré, a student of Froeschels and Flatau, who settled in Buenos Aires and played a seminal role in the establishment of medical voice care in South America. The development of phoniatrics has been narrated in a volume edited by J. Wendler (1980).

A parallel growth occurred in specialized phonatory and laryngeal research. Distinguished voice specialists in speech pathology, such as Svend Smith of Denmark (1907–1986) and S. Borel-Maisonny of Paris, emerged in relation to the development of phoniatrics. Smith's membrane-cushion notion of vocal fold vibration, like the mucosal wave theory of J. Perello (1962, 1967), was one of a number of important predecessors of body-cover notions usually associated with the name

of M. Hirano (1975). After the first demonstration of laryngeal electromyography by G. B. Weddell, B. Feinstein, and R. E. Pattle (1944), a classic Danish contribution was made by K. Faaborg-Anderson in the research summarized in his monographs on laryngeal electromyography (1957, 1964). The works of R. Husson (1952, 1962) on phonatory physiology, perhaps still not thoroughly evaluated even today, evoked a critical response that brought a broad renewal of phonatory physiology in works such as those of the Dutch medical physicist Janwillem van den Berg (1953, 1962). van den Berg created a broad physical conceptualization of voice production as part of what he called experimental phoniatrics, invoking concepts of fluid mechanics such as the Bernoulli effect, which has widened the physical aspect of modern phonatory research (Cooper, 1989b, 1993).

Laryngological specialization of surgeons in the United States goes back as far as the practice of Horace Green of New York in the early nineteenth century, who used indirect laryngoscopy in 1858, only 3 years after the demonstration of the laryngeal mirror by M. Garcia; however, this early development had little specific relation to voice physiology and voice disorders. The basic research of individuals such as Franklin Hooper of Boston on laryngeal nerve and muscle physiology (1883, 1887) and Thomas French of Brooklyn on laryngeal photography (1883) and voice production was isolated. The growth of the laryngological armamentarium as in the extension of optical techniques by Chevalier Jackson of Philadelphia (1852–1958) supposed the potential of, but did not bring an actual focus on, voice disorders. Contributions from fields as diverse as physiological psychology (E. W. Scripture, 1902), communication engineering (R. L. Wegel, 1930), anatomy (F. Lemere, 1932), experimental phonetics (G. E. Peterson, 1937), speech pathology

(G. P. Moore, 1936; R. T. Carhart, 1938), and musical acoustics (C. Seashore, 1942) outnumbered medical contributions to laryngeal and voice research (Pressman, 1942; Pressman & Kelemen, 1955; Kirchner, 1970), but at first lacked an organizational focus.

The two interwar decades which witnessed the creation of speech pathology as a profession in the United States and elsewhere (Rieber & Brubaker, 1966; Eldridge, 1968), and which partly provided this focus, only rarely found a complementary medical specialization on voice disorders. However, the Nazi persecutions in Europe before and during World War II created an influx of emigre physicians and scholars schooled in the European medical traditions of voice care sketched above. von Leden (1990) has noted the contributions to the growth of voice-related laryngology in the United States from members of this immigrant group, particularly from phoniatrists such as E. Froeschels and his pupils, D. Weiss, P. Moses, and G. E. Arnold, and otolaryngologists such as F. Brodnitz and G. Kelemen.

The developments that have brought Japan to a prominent position in laryngeal studies and phonosurgery have been sketched by Kirikae (1966) and Isshiki (1980). The foundations were laid early; Japanese contributions to laryngeal neuroanatomy in the early part of this century were noted above. Voice-related laryngology in Japan arose partly as a native medical development, in the person of K. Satta of Tokyo and his students (I. Kirikae, T. Shiraiwa, S. Horiguchi, K. Fujita), and partly under external stimuli, first particularly of German, and after World War II particularly of American training and collaboration. Japanese specialists have gained distinction especially in surgically related areas and physically oriented studies of voice, while practice and research in medical and behavioral areas related to voice has been limited.

BEHAVIORAL, SURGICAL, AND MEDICAL DIRECTIONS

It will be apparent that the basic and clinical fields of voice include specialists from many fields. Apart from particular cases of personal collaboration to bring together varied skills, sometimes this multifacetted aspect of voice studies has assumed institutional form, as in the pioneer multidisciplinary voice clinic and institute for voice care and voice research which Hans von Leden and Paul Moore created at Northwestern University Medical School in 1954. This approach was continued after their respective moves to Los Angeles and the University of Florida in Gainesville. A logical conclusion from the multifacetted character of the field of voice is that optimal clinical practice for patients with voice disorders requires the cooperation of specialists who bring training from medical, surgical, and behavioral specialties. This point of view is not accepted by all, and questions of respective dominance, independence, or even reciprocal exclusion of practitioners in other specialties may arise. Analogous issues arise more rarely in voice research. In fact, although this multidisciplinary approach is regarded by some as the most important contribution in recent decades to the care of voice and the larynx, at times it has been the subject of bitter dispute.

During recent decades, the Voice Foundation, based in New York and Philadelphia, first under the chairmanship of W. J. Gould and then under R. T. Sataloff, has undertaken to bring together the interests of specialists in the basic and medical sciences relating to voice with those of voice professionals, their teachers, and clinicians specializing in related problems at annual meetings and scientific forums, and in resulting publications (*The Journal of Voice* and *Proceedings of Symposia on Vocal Fold Physiology*). A number of national and international organizations in the fields of otolaryngology, speech pathology, musical performance and pedagogy, and so on have corresponding interdisciplinary committees.

The specialty of laryngology has had an inherent duality in that in some traditions it has constituted a subdivision of medicine rather than one of surgery. It is largely from this medical aspect that the primarily European field of phoniatry as a specialty which deals with disorders of speech and voice from a medical point of view has developed (Wendler, 1980). In the United States, and partly in British otolaryngology, specialization of otolaryngologists and other medical specialties regarding phonatory aspects of the larynx has been exceptional, and laryngology has usually had a more surgical emphasis. von Leden has described the development of phonosurgery (von Leden, 1993a, 1993b), the surgical modality for the maintenace and improvement of voice. After the introduction of laryngectomy by T. Billroth of Vienna in 1873, removal of the larynx for cancer long dominated the scene in laryngeal surgery, although isolated progress in surgical techniques for the improvement of voice can be noted. Until after World War II, this was at first overwhelmingly a Central European specialty, and a significant role in its expansion in the United States during the 1950s amd 1960s was played by specialists with Central European roots. Phonosurgery for such problems as vocal fold paralysis, microsurgical techniques, restorative surgery of the laryngeal nerves, surgery for spastic dysphonia, external framework surgery of the larynx, construction of an alternative voice source after laryngectomy, and, potentially, laryngeal transplantation has extended the range of voice-related laryngology.

SUMMARY

Although the training of American clinical specialists in speech and voice pathology traditionally has emphasized behavioral clinical techniques, research and training in the field have gradually expanded to include most basic scientific aspects of their subject matter, sometimes with a resulting partial overlap of expertise with physicians and other professionals. As for the medical specialists in voice and the larynx, this multifaceted aspect of speech and voice disorders was inherent in the founding group which eventually matured into the American Speech and Hearing Association, as described by Lee Travis: "We had phoneticians, psychiatrists, psychologists, speech people, two or three M.D.'s" (Moeller, 1975) at the organizational meeting in 1925.

A significant common ground between physicians and speech pathologists has been created in terms of the development of functional measurements of voice, capable of application for both basic research and demonstrating the effects of surgical, medical, or behavioral intervention in relation to voice disorders. Although their earlier application in research is described above, these procedures have come into practical clinical use progressively during the decades since World War II. The most significant ones have been stroboscopy and related optical techniques, with assistance from photoglottography and electroglottography, aerodynamic techniques, and acoustic techniques (Hirano, 1981; Baken, 1987).

Just as teachers of rhetoricians, singers, and actors were among the first to develop pedagogic techniques for their students over two millenia ago, in our own time voice professionals and their teachers have at times developed skills and knowledge which speech pathologists and physicians must either learn or access for the good of their patients. These have been complemented by both physicians who have focused on the professional voice, such as M. Nadoleczny (1912, 1925), T. Flatau (1898, 1929), J. Tarneaud (1935, 1946, 1961), and R. Leanderson (1972, 1984), and voice teachers who have made noteworthy contributions to voice acoustics (e.g., W. Vennard, R. Appleman, J. Large, T. Cleveland). The laryngologist who is also an accomplished singer or is skilled with behavioral techniques, the teacher of singing who has qualified in speech pathology or voice acoustics, the speech pathologist who has acquired skills in physiological and acoustical measurements of the voice and its disorders, and many other individual combinations remind us that the complex of individuals who best serve the interests of patients with voice disorders need have no specific form and will be most effective if it includes the demonstrated skills of various specialties.

REFERENCES

EDITORS' NOTE: Items listed in the text but not in the reference refer to historical dates which reflect either the prime period of active research for the individual, or the life span of the individual.

Allen, W. S. (1953). *Phonetics in ancient India.* London: Oxford University Press.

Baken, R. J. (1987). *Clinical measurement of speech and voice.* Boston-Toronto-San Diego: College-Hill Press.

Blitzer, A., Brin, M. F., Sasaki, C. T., Fahn, S., & Harris, K. S. (1992). *Neurologic disorders of the larynx.* Stuttgart-New York: Georg Thieme Verlag.

Brodnitz, F. S. (1954). One hundred years of laryngoscopy: To the memory of Garcia, Tuerck, and Czermak. *Transactions of the American Academy of Ophthalmology and Otolaryngology,* 663–669.

Cooper, D. S. (1989a). Antoine Ferrein and the formation of the human voice. *Journal of Voice, 3*(3), 187–203.

Cooper, D. S. (1989b). Woldemar Tonndorf and the Bernoulli effect in voice production. *Journal of Voice, 3*(1), 1–6.

Cooper, D. S. (1991). Leopold Rethi and laryngeal muscle mechanics. *Journal of Voice, 5*(4), 354–359.

Cooper, D. S. (1993). Research in laryngeal physiology with excised larynges. In C. W. Cummings (Ed.), *Otolaryngology—Head and neck surgery, 3,* 1728–1737. St. Louis: Mosby Year Book.

Daoud, S. A. (1965). Voice and speech in the writings of three medical writers of the 10th century: Rhazes, Haly-Abass, and Avicenna. *Proceedings of the 13th International Congress of Logopedics and Phoniatrics, 2,* 237–239

Eldridge, M. (1968). *A history of the treatment of speech disorders.* Edinburgh and London: E. & S. Livingstone Ltd.

Ernout, A., & Meillet, A. (1967). *Dictionnaire etymologique de la langue latine* (4th ed.). Paris: Klincksieck.

Fink, B. R. (1975). *The human larynx.* New York: Raven Press.

Ford, C. N., & Bless, D. M. (Eds.). (1991). *Phonosurgery: Assessment and surgical management of voice disorders.* New York: Raven Press.

Garrison, D. H., & Hast, M. H. (1993). Andreas Vesalius on the larynx and hyoid bone: An annotated translation from the 1543 and 1555 editions of De humani corporis fabrica. *Medical History, 37,* 3–36.

Habermann, G. (1987). Zur Stimme und ihrer Heilbehandlung in der Geschichte der Medizin. In H. Gundermann (Ed.), *Aktuelle probleme der Stimmterapie* (pp. 69–82). Stuttgart, New York: Gustave Fischer Verlag.

Hast, M. H., & Holtsmark, E. R. (1969). The larynx, organ of voice, by Julius Casserius. *Acta Oto-Laryngologica,* Suppl. 261.

Helmholtz, H. L. F. (1877, reprint 1954). *On the sensations of tone* (4th ed.). Translated by A. J. Ellis. New York: Dover.

Heseler, B. (1959). Andreas Vesalius' first public anatomy at Bologna 1540. An eyewitness report. R. Eriksson (Ed.). Uppsala and Stockholm: Almqvist & Eriksells Boktryckeri AB.

Hirano, M. (1981). Clinical examination of voice. Wien/New York: Springer-Verlag.

Höfler, H., & Major, E. H. (1980). Österreich. In J. Wendler (Ed.), *75 Jahre Phoniatrie* (pp. 134–142). Berlin: Humboldt-Universität.

Huard, P., & Wong, M. (1959). *La médecine chinoise au cours des siècles.* Paris: Les Éditions Roger Dacosta.

Hubotter, F. (1929). *Die chinesische Medizin.* Leipzig: Verlag der "Asia Major."

Hunt, F. V. (1978). *Origins in acoustics.* New Haven and London: Yale University Press.

Isshiki, N. (1980). Japan. In J. Wendler (Ed.), *75 Jahre Phonaitrie* (pp. 114–122). Berlin: Humboldt-Universiät.

Kirchner, J. A. (1986). *Pressman and Kelemen's physiology of the larynx* (3rd ed.). Washington, DC: American Academy of Ophthalmology and Otolaryngology.

Kirikae, I. (1966). Speech pathology in Japan and Formosa. In R. W. Rieber & R. S. Brubaker (Eds.), *Speech pathology* (pp. 561–570). Philadelphia: Lippincott.

Kleiweg de Zwaan, J. P. (1917). Völkerkundisches und geschichtliches uber die Heilkunde der Chinesen und Japaner. Naturkundige Verhandelingen van de Hollandsche Maatschappij der Wetenschappen. *Derde Verzameling, Deel VII.* Haarlem: De Erven Loosjes.

Kutumbiah, P. (1962). *Ancient Indian medicine.* Bombay-Calcutta-Madras-New Delhi: Orient Longmans Ltd.

Lesky, E. (1965). *Die Wiener medizinische Schule im 19. Jahrhundert.* Graz-Köln: Hermann Bohlaus Nachf.

Luchsinger, R. (1970). *Handbuch der Stimm- und Sprachheilkunde. Vol. I. Die Stimme und ihre Störungen.* Wien-New York: Springer-Verlag.

Lullies, H. (1953). Physiologie der Stimme und Sprache. In O. Ranke & H. Lullies, (Eds.), *Gehör Stimme Sprache* (pp. 163–293). Berlin-Göttingen-Heidelberg: Springer Verlag.

May, M. D. (1968). *Galen on the usefulness of the parts ofthe body.* I, II. Ithaca: Cornell University Press.

Moeller, D. (1975). *Speech pathology and audiology. Iowa origins of a dicipline.* Iowa City: The University of Iowa.

Moore, G. P. (1937). A short history of laryngeal investigation. *Journal of Speech, 23,* 531–564.

Moore, G. P. (1991). A short history of laryngeal investigation. *Journal of Voice, 5*(3), 266–281.

O'Malley, C. D. (1964). *Andreas Vesalius of Brussels.* Berkeley and Los Angeles: University of California Press.

O'Malley, C. D., & Saunders, J. B. de C. M. (1952). *Leonardo da Vinci on the human body.* New York: H. Schuman.

O'Neill, Y. V. (1980). *Speech and speech disorders in Western thought before 1600.* Westport, CN: Greenwood Press.

Panconcelli-Calzia, G. (1940). *Quellenatlas zur Geschichte der Phonetik.* Hamburg: Hansischer Gildenverlag.

Panconcelli-Calzia, G. (1941). *Geschichtszahlen der Phonetik. 3000 Jahre Phonetik.* Hamburg: Hansischer Gildenverlag.

Panconcelli-Calzia, G. (1942). *Die phonetik des Aristoteles.* Hamburg: Hansischer Gildenverlag.

Panconcelli-Calzia, G. (1943). *Leonardo als Phonetiker.* Hamburg: Hansischer Gildenverlag.

Panconcelli-Calzia, G. (1957a). Entstehung und Entwicklung der bildlichen Darstellung des Kehlkopfes. *Folia Phoniatrica, 9*(1), 1–10.

Panconcelli-Calzia, G. (1957b). Earlier history of phonetics. In L. Kaiser (Ed.), *Manual of phonetics.* Amsterdam: North-Holland Publishing Co.

Panconcelli-Calzia, G. (1961). *3000 Jahre Stimmforschung.* Marburg: N. G. Elwert Verlag.

Pressman, J. J. (1942). Physiology of the vocal cords in phonation and respiration. *Archives of Otolaryngology, 35*(3), 355–398.

Pressman, J. J., & Kelemen, G. (1955). Physiology of the larynx. *Physiological Reviews, 35,* 506–554.

Reich, W. (1950). Historische und ästhetische Grundlagen der Stimmkunst. *Ciba-zeitschrift, 11*(123), 4509–4513.

Rieber, R. W., & Brubaker, R. S. (Eds.). (1966). *Speech pathology.* Philadelphia: Lippincott.

Rothenberg, M. (1981). Some relations between glottal air flow and vocal fold contact area. In C. L. Ludlow & M. O. Hart (Eds.),

Proceedings of the Conference on the Assessment of Vocal Pathology (pp. 88–96). American Speech-Language-Hearing Association Reports, No. 11.

Sarton, G. (1955). *Appreciation of ancient and medieval science during the renaissance.* New York: A. S. Barnes & Co.

Savithri,S. R. (1988). Speech and hearing science in ancient India—a review of Sanskirt literature. *Journal of Communication Disorders, 21,* 271–317.

Scherer, R. C. (1981). *Laryngeal fluid mechanics: Steady flow considerations using static models.* Doctoral dissertation, University of Iowa: Iowa City.

Scherer, R. C. (1991). Physiology of phonation: A review of basic mechanics. In C. N. Ford & D. M. Bless (Eds.), *Phonosurgery: Assessment and surgical management of voice disorders* (pp. 77–93). New York: Raven Press.

Schönhärl, E. (1960). *Die Stroboskopie in der Praktischen Laryngologie.* Stuttgart: Georg Thieme Verlag.

Singer, C. (1959). *A short history of scientific ideas to 1900.* Oxford: Oxford University Press.

Stumpf, C. (1926). *Die Sprachlaute.* Berlin: Julius Springer.

Sundberg, J. (1987). *The science of the singing voice. Dekalb:* Northern Illinois University Press.

Titze, I. R. (Ed.). (1993). *Vocal fold physiology.* San Diego: Singular Publishing Group.

Titze, I. R. (1994). *Principles of voice production.* Englewood Cliffs, NJ: Prentice-Hall.

Ungeheuer, G. (1962). *Elemmente einer akustischen Theorie der Vokalartikulation.* Berlin: Springer-Verlag.

von Leden, H. (1990). Pioneers in the evolution of voice care and voice science in the United States of America. *Journal of Voice, 4*(2), 99–106.

von Leden, H. (1993a). The cultural history of the larynx and voice. In W. J. Gould, R. T. Sataloff, & J. R. Spiegel, (Eds.), *Voice surgery* (pp. 3–63). St. Louis: Mosby.

von Leden, H. (1993b). The history of phonosurgery. In W. J. Gould, R. T. Sataloff, & J. R. Spiegel, (Eds.), *Voice surgery* (pp. 65–95). St. Louis: Mosby.

Weir, N. (1990). *Otolaryngology, an illustrated history.* London: Butterworths.

Wendler, J. (Ed.). (1980). *75 Jahre Phoniatrie.* Berlin: Humboldt-Universität.

Wyke, B. D., & Kirchner, J. A. (1976). Neurology of the larynx. In R. Hinchcliffe & D. Harrison (Eds.), *Scientific foundations of otolarygology* (pp. 546–574). London: Heinemann.

Zehmisch, H., Siegert, C., & Wendler, J. (1980). Deutschland bis 1945. In J. Wendler (Ed.), *75 Jahre Phoniatrie* (pp. 11–41). Berlin: Humboldt-Universität.

CHAPTER 2

THE ANATOMY OF THE VOCAL MECHANISM

G. PAUL MOORE, PH.D.

Most adults are aware, in a general way, of the function of the respiratory tract, through which air flows to and from the lungs. They recognize that this airway is composed of the mouth, nose, pharynx, larynx, trachea, and lungs. Observation and incidental study have revealed that vocal sound is produced when the vocal folds, which are located in the larynx, are set into vibration by the breath during exhalation. Most people have felt the vibration of the vocal folds upon touching their "Adam's Apple" on the anterior part of the neck while they are speaking. This common information is a valuable reference point when the speech-language pathologist is called upon to aid an individual who has a voice disorder.

When such a person presents himself to a speech-language pathologist for help, a professional relationship is established and the clinician is expected to know how to evaluate and treat the voice disorder. The steps would be routine if each voice defect were related directly to a specific structural or functional cause; diagnosis would be unnecessary and therapy could be guided by recipe or computer! It is un-

fortunate, perhaps, that defects of voice cannot be managed with such precision, but the audible factor, the symptom, does not reveal its etiology; its possible causes are frequently hidden in heredity, disease, trauma, environmental models, and surgical alteration. Diagnosis and treatment of organic voice disorders usually involve medical specialists in various fields, and it is not only desirable but necessary to combine the professional skills and information of these related disciplines with speech pathology. However, to do so successfully requires meaningful communication among these specialties which demands insight and knowledge within each group as well as a common vocabulary. One of the minimal expectations is that the speech-language pathologist understand and be conversant with the anatomy and physiology of the organs used in voice production.

Such knowledge is equally important as a basis for the voice evaluations and therapy carried on by the speech pathologist. Many strange ideas about voice disorders have been constructed on foundations of misinformation, and no one can

23

know the number of errors in therapy that have been practiced because the clinician did not understand the mechanism with which he or she was working.

Persons who are already familiar with the anatomy and physiology of the vocal organs can use this chapter as a review outline. Those who have not studied this area should look upon the chapter as a base from which to explore the detailed literature.

STRUCTURE OF THE LARYNX

Because vocal sound and the phonatory disorders are generated in the larynx, this organ offers an appropriate place to begin a detailed description of the mechanisms of voice production. It will be observed in the subsequent presentations that the larynx has been featured much as is the jewel in a ring; the adjacent supports are independently important, but they are relatively subordinate to the central stone. This focal emphasis results from the subject being discussed and should not imply that the larynx is more important to oral communication than the tongue, soft palate, or any other essential structure.

The larynx is a midline organ located in the anterior part of the neck, immediately deep to the skin and a few thin muscles. It extends approximately from the jaw-neck angle downward to within a short distance above the sternal notch and can be palpated readily. If a finger is placed on the Adam's apple, which is the prominence of the thyroid cartilage, and moved upward a fraction of an inch, a small v-shaped notch can be felt. This region has no functional significance in phonation but is useful as a reference point for the identification of other structures. It may be seen in Figure 2–1.

Immediately above the thyroid notch there is a small soft area which is bordered above by what feels like a hard horizontal ridge. This structure is the anterior part of the hyoid bone, a u-shaped member which is represented in the Figure 2–1 and is usually considered to be the upper boundary of the larynx.

If the finger is moved directly downward from the thyroid notch along the cartilage, a distance of one-half to three-quarters of an inch, another soft area will be felt which is bordered below by another prominent hard ridge. This soft region represents the separation between the lower border of the thyroid cartilage and the upper part of the anterior section of the cricoid cartilage. The lower border of the cricoid ring is designated as the limit of the larynx and also the division between the larynx and the trachea. However, examination of the structures demonstrates that one or more of the tracheal rings may be continuous with the cricoid cartilage and explains why that is sometimes referred to as the upper limit of the trachea.

Laryngeal Cartilages

Two of the five major cartilages of the larynx have been encountered in the preceding reference to the external features of the anterior section of the neck. These two, the thyroid and the cricoid, are unpaired midline structures that lie across the median sagittal plane. Another single cartilage that crosses the median plane is the epiglottis. This member is shaped somewhat like a leaf and rests almost vertically above the vocal folds with its stem end attached just above the anterior commissure. The two other major cartilages are the arytenoids, which are paired and rest on the cricoid cartilage approximately at the junction of its posterior plate and the lateral portion of its arch. There are also two pairs of minor cartilages, the corniculate and cuneiform, which are unimportant in phonation and consequently will not be discussed here. The arytenoid car-

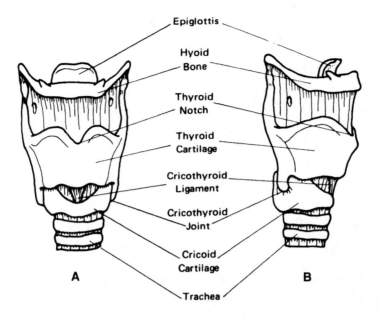

FIGURE 2–1. Hyoid bone and cartilages of the larynx. **A.** Front view. **B.** Lateral view from the right side.

tilages, the epiglottis, and the corniculate cartilages can be identified in Figures 2–1 and 2–2. These figures can serve as a useful reference throughout the subsequent portions of this book. Because the major cartilages provide the supporting framework of the larynx and its muscle attachments and they are functionally important in phonation, it is desirable to examine certain features in some detail.

Thyroid Cartilage

The thyroid cartilage is the largest of the group, and although its size varies considerably among individuals in conformity with their other structures, some concept of its dimensions can be gained from the following measurements: the angle formed by the two alae is about 90° in men and up to 120° in women; the vertical midline junction between the wings is about three-quarters of an inch long, and the distance between the line of junction and the posterior border of each ala is ap-

proximately 1.5 inches; the vertical dimension of each ala also averages about 1.5 inches along a line in front of the inferior and superior cornua, which, in turn, measure vertically about 2 inches from tip to tip. These dimensions are given to help those who work with voices to realize the relatively small size of the structures involved. Photographs, drawings, and motion pictures are apt to create distorted concepts for those who do not have an opportunity to dissect or directly observe human anatomical material.

The internal structures of the larynx are enclosed on two sides by the thyroid cartilage, which forms a triangular area that is open posteriorly. This arrangement and the dimensions further reflect the diminutive size of the laryngeal parts and indicate the protection which the thyroid cartilage gives to the interior larynx and airway. On the outer surface of each ala is a low ridge which extends from the base of the superior cornu downward and forward to the lower border. This

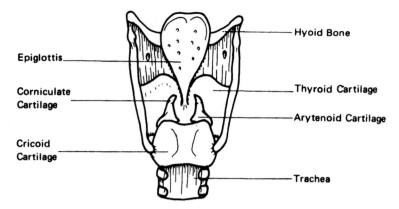

Epiglottis

Corniculate
Cartilage

Cricoid
Cartilage

Hyoid Bone

Thyroid Cartilage

Arytenoid Cartilage

Trachea

FIGURE 2-2. Hyoid bone and laryngeal cartilages: posterior view.

oblique line provides attachment for certain extrinsic laryngeal muscles which are described below.

Cricoid Cartilage

The cricoid cartilage is partially surrounded by the lower portions of the thyroid cartilage, to which it is attached at joints located at the junction of the inferior cornua of the thyroid and the articular facets on the cricoid. The contacting areas of the cricothyroid joints are relatively flat and usually ovoid, indicating that the cartilages are capable of limited rotational and some anterior-posterior sliding movements. The location of the articular facets on the cricoid cartilage should be noted in relation to the margins of the cartilages. The significance of the motions of the two cartilages in relation to each other during phonation is discussed below.

The cricoid cartilage is a ring that completely surrounds the airway at the top of the trachea. It is thick in cross-section, wide posteriorly in the vertical dimension, and narrow anteriorly. It resembles a signet ring, as can be observed in Figure 2-3. The cricoid facets of the cricoarytenoid joints are located posterolaterally on the upper angular rim of the cricoid cartilage and not on top of the

broad posterior plate where they sometimes appear in anatomical illustrations. The joint surfaces are shaped somewhat like the side of a bean with the long dimension following the underlying cartilage. The axis of each facet has been represented in Figure 2-3; it is apparent that the axes extend downward and laterally from a point that is above, medial, and posterior to the facets. The angles of these axes determine the gross movements of the arytenoid cartilages.

Arytenoid Cartilages

The arytenoid cartilages rest on the cricoid cartilage at the cricoarytenoid facets mentioned previously. Each of these cartilages has a base and three sides which taper to a peak somewhat like a pyramid (see Figures 2-2, 2-4, and 2-10). The posterior face is triangular with the upper angle rising at the medial side; it is concave along its vertical dimension and its surface is smooth. The medial face is also triangular, having its apex curving posteriorly; the surface is relatively flat and smooth. The lower portion of the medial face projects forward in combination with extensions of the base and anterior face to form the vocal process. The frontal or, more accurately, the antero-lateral face,

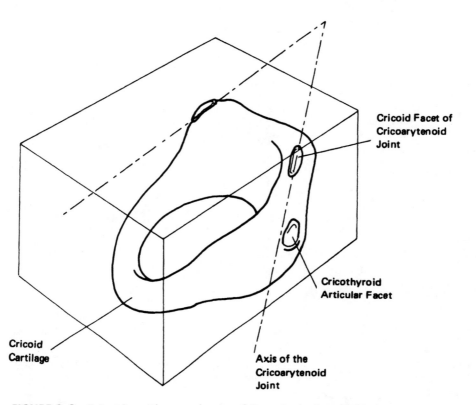

FIGURE 2-3. Cricoid cartilage and axes of the cricoarytenoid joints.

extends from the anterior border of the medial face to the lateral border of the posterior face, somewhat like the widest side of a right angle pyramid. This face has an irregular contour which is distinguished by two large depressions separated by a horizontal ridge. The lower indentation or fovea is identified later as the site of attachments for vocal fold muscles. The arytenoid base, or under surface, is relatively broad and contains a prominent concavity toward its lateral aspect. This depression contains the smooth joint surface that rests on and articulates with the cricoid facet. Immediately beyond the lateral aspect of the arytenoid joint surface, the base of the cartilage terminates in a blunt, rounded projection which is the muscular process. The upper surface of this prominence provides attachment for the lateral and posterior

cricoarytenoid muscles. The shape of the arytenoid cartilage gives it great strength at its areas of stress and provides a minimum of size and weight. These factors undoubtedly contribute to the speed and efficiency of the cartilage movement that occurs during adduction and abduction associated with protection of the airway and the voicing and unvoicing of sounds in speaking.

Epiglottic Cartilage

The cartilage of the epiglottis is the fifth major cartilage of the laryngeal complex. This structure is shaped somewhat like a leaf, narrow at its stem and widening to a broad rounded extremity. It is attached by a ligament at its narrow end to the inner surface of the thyroid cartilage at the midline, a short distance below the

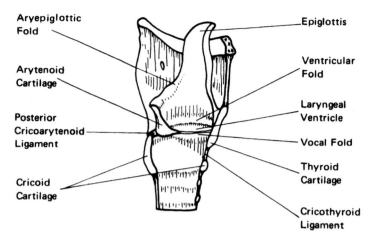

Aryepiglottic Fold

Arytenoid Cartilage

Posterior Cricoarytenoid Ligament

Cricoid Cartilage

Epiglottis

Ventricular Fold

Laryngeal Ventricle

Vocal Fold

Thyroid Cartilage

Cricothyroid Ligament

FIGURE 2–4. Left half of the larynx viewed from the right side. The structures are exposed by a median sagittal section.

thyroid notch. It projects upward and backward into the pharyngeal area and is supported partly by an elastic ligament extending from its anterior surface to the posterior surface of the body of the hyoid bone. The primary function of the epiglottis is the protection of the airway during swallowing; it helps to close the laryngeal opening into the pharynx and assists in channeling food and water into the esophagus. Because it is relatively unimportant in the production of voice and is not the direct source of voice disorders, it need not be discussed further.

Laryngeal Ligaments and Membranes

Some of the ligaments and membranes of the larynx are important in the functioning of the various parts and consequently contribute to voice production. The moving members of the two laryngeal joints, cricothyroid and cricoarytenoid, are held in place by ligaments. These bands of tissue maintain the joint surfaces in proper operational relationships to each other and limit motion, thus preventing functional dislocations. Deep to the ligaments, each joint is surrounded by a synovial

membrane which supplies and holds the lubricant for the sliding surfaces. The ligaments and membranes of the cricoarytenoid joint are arranged to allow great freedom of motion.

Posterior Cricoarytenoid Ligament

The posterior cricoarytenoid ligament is not directly adjacent to the cricoarytenoid joint, but it is intimately involved with the motion of the arytenoid cartilage. This tissue band extends from the internal face and upper border of the posterior section of the cricoid cartilage to the lower portions of the posterior face of the arytenoid cartilage (see Figures 2–4 and 2–5). It prevents the arytenoid from sliding too far forward on its facet, and provides a complex radius that regulates the arc of the adductive and abductive motions of the arytenoid cartilages. Furthermore, and perhaps most importantly, it offers an anchor for the attached arytenoid cartilages when the muscles in the vocal fold contract for phonatory and valvular adjustments. If this posterior anchoring were not present, the contraction of the vocal fold muscles could disarticulate the arytenoid cartilages (von Leden & Moore, 1961).

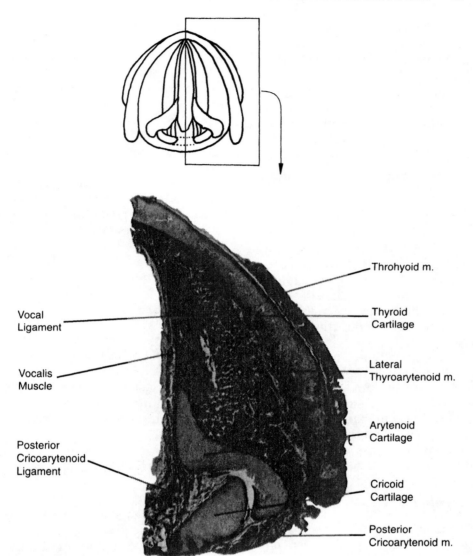

FIGURE 2-5. Horizontal section through the right half of the larynx at the level of the vocal ligament.

Vocal Ligaments

The vocal ligament is a threadlike structure extending from the vocal process of each arytenoid cartilage to an anterior attachment on the inner surface of the thyroid cartilage just lateral to the midline. This strand usually parallels the vocalis muscle, supplies substance to the glottal margins of the vocal folds, and probably limits their elongation. The vocal ligament is strongly adherent to the mucosal covering of the vocal folds and is formed as the thickened upper border of the conus elasticus. The latter structure is a tough membrane that lies immediately deep to the mucosa in the larynx from the level of the vocal folds down to the lower border of the cricoid cartilage. Anteriorly, in the area between the thyroid and cricoid cartilages, the membrane is continuous with a thickened band called the cricothyroid ligament. The conus elasticus protects the vocal fold muscles from below and may influence vibrational pattern; the anterior ligament limits the separation of the thyroid and cricoid cartilages and indirectly influences the rotational and sliding motion of the cricothyroid joint, which could affect pitch range.

Muscles That Support and Position the Larynx

It is general knowledge that muscles function actively in only one way: they shorten by contraction and consequently tend to draw the structures that are fastened to them toward each other. Because muscles cannot push, there are opposing groups of muscles that draw their associated structures first in one direction and then in another.

Muscles usually are named for the structures to which they are attached, but some are labeled to denote a particular characteristic or position. The student who has not become familiar with anatomical terms will find the names easy to learn if he visualizes each structure clearly and traces the interconnecting tissues.

Suprahyoid Muscles

All of the bones in the body except one articulate in some manner with other bones; the exception is the hyoid bone situated at the angle of the neck. The larynx is suspended from this bone, which is itself supported by many muscles from the tongue, mandible, pharynx, and skull. However, there are four muscles that operate synergistically to shift the hyoid bone in a forward, upward, or backward direction and consequently contribute importantly to the positioning of the larynx. These are the focus of the immediate discussion.

Digastric Muscle

The digastricus, as its name indicates, is a muscle with two bellies or sections that

are joined by an intermediate tendon which is itself attached to the hyoid bone by a sling of connective tissue (Figure 2–6). The anterior belly runs forward to attach to the inner surface of the mandible near its lower border and slightly lateral to the midline. The posterior belly is longer than its counterpart and extends backward and downward from the ear to its origin on the mastoid process. The contraction of the anterior belly shifts the hyoid bone forward and upward; contraction of the posterior belly moves the bone backward and upward; when both bellies contract simultaneously, the motion is more or less vertical, depending on the relative pull from the two sections.

Stylohyoid Muscle

The stylohyoideus is a slender muscle that originates on the styloid process (a bony projection that extends downward from the region of the ear canal) and travels to the anterior portion of the greater cornu of the hyoid bone. Contraction of this muscle lifts and retracts the hyoid.

Mylohyoid and Geniohyoid Muscles

The remaining two suprahyoid muscles, the mylohyoideus and the geniohyoideus, arise along the inner surface of the lower border of the mandible and insert in the body of the hyoid bone. The mylohyoideus forms the floor of the mouth, and its posterior fibers tend to lift the hyoid bone. The geniohyoideus is paired and runs beside the anterior belly of the digastricus directly from its attachments on either side of the symphysis of the mandible to the hyoid bone. Its contraction draws this bone forward.

Infrahyoid Muscles

The muscles which reach the hyoid bone from below exert a pull in a downward direction. It is evident that the lifting and

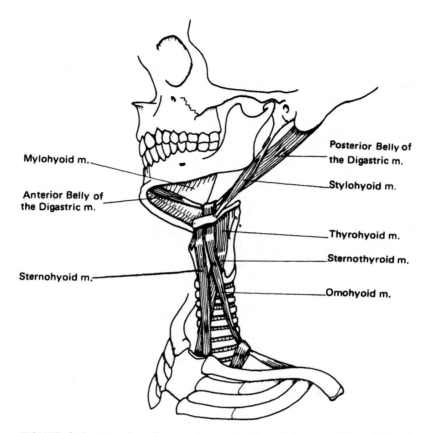

FIGURE 2–6. Muscles that support the hyoid bone superiorly and inferiorly.

shifting by the suprahyoid muscles, combined with a downward pull from the infrahyoid group, could place the hyoid bone and the larynx in a variety of positions. There is some clinical evidence that adjustments in hyoid position are associated with voice quality and pitch. Whether these modifications contribute to phonation or simply accompany it is not known at this time.

Omohyoid Muscle

The omohyoideus is a long, thin, narrow, two-bellied muscle that originates along the upper border of the scapula (shoulder blade) and inserts in the lateral aspect of the body of the hyoid bone. Between these two attachments the inferior belly ex-

tends across the lower part of the neck to the region above the medial end of the clavicle (collar bone), where it is encased by a sheath of connective tissue that tethers it to the clavicle and first rib. The superior belly forms an angle with the inferior section at the sheath and passes almost vertically to the hyoid bone. The omohyoideus usually contracts to lower the hyoid at the time of inhalation, but it is often active during phonation when low pitches are attempted.

Sternohyoid Muscle

The sternohyoideus is one of the so-called strap muscles that extend upward from the superior border of the sternum, or breast bone, along the anterior part of the neck over the thyroid cartilage to the body of the hyoid bone. The label "strap" is applied descriptively because the muscles are relatively long, thin, and of uniform width throughout their length. The descriptive term is found frequently in the literature dealing with laryngectomy.

Sternothyroid Muscle

Another strap-like infrahyoid muscle, similar in structure to the sternohyoideus, is the sternothyroideus, which originates from the cartilage of the first rib and the posterior surface of the upper part of the sternum. It ascends under the sternohyoideus to the thyroid cartilage, where it inserts along the oblique line. Upon contraction it draws the thyroid cartilage downward.

Thyrohyoid Muscle

A relatively short muscle, having approximately the same width and thickness as the sternothyroideus, extends upward from the oblique line on the lamina of the thyroid cartilage and inserts into the greater horn of the hyoid bone. As might be guessed, it is called the thyrohyoideus. Contraction of this muscle lifts the larynx if the hyoid bone is fixed, or lowers the hyoid bone if the larynx is fixed. The implications of this deceptively simple statement are extremely complex when one contemplates the infinite number of possible adjustments between the suprahyoid muscles and the combined or independent actions of the thyrohyoid, the sternothyroid, and the sternohyoid muscles.

Inferior Pharyngeal Constrictor Muscle

The inferior constrictor muscle of the pharynx is the principal contractile tissue of the lower one-third of the pharynx. This muscle arises from the sides of the cricoid cartilage, the inferior cornua, and posterior areas of the thyroid cartilage. The lower muscle fibers are horizontal and join with the circular fibers of the upper end of the esophagus. This section of the constrictor is sometimes referred to as the cricopharyngeus muscle. The upper fibers of the inferior constrictor become increasingly oblique from below upward as they sweep around both sides of the pharynx to their medial attachments along the posterior pharyngeal wall. Contraction of the inferior constrictor muscle lifts and retracts the larynx to hold it against the posterior surface of the hypopharynx. During swallowing the inferior constrictor relaxes when the suprahyoid muscles draw the larynx forward to enlarge the pharynx. There is some clinical evidence to suggest that persons who appear to exert extreme muscular effort in the neck area and pharynx during speaking are contracting the inferior constrictor muscle and probably most of the other extrinsic muscles also. However, the major reason for the student of voice disorders to understand the role of the inferior constrictor, and particularly the part called the cricopharyngeus, is its relationship to laryngectomy and esophageal speech. This latter group of muscle fibers often plays an important role in the development of alaryngeal voice.

With the exception of the lower fibers of the inferior constrictor, the extrinsic muscles of the larynx are attached to the thyroid cartilage. This arrangement permits positioning and stabilizing of the larynx, allows the cricoid cartilage to perform a limited rotatory type movement in which the front arch of the cartilage lifts upward toward the thyroid cartilage and simultaneously the posterior segment of the cartilage tilts backward. This backward tilt carries the arytenoid cartilages in the same direction. An imaginary axis for this rotatory adjustment passes through the cricothyroid joints. With normal relaxation of the inferior constrictor muscles, the thyroid and cricoid cartilages can also shift anteriorly and posteriorly in opposite directions. These rotatory and sliding adjustments move the anterior and posterior attachments of the vocal folds alternately away from and toward each other thereby lengthening and shortening the vocal folds. These adjustments assist in the changes of vocal pitch.

Muscles That Compose and Adjust the Vocal Folds

The intrinsic laryngeal musculature can be presented more meaningfully when the topography and arrangement of the laryngeal interior is known. Figure 2–4 represents the left half of a larynx and reveals not only the location of the cartilages but also some of the muscles and other structures. In the upper part of the diagram a vertical, medial section of the epiglottis is shown, from the lateral border of which the aryepiglottic fold can be seen extending to its attachment at the arytenoid cartilage. Anterior to this latter structure, two ridges are shown separated by a deep recess. The upper ridge marks the ventricular or false vocal fold; the lower represents the true vocal fold; and the recess denotes the laryngeal ventricle (sometimes called the ventricle of Morgagni). At the anterior ends of the ventricular and vocal folds, a median sagittal section of the thyroid cartilage is shown, and below it there appears a section through the anterior arch of the cricoid cartilage. On the opposite or posterior side of the airway, this same diagram reveals the relative height of the posterior cricoid lamina and demonstrates the placement of the arytenoid cartilage. The lower part of this latter member is below the upper posterior border of the cricoid cartilage, which demonstrates again that the arytenoid cartilage does not sit upon the signet portion of the cricoid. The location of the ary-

tenoid also indicates the manner in which the posterior cricoarytenoid ligament can secure the arytenoid cartilage to the cricoid cartilage and thereby provide a firm anchor for the muscular contraction of the vocal fold.

The appearance of the internal laryngeal structures, as seen from above, is represented in Figure 2–7. For orientation purposes, the following structures should be cross-referenced in Figures 2–2 and 2–4, and visualized clearly for quick recognition: epiglottis, aryepiglottic folds, ventricular folds, vocal folds, glottis, arytenoid cartilages, and trachea.

The intrinsic laryngeal muscles open and close the glottis, adjust the length of the vocal folds, and establish their internal tension and elasticity. (It should be understood that muscle functions of the type indicated are regulated by neural impulses traveling through the nerves attached to the muscles. A subsequent section of this chapter reviews the nerve supply to the larynx.) These functions may combine to form a protective valve to keep food, water, and foreign objects out of the lungs; or they may be synthesized into the delicate adjustments of phonation. The ability of the intrinsic muscles to accomplish these diverse feats is directly related to their size, shape, and location, an account of which is the intent of this immediate presentation. The muscles that will be described are the thyroarytenoid (including the vocalis), lateral cricoarytenoid, two types of interarytenoids, posterior cricoarytenoid, and the cricothyroid.

Thyroarytenoid and Vocalis Muscles

The mass of muscle fibers that constitute the body of the vocal folds has been described in various ways by different anatomists. Some consider the structure to be a single muscle with two or more parts, whereas others describe the separate divisions as distinct muscles. For the speech-

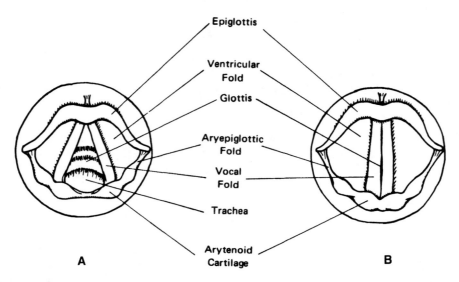

FIGURE 2–7. Views of the interior of the larynx as seen from above with the aid of a laryngeal mirror. **A.** Vocal folds abducted for respiration. **B.** Vocal folds adducted for phonation.

language pathologist and teacher, the different concepts are not important; the variations that are evident in the literature are pointed out here in an effort to reduce confusion in related reading.

The muscle fibers composing the vocal folds originate on the thyroid cartilage and insert at the arytenoid cartilages. In consequence, they are called the thyroarytenoid muscle or muscles. A medial bundle of fibers that arises from the inner surface of the thyroid cartilage just lateral to the median line and about midway between the upper and lower edges of the cartilage is often designated as the vocalis muscle (see Figure 2–5). This group of fibers, or fasciculus, passes backward parallel with and attached to the vocal ligament and is inserted along the superior and lateral aspects of the vocal process of the arytenoid cartilage. Other muscle bundles originate on the thyroid cartilage beside and below the vocalis along a line that extends downward over the lower half of the thyroid cartilage and onto the upper portion of the central cricothyroid

ligament as seen in Figure 2–8. These fibers pass posteriorly in an upward and lateral direction with the strands that are adjacent to the vocalis, inserting on the lower and lateral aspects of the vocal process. Other fibers, originating from above and running downward, attach progressively along the anterolateral face of the arytenoid, particularly in the inferior fossa. Some of the lateral-most fibers course behind the laryngeal ventricle; others pass through the ventricular folds to attach to the prominent ridge about half-way up the anterolateral face of the arytenoid cartilage. The muscle fibers in the ventricular fold are designated by some anatomists as the ventricular muscle. Frequently, fibers of the lateral or external thyroarytenoideus also run to the ridge above the muscular process of the arytenoid cartilage and pass beyond as part of the transverse arytenoideus. The length of the thyroarytenoid muscle mass in adult larynges varies from approximately 0.5 inch in small females to 1 inch in large males. The relatively small size of

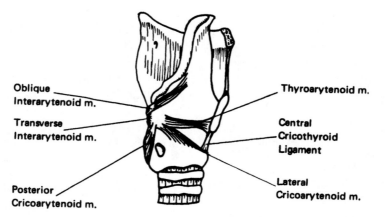

FIGURE 2–8. Muscles of adduction and abduction. View of the larynx from the right side with the right ala of the thyroid cartilage removed.

the vocal folds makes the complexity of this structure and its function seem even more remarkable.

Contraction of the vocalis and the thyroarytenoid muscles has varying effects, depending on the positions of the arytenoid cartilages. These cartilages, and consequently the vocal folds, are approximated by contraction of the muscles of the folds. However, when the glottis is closed, additional muscle tension presses the folds together more tightly and also tends to draw the anterior and posterior attachments toward each other, thereby shortening the vocal folds. Activation of the lateral fibers behind the ventricle and the muscle elements of the false vocal folds moves these structures toward the midline to constrict the supraglottic space of the larynx. There is no direct evidence that the vocalis and the thyroarytenoideus operate independently of each other, but the possibility is expressed frequently in the literature and seems to be supported in laryngeal studies. This concept contends that contraction of the lateral portions of the thyroarytenoid muscle shortens the anterior-posterior dimension of the larynx and thereby allows the vocalis to relax and to be shortened passively. This

difference of behavior may account for the flaccid appearance of the vocal folds observed in high speed motion pictures when low pitches are being produced.

Lateral Cricoarytenoid Muscle

The lateral cricoarytenoid muscle arises along the upper border of the arch of the cricoid cartilage and extends posteriorly to insert into the anterior segment of the muscular process of the arytenoid cartilage (see Figure 2–8). When the arytenoid cartilage is in an adducted position, the pull of the lateral cricoarytenoid muscle almost parallels the axis of the cricoarytenoid joint. In this relationship the force of the muscle is exerted primarily along the axis of the joint to pull the cartilage anteriorly. However, when the arytenoid cartilage is abducted, the muscular process, and hence the muscle attachment, lies farther laterally; consequently, the angle between the muscle and joint axis is greater and the medial component of the muscle action is increased. The combination of the medial and anterior forces creates the possibility of a spiral motion of the arytenoid cartilage on the cricoarytenoid joint. However, the word "possibility" should be stressed because the effects of other muscles, combined with the constraints of the cricoarytenoid ligament, alter the movement in conformity with the kinds of laryngeal behavior needed.

Transverse Arytenoid Muscle

The transverse interarytenoideus is an unpaired, relatively thick muscle, oval in cross section, that rests in the concavity of the posterior surfaces of the arytenoid cartilages (see Figures 2–8 and 2–9). It passes from a continuous attachment along the lateral ridge and adjacent face of one arytenoid to similar positions on the other.

Electromyographic investigations have demonstrated that this muscle relaxes during abduction of the vocal folds and contracts during adduction (Faaborg-Anderson, 1957). Contraction affects both of the arytenoid cartilages simultaneously and causes each to sweep through a small arc around its cricoarytenoid joint axis and concurrently to slide in a posterio-medial-cranial direction along the joint axis. This combined motion approximates the medial faces of the arytenoid cartilages at the median sagittal plane and consequently adducts the vocal folds.

The action just presented postulates cooperative behavior by the lateral cricoarytenoid and thyroarytenoid muscles previously described. These muscles facilitate adduction and subsequently help to stabilize the arytenoid cartilages on their joint surfaces and to maintain approximation of the vocal processes.

The lateral cricoarytenoid muscle, in a synergistic relationship with the interarytenoideus, probably also accomplishes the variation in posterior closure of the glottis that occurs with rapid variation of voice pitch. If both lateral cricoarytenoid muscles pull the arytenoid cartilages anterolaterally along the joint axis, the car-

tilages will separate slightly and the vocal folds will be shortened. These two adjustments appear to occur when the vocal pitch is lowered.

Ultra high speed motion pictures suggest the possibility that the so-called chest register is created in part by loosely approximated arytenoid cartilages that are vibrated by the movements of the membranous portions of the vocal folds. The effect of the additional mass of the cartilages would be a reduction in frequency of the vibrator and a modification of vibratory pattern.

During phonation at the higher vocal pitches the interarytenoideus and lateral cricoarytenoideus hold the medial surfaces of the arytenoid cartilages together tightly and thereby help to provide a firm anchor for the strong contractions of the vocalis and thyroarytenoid muscles. At the same time this tight approximation of the cartilages impedes their vibratory motion and limits phonatory vibration to the membranous portions of the vocal folds.

Oblique Arytenoid Muscle

Some of the adjustments of the arytenoid cartilages that have been associated with the transverse interarytenoideus are aided also by the oblique interarytenoid muscles. These muscles are paired, originate near the muscular processes of both arytenoid cartilages, pass upward and medialward across each other at midline, and insert near the top of the opposite cartilage (refer to Figure 2–9). Some fibers continue beyond the upper attachments into the aryepiglottic folds.

The oblique muscles facilitate adduction by drawing the apices of the arytenoid cartilages medially, thereby helping to slide the cartilages around their axes. The direction of pull of these muscles and the mechanical advantage that they obtain by their attachments at the upper ends of the cartilages enable them

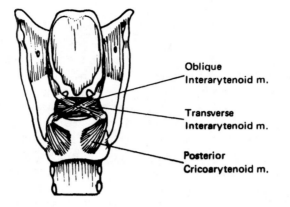

FIGURE 2-9. Posterior view of the larynx.

to exert relatively great power and to move the cartilages rapidly in the closure of the larynx. Although the oblique muscles normally function in concert, each acts independently on the cartilage to which it has its apical attachment. This arrangement is in contrast to the single transverse arytenoid muscle which affects both arytenoid cartilages equally. The capacity for separate functioning of the oblique muscles probably determines some of the adductory motion of the arytenoid cartilage on the healthy side in unilateral paralysis.

The fibers of the oblique interarytenoideus that continue beyond the upper border of the cartilage into the aryepiglottic folds help to pull the epiglottis backward as part of the mechanism of protective laryngeal closure. Concurrently, the aryepiglottic folds are drawn medially as part of the generalized closure pattern.

Posterior Cricoarytenoid Muscle

The intrinsic laryngeal muscles that have been described above close the larynx for phonation and protection of the airway. The posterior cricoarytenoid muscle, which is paired, is the only one that opens the larynx; it is the abductor. Its fibers arise over a broad area on the posterior aspect of the cricoid lamina, extend upward and

laterally, as illustrated in Figure 2–9, and converge to terminate on the lateral part of the muscular process of the arytenoid cartilage. If a plane is drawn through the middle of the muscle parallel to the longest fibers and perpendicular to the muscle mass, it will intersect the axis of the cricoarytenoid joint at an angle of approximately 90°. When the muscle contracts, it draws the muscular process of the arytenoid cartilage around the axis of the joint in a downward and backward direction.

This motion describes a circular arc around the joint axis, at right angles to it, and represents a simple type of rotation. The muscle contraction produces a direct and immediate response of the arytenoid cartilage and undoubtedly accounts for the rapid abduction of the vocal folds. High speed photographs reveal that the glottis can open within small fractions of a second, which provides physiologic support for the common observation that voiced sounds can become unvoiced almost instantaneously. It is probable that the arytenoid cartilage is capable of quicker movement than any other articulated body structure (Mårtensson, 1968).

Two physical factors are primarily responsible for the speed and extent of vocal fold abduction and deserve recognition. First, the posterior cricoarytenoid muscle is attached to the muscular process of the arytenoid cartilage close to the joint facet which serves as the fulcrum of cartilage movement. Second, it is the largest intrinsic laryngeal muscle and is, relatively, quite powerful. Because the arytenoid cartilage approximates a lever and fulcrum system, it is appropriate to apply the principles of such systems to the motions of the cartilage. It is well known that a small movement of the shorter arm of a lever will produce a proportionately larger motion in the longer arm. It is also true that the force exerted at the end of the shorter arm must be proportionately greater to move a load than the force applied at the end of the longer arm. When these principles are associated with the arytenoid cartilages, it can be said that a strong muscle acting on the arytenoid cartilage close to its fulcrum will produce a large motion at the vocal process, which is at the end of the longer arm of the lever. The physiologic effect of this mechanical system is a quick, wide opening of the airway resulting from a powerful short-stroke contraction of the posterior cricoarytenoid muscle.

The primary movements of the arytenoid cartilages are represented in Figure 2–10 by views of an animated model photographed simultaneously from the front and from above. Figure 2–10A shows the arytenoid cartilages in an abducted position; Figure 2–10B is a multiple expo-

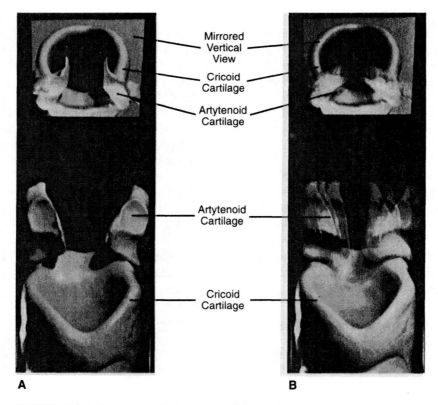

Mirrored Vertical View

Cricoid Cartilage

Artytenoid Cartilage

Artytenoid Cartilage

Cricoid Cartilage

A   **B**

FIGURE 2–10. Motions of the arytenoid cartilages illustrated by photographs of an animated model. The upper images are mirrored views of the cricoid and arytenoid cartilages shown below. **A.** Arytenoid cartilages in an abducted position. **B.** Multiple exposures to illustrate excursions of arytenoid cartilages.

sure that demonstrates the excursion of these cartilages. The upper image in both parts of the figure is a vertical view, obtained by reflection in a mirror comparable to a laryngeal mirror placed in the pharynx. The movements of the arytenoid cartilages presented in the preceding paragraphs differ in several respects from the descriptions found in many of the textbooks of anatomy and speech pathology. These works describe a rotation of the arytenoids around a vertical axis combined with a horizontal sliding motion toward and away from the glottis. Several investigators (Mårtensson, 1968) have demonstrated conclusively that a vertical axis of the type described does not exist and that the gliding motions occur in the direction of the joint axis with a maximum excursion of 2–3 mm. The preceding discussion attempted to present the concepts of the research cited.

Cricothyroid Muscle

It will be recalled from previous descriptions that the thyroid and cricoid cartilages articulate with sliding and rotatory motions at the cricothyroid joints. The muscles that are responsible for these movements are the cricothyroid muscles and their antagonists, the thyroarytenoids,

that compose the vocal folds. The cricothyroid muscles are paired and each one has two segments, both of which arise on the outer surface of the cricoid ring along the arch and forward nearly to the midline. One segment passes backward to the front edge of the inferior cornua of the thyroid cartilage; the other sends fibers in a more vertical direction to insert along the margin and lower inner face of the thyroid cartilage as illustrated in Figure 2–11. Contraction of the more horizontal fibers tends to pull the inferior cornua forward and the cricoid ring backward, thereby sliding the cartilages in opposite directions and increasing the distance between the inner surface of the thyroid cartilage and the arytenoid cartilages, an adjustment that elongates the vocal folds. Activation of the more vertically placed segment of the muscle draws the cricoid and thyroid cartilages toward each other anteriorly, causing a limited rotation at the cricothyroid articulation. When the thyroid cartilage is being actively supported by the extrinsic muscles, the rotational movement will be confined to the cricoid cartilage. However, if the thyroid and cricoid cartilages are equally free or restricted, their anterior parts will move toward each other uniformly. In either situation the rotary motion increases the

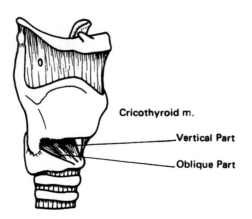

Cricothyroid m.

Vertical Part

Oblique Part

FIGURE 2-11. Cricothyroid muscle.

anterior-posterior distance in the larynx, thereby elongating the vocal folds, decreasing their cross-sectional dimension, and increasing their tension. The audible result of the functional elongation of the vocal folds is a rise of pitch. Since the cricothyroid muscles accomplish this adjustment they are sometimes referred to as the "pitch muscles."

NERVE SUPPLY TO THE LARYNX

Detailed description of the motor and sensory innervation of the larynx can be found in all books on general anatomy, and reading such literature is strongly recommended for greater clinical insight. Familiarity with the function and distribution of the major nerves to the larynx is basic to an understanding of laryngeal performance and disease. The brief sketch presented in the following paragraphs is intended as an introduction and focuses on the superior laryngeal and the recurrent laryngeal nerves, both of which are paired and supply structures on their respective right and left sides.

Superior Laryngeal Nerve

The superior laryngeal nerve branches from the vagus nerve (cranial nerve X) high in the neck, passes downward close to the carotid artery (in which the pulse can be felt at the side of the neck just back of the larynx), and subdivides into internal and external branches at a point a little above the level of the hyoid bone. The internal portion, which is sensory, enters the larynx through the membrane between the hyoid bone and the thyroid cartilage, after which it branches profusely to supply sensory fibers to glands and membranes of the epiglottis and interior of the larynx.

The external branch of the superior laryngeal nerve continues downward along the outside of the larynx to provide motor fibers to the cricothyroid muscle and to the lower section of the inferior pharyngeal constrictor, sometimes designated as the cricopharyngeus muscle.

Recurrent Laryngeal Nerve

After giving off the superior laryngeal nerves, the vagus nerve continues downward through the neck, supplying branches to many structures. When the nerve on the right side reaches the base of the neck, it crosses the subclavian artery where the right inferior or recurrent nerve emerges.

This recurrent nerve loops posteriorly around the subclavian artery, where it encounters the esophagus and trachea which it follows upward to the larynx. On the left side the vagus nerve passes downward to the level of the aorta (just above the heart) before giving off its recurrent laryngeal branch, which swings around the artery posteriorly and passes beside the esophagus and trachea to the larynx.

Both recurrent nerves enter the larynx just posterior to the inferior cornua of the thyroid cartilage and proliferate motor fibers to all of the intrinsic muscles except the cricothyroid. Research reveals that the density of nerve endings on the intrinsic laryngeal muscles is quite great, second only to that of the eye muscles. The implication is that the laryngeal musculature is capable of almost the same order of speed and adjustment as the muscles of the eye (Konig & von Leden, 1961).

The pathways and attachments of the laryngeal nerves have clinical significance in both diagnosis and rehabilitation of certain voice disorders. The longer course of the left recurrent nerve into the thoracic area subjects it to greater hazards, and its location in the region of the heart may also account for greater involvement of the left side of the larynx. It has been clinically observed by Moore that some phonatory distress is often the first evidence of a circulatory problem.

RESPIRATORY STRUCTURES RELATED TO VOICE

Professional interest in training and rehabilitation of speech requires a constant alertness to signs and symptoms that may relate to a particular disorder. It is presumed that the student of the study of voice has a working knowledge of the structures comprising the respiratory tract. However, experience has demonstrated that some reemphasis of the mechanisms and their functions as they related to the specific disorders is appropriate. The varied and subtle organic deviations that may underlie voice problems stress the need for sensitivity to every variation from the normal; and, by implication, this requires a familiarity with all aspects of the normal respiratory anatomy.

Airflow through the larynx is necessary for the production of vocal sound; the breath sets the vocal folds into vibration, and this process creates a series of pressure waves in the air which are heard as sounds. The importance of air stream to phonation makes it necessary for persons working with voice to understand the basic structures of respiration and their functions.

The fundamental principle of air motion that pertains to breathing is that air flows from regions of higher pressure toward areas of lower pressure. Air pressure may be decreased by expanding its container and increased by compressing the container. When the principle is applied to the thorax, it is evident that, as the chest cavity is enlarged, air pressure inside is decreased, and if there are no obstructions, air will flow in; by reversing the process, contraction of the thorax increases the intrathoracic pressure, causing exhalation. The means by which these changes in thoracic volume and air pressure are accomplished constitute the focus of this section.

The Trachea

Previous statements associated the larynx with the trachea, which extends from the cricoid cartilage into the thorax toward the lungs. It is the tube through which the air travels during both inhalation and exhalation. The trachea is held open by a series of closely spaced u-shaped cartilages spaced along this membranous tube. The open sections of the tracheal cartilages point toward the back and provide a flexible posterior wall that lies adjacent to the esophagus. At the lower end of the trachea, which is about 4 inches long in adults, there is a bifurcation into a right and a left bronchus, both of which continue to subdivide into bronchial tubes within the confines of the lungs until the airway eventually terminates in bronchioles and alveoli, where the gaseous interchanges with the blood take place. The lung spaces expand and contract with the ebb and flow of the air, but they have no power within themselves beyond their elasticity to move the air. Respiration is accomplished solely by the radial and vertical expansion and contraction of the thorax.

The Thorax

The thorax, or chest, is somewhat conical in shape, tapering toward the top and is wider from side to side than from front to back, as illustrated in Figures 2–12 and 2–13. The walls of the thorax are formed primarily by the 12 pairs of ribs which sweep in a downward direction from the spinal column around the cavity to the front. The ribs are attached posteriorly at joints on the vertebrae and by ligamentous connections on the lateral vertebral processes. The significance of the slope of the ribs and the arrangement of the posterior attachments is that the ribs are forced to move outward when they are lifted, which produces a radial-type ex-

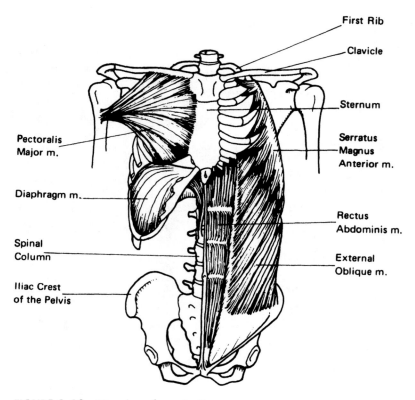

FIGURE 2-12. Muscles of respiration.

pansion of the thorax that contributes to inhalation.

The seven upper pairs of ribs are connected individually in front to the sternum, or breast bone, by means of costal cartilages; the next three pairs are attached to cartilages which join similar structures of the ribs above; and the last two, the so-called floating ribs, terminate anteriorly in the muscle walls of the abdomen. The costal cartilages in conjunction with the posterior joints permit rib movements and general flexibility of the chest wall.

The ribs are raised and lowered by several sets of muscles, some of which extend from one rib to another while others connect a rib to an external structure. The muscles that lie between the ribs extend from the lower border of one to the upper border of the one below and are or-

ganized into two groupings called the external and internal intercostal muscles. The fibers of the external muscles extend in a downward and forward direction; the internal fibers travel downward and backward. Another intrinsic muscle, the triangularis sterni, extends vertically across several ribs and the sternum on the inner surface of the thorax. External muscles attach the ribs to the vertebrae, to the bones and ligaments of the neck and shoulder region, and to the iliac crest of the pelvis and associated ligaments. The extrinsic muscles include the costal elevators, the subcostals, the superior and inferior posterior serratus, the major and minor pectoralis, the anterior serratus, the latissimus dorsi, and the quadratus lumborum. A clear visualization of their locations and functions is helpful in the diagnosis and treatment of voice disorders.

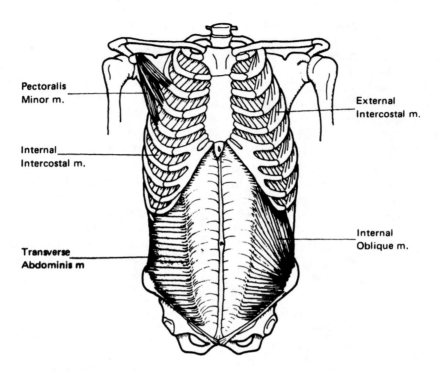

Pectoralis
Minor m.

External
Intercostal m.

Internal
Intercostal m.

Internal
Oblique m.

Transverse
Abdominis m

FIGURE 2-13. Muscles of respiration.

The Diaphragm and Abdominal Muscles

The floor of the thorax is the diaphragm, a musculotendinous partition between the thorax and abdominal cavity that bulges upward, forming an irregular dome which is somewhat higher on the right side than on the left. The central part of the diaphragm is a flat tendon with an irregular contour that is pierced by large blood vessels and the esophagus, the latter going to the stomach, situated immediately below the tendon. The peripheral parts of the diaphragm are composed of muscle fibers extending radially in a downward curve from their insertions in the central tendon to their origins, which circle the lower internal wall of the thorax. The attachments of the diaphragm are located in front on the xiphoid process of the sternum, at the sides on the lower six ribs, and posteriorly on aponeurotic arches and ligaments that connect with the spinal column and posterior ribs. When the muscle fibers contract, they draw the diaphragm downward, thereby enlarging the thoracic area in a vertical direction. However, the actual movement of the diaphragm is more complex than just implied; the excursions of parts of the central tendon are limited by its attachments to the pericardium and esophagus, thereby causing the major movements of the diaphragm to be lateralized. Furthermore, the posterior muscle fibers are longer and their insertions are lower than those of the other fibers; consequently the effective motion of the diaphragm is downward and forward. This movement does not alter the fact of vertical expansion of the thorax with contraction of the diaphragm, but it does account for the concurrent forward bulge of the abdominal wall. The diaphragm displaces the content of the viscera downward and forward.

It is this last fact that enables the abdominal muscles to function in opposition to the diaphragm. The coordinated contraction of the four principal abdominal muscles (the external oblique, internal oblique, transverse, and rectus abdominus) compresses the viscera, causing it to press against all the abdominal surfaces, including the diaphragm. If the fibers of the latter are relaxed, the visceral pressure will push the diaphragm upward to decrease the thoracic area, increase the internal pressure, and force the air out.

THE PHARYNX AND VELOPHARYNGEAL CLOSURE

As the breath is exhaled and the vocal folds are set into vibration, the air and sound flow from the larynx into the pharynx, an irregular tubular space that is shared by both the respiratory and alimentary tracts. The pharynx extends from the esophagus below to the nasal cavities and is continuous not only with those channels, but also with the larynx, mouth, and eustachian tube. In its lower two-thirds, the pharynx is capable of great change of dimension from front to back and from side to side, a factor that contributes to the act of swallowing and influences vocal resonance. The pharynx is divided into three functional sections that are from above downward: nasopharynx, oropharynx, and laryngopharynx. The nasopharynx reaches from the posterior end of the nasal passages to the level of the palate; the oropharynx extends to the hyoid bone; and the laryngopharynx continues to the esophagus, which begins at the lower border of the cricoid cartilage.

The soft palate and its associated structures are contiguous with the pharynx. Because they contribute importantly to certain organic voice disorders, the region of the pharynx and velum is discussed here in its functional continuity.

The Muscles of the Pharynx

The muscles of the pharynx serve three major functions: (1) transporting and propelling food and liquid to the esophagus; (2) maintaining an airway to the larynx; and (3) regulating the size and shape of the pharyngeal area for phonemic and voice quality resonances. The six muscles of the pharynx include the superior, middle, and inferior constrictors, the stylopharyngeus, the salpingopharyngeus, and the palatopharyngeus. The three constrictor muscles surround the pharyngeal space and constitute the principal substance of the walls of the pharynx. The other three pairs of pharyngeal muscles run more or less vertically, and although they help the constrictor muscles to vary the dimensions of the lower part of the pharynx, their primary function is the lifting of the larynx and hypopharynx.

The inferior constrictor muscle was introduced earlier in the discussion of the extrinsic muscles of the larynx, where its several attachments to the thyroid and cricoid cartilages were mentioned. The middle constrictor also has multiple originating attachments, including the lesser and greater horns of the hyoid bone, the stylohyoid ligament, and, minimally, the tongue. The fibers spread fan-like backward and medially around the pharynx to meet their opposite members and to insert along the median raphe that lies anterior to the cervical portion of the vertebral column. The lower border of the muscle overlaps and rests in front of the superior portion of the inferior constrictor, while the upper border, which is approximately at the level of the palate, lies behind the lower fibers of the superior constrictor. The multiple origins of this latter muscle are located on the alveolar process of the mandible, the pterygomandibular raphe, the lower part of the posterior border of the medial pterygoid plate, and among the muscles of the soft palate. The superior constrictor muscle follows the general contour of its fellows and inserts along the median raphe of the pharynx. The upper fibers extend into the nasopharynx almost to the base of the skull.

The stylopharyngeus muscle arises on the styloid process just above the origin of the stylohyoid muscle and travels downward in the lateral wall of the pharynx to terminate among the fibers of the inferior constrictor muscle and on the posterior border of the thyroid cartilage.

The salpingopharyngeus muscle originates from the cartilage of the auditory tube near its pharyngeal orifice and passes downward in the lateral wall of the pharynx, where it attaches among the inferior constrictor muscle fibers along with part of the pharyngopalatal muscle. It also sends some fascicles to the posterior border of the thyroid cartilage in company with fibers from the stylopharyngeus.

The pharyngopalatal muscle is appropriately considered to be a part of the soft palate, but because it terminates in the pharynx, it is equally part of that structure. This arrangement emphasizes both the continuity of body structure and the arbitrariness of the divisions that have been established to simplify description and study.

The Muscles of the Soft Palate

The soft palate, or palatal velum, is a complex muscular structure containing five muscles, two of which originate above the palate, two are attached below the palate, and the remaining muscle, which is unpaired, lies completely within the palate, where it extends from its origin on the posterior border of the hard palate to its termination in the uvula. The two muscles that travel superiorly are the palatal elevator and palatal tensor; those that project downward are the glossopalatal and pharyngopalatal. The elevator and tensor muscles and the uvular muscle

function synergistically to close the pharyngeal space at the junction of the nasal and oral portions of the pharynx; the glossopalatal and pharyngopalatal muscles oppose the former and contribute to other adjustments described below (Gray, 1959).

The pharyngopalatal muscle (also frequently called the palatopharyngeus) passes upward in the lateral wall of the pharynx from its attachments on the thyroid cartilage and among the fibers of the inferior pharyngeal constrictor muscle to its insertion in the soft palate. The palatopharyngeus muscle, with its overlying mucous membrane, forms the pharyngopalatine arch that is often called the posterior pillar of the fauces. It can be seen by looking into the mouth and is recognized as the fold leading from the palate downward and laterally behind the palatine tonsil. The muscle terminates (or arises) near the midline of the velum and forms much of the body of that structure. When the palatopharyngeus muscle contracts, it draws the soft palate downward to open the velopharyngeal valve, an action that occurs rapidly in the production of nasal sounds during speech.

The other palatine muscle that joins the velum from below is the palatoglossus. It originates on the anterior surface of the soft palate, from there it passes in a downward, forward, and lateral direction to its insertion in the side of the tongue. This muscle is covered by mucous membrane and forms the glossopalatine arch, or the anterior pillar of the fauces, which can be observed as the ridge in front of the palatine tonsil. When the tongue is protruded, it draws the anterior pillar forward and makes it more prominent. If the /ŋ/ sound is produced while the tongue is extended, the glossopalatine arches can be seen to grasp the sides of the tongue tightly to provide posterior closure of the mouth.

The palatal elevator and the palatal tensor muscles, as their names indicate, lift and tense the velum. The former originates at both the cartilage of the auditory tube and the temporal bone, from which it passes downward to the upper mediolateral surface of the palate, where the fibers spread posteriorly and medially to join those of the opposite side.

The palatal tensor arises from the auditory tube also and from several somewhat scattered locations on the bones of the skull, from which it descends to the base of the medial pterygoid lamina. At this point it attaches to a tendon that passes around a small bony projection, the hamular process, and continues medially to its insertions in the palatine aponeurosis and posterolateral part of the palatine bone.

The elevator and tensor muscles normally function in concert with the uvular muscle and the superior pharyngeal constrictor to produce the velopharyngeal closure. The elevator draws the palatal structure upward and backward toward the posterior pharyngeal wall, while the simultaneous contraction of the tensor distributes the lift of the elevators throughout the velum and prevents peaking of the palate where the elevators enter the structure. The uvular muscle shortens the uvula and produces a slight bulging of muscle tissue in the central area of contact between the velum and posterior pharyngeal wall, thereby contributing to the closure. It also is probable that the contraction of the uvular muscle increases the tautness of the velum by pulling against the elevators and tensors. The superior pharyngeal constrictor contributes to the valving action by drawing the lateral walls of the pharynx medially. When the closure is viewed from above, its sphincteric nature is evident, particularly at the sides where the puckering is prominent.

Nerve Supply to the Muscles of the Pharynx and Palatal Velum

The sensory and motor innervations of the pharynx and soft palate involve four of the twelve pairs of cranial nerves: trigeminal (cranial nerve V), glossopharyngeal (cranial nerve IX), vagus (cranial nerve X), and accessory (cranial nerve XI). Each one branches complexly and all are intermingled through ganglia and common nerve trunks, but even rudimentary knowledge of this multiple network can provide clinical insight into certain patterns of disability and sensory involvement. For example, tickling one or both external ear canals will often produce a cough, and, conversely, sharp pain in an ear may indicate the presence of a tumor or infection in the larynx. Such associations can be diagnostically significant to the person working with voice disorders. The four great cranial nerves referred to previously travel to many structures, and their contributions to voice production may be insignificant compared to their life functions, but the special objective of this book necessarily focuses the discussion on the relationship of these nerves to voice disorders. This apparent distortion of emphasis should be recognized as such and not interpreted as myopia of speech-language pathology.

The trigeminal nerve (V), as part of its distribution, supplies sensory fibers to the mucosa of the mouth, including the soft palate, and sends a motor nerve to the palatal tensor muscle. It also carries some of the sensory fibers to the external auditory meatus.

The glossopharyngeal nerve (IX), as indicated by its name, is associated primarily with the tongue and the pharynx. It is composed almost entirely of sensory fibers, but it also carries motor fibers to the stylopharyngeus muscle.

The vagus nerve (X) was mentioned in the previous discussion of the larynx, at which time it was associated nonspecifically with other structures in the neck and thorax. This great wandering nerve also sends sensory connections to the external ear canal and to the pharyngeal constrictor muscles by way of various ganglial connections with the glossopharyngeal nerve. It is probable that the sensory affiliation of the external auditory canal and the larynx is the same structural basis for the cough and pain relationship mentioned above.

The earlier reference to the vagus nerve indicated that it was the source of the motor connections to the laryngeal muscles. This is true, but the accessory (XI), which is a motor nerve, gives off many fibers to the vagus nerve at a connection high in the neck, and it is these that branch to the larynx. The accessory nerve also sends motor fibers by way of the pharyngeal branch of the vagus to the pharyngeal constrictors, the palatal elevators, and the uvular muscle.

The complex nerve supply to the pharynx and velum can be summarized and simplified by indicating that the sensory or afferent impulses are carried primarily by nerves V and IX, while the efferent impulses are supplied by nerves X and XI.

SUMMARY

The cartilages, muscles, bones, and nerves that compose the mechanisms used in the process of phonation, breathing, and resonation have been described from the point of view of communication. Little has been said about the larynx as a valve protecting the lungs or about respiration as a basic life process or about the role of the pharynx and its associated structures in swallowing. However, it is evident that these biological functions are performed and that the mechanisms used are shared with the communication function. The biological types of activity are primarily reflexive and intuitive; the communication functions are almost entirely learned. This dual use presents very few conflicts and instead demonstrates the responsiveness and adaptability of the structures involved. These characteristics indicate that the processes are subject to modification and learning, a fact that is basic in vocal rehabilitation.

REFERENCES

Faaborg-Anderson, K., (1957). Electromyographic investigation of intrinsic laryngeal muscles in humans. *Acta Physiological Scandinavica*, Suppl. 140, 1–148.

Gray, H. (1959). *Anatomy of the human body* (27th ed.). Philadelphia: Lea and Febiger.

Konig, W. F., & von Leden, H. (1961). The peripheral nervous system of the human larynx. III. The development. *Archives of Otolaryngology, 74*, 494–500.

Mårtensson, A. (1968). The functional organization of the intrinsic laryngeal muscles. *Annals of the New York Academy of Science, 155*, 91–96.

von Leden, H., & Moore, G. P. (1961). The mechanism of the cricoarytenoid joint. *Archives of Otolaryngology, 73*, 541–550.

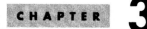

PHYSIOLOGY OF VOICE QUALITY

RAYMOND H. COLTON, PH.D.

NORMAL VOICE QUALITY

The Study of Voice Quality

The quality of the voice is determined by the physiological and acoustic characteristics of the sound source (i.e., the vocal folds) and the resonating system above the vocal folds. Although we think of the vocal tract as a resonator for individual speech sounds such as vowels and consonants, it affects and determines the overall quality of an individual's voice. Therefore, both the vocal folds and the vocal tract must be considered in any discussion of voice quality. However, the focus in this chapter will be on the contributions of the vocal folds to the production of voice quality. In a later section, a brief consideration of vocal tract effects will be considered.

Phonation can be investigated on one of three possible levels: physiological, acoustical, and perceptual. A complete understanding of phonation can be gained only from the integration of all three levels. In the following sections, techniques used to study phonation on each of the three levels will be reviewed.

TECHNIQUES FOR THE STUDY OF THE PHYSIOLOGY OF PHONATION

Normal and High Speed Photography

With the development of the motion picture camera in the late nineteenth century, it became possible to capture and study the normal, although slow motion, characteristics of the vocal folds. With the development of high speed cameras, it became possible to capture and analyze the details of the vocal fold vibratory cycle. Professor G. Paul Moore is one of the foremost leaders in the development and application of this technology.

Normal speed photography permits the recording and analysis of the slow motion of some of the structures in the larynx, specifically the arytenoids. The motion of the vocal folds during adduction and abduction can be analyzed from such images. In addition, this technique can be used to document the location, size, and extent of any lesions visible on the upper surface of the vocal folds. It also has been used to measure the length of the vocal folds at different pitches.

High speed motion pictures photograph the vocal folds at rates exceeding 5,000 frames per second. When projected at normal speed (about 24 frames/sec), the details of the vocal fold vibratory cycle can be observed. Analysis of each frame yields information about vibratory details. The effects of pathology on the vibratory motion of each vocal fold can also be observed and studied.

Unfortunately, high speed photography is very expensive and technically difficult to use, particularly in a clinic setting. Due to the difficulty of the procedure, not all patients can be studied successfully and considerable time is required to analyze the films.

Videoendoscopy and Stroboscopy

The development of video technology can largely supplant motion pictures of the vocal folds. Endoscopy with either a rigid or a flexible endoscope enables investigators and clinicians to obtain excellent views of the normal, slow motions of the larynx and visualization of any pathology. The pictures can be viewed immediately and are relatively inexpensive to obtain.

Stroboscopy is a technique to obtain slow motion pictures of the vocal fold vibration although considerable details of the actual vibratory cycle are missed. The technique can be used in the clinic with most patients and provides information about the motion characteristics of the vocal folds and the effects of pathology on vibration. Further information about the use of the stroboscopy for the quantification of vibratory function will be presented later (see Stroboscopy: A Clinical Tool for the Analysis of Vibration).

Photoglottography

Photoglottography is a technique for indirectly obtaining information about the vocal fold vibratory cycle. A light is directed through the vocal folds either from below or most often from above (usually from an endoscope). On the other side of the vocal folds, a light sensitive electronic device records the light transmitted through the vocal folds during vibration. The amount of light is proportional to the area of opening of the vocal folds and can be used to estimate the vocal fold area versus time pattern. It is easy to use clinically and relatively easy to obtain reliable and valid data. From it, measurements of vibratory function, vocal fold amplitude and fundamental frequency can be obtained.

Inverse Filtering

Inverse filtering is a technique for deriving amplitude versus time or the airflow versus time waveform produced at the vocal folds. Two general approaches are used: in one the acoustic signal recorded at the lips is analyzed; in the other, the orally emitted airflow waveform is analyzed. Both approaches assume that the acoustic (or airflow) output of the vocal tract is the product of the acoustic pressure waveform (or air flow waveform) and the resonant characteristics of the vocal tract. By removing the resonant effects via inverse filtering of the oral waveform, the approximate waveform at the vocal folds can be estimated. The advantage of using the airflow waveform is that a meaningful zero level can be obtained. However, the acoustic signal may yield a much larger frequency response.

The results of inverse filtering of the oral airflow waveform is called the flowglottogram, or simply glottogram. Measurements of fundamental frequency, opening time, closing time, and closed time can be obtained from the inverse glottogram. Measurements of mean airflow rate, ac or peak airflow rate (airflow modulated by the vocal folds) and dc, leakage or minimum[1] airflow rates can be made.

Electroglottography

Electroglottography is a technique for obtaining an estimate of the vocal fold contact pattern during vibration. A small current is passed from two electrodes located on the two sides of the thyroid cartilage and modulated by the movements of the vocal folds. The waveform obtained reproduces the pattern of vocal fold contact. In most cases, increasing contact is shown as a positive deflection of the waveform. In other portrayals, increased vocal fold contact is shown as a downward deflection of the waveform, especially when compared to other methods used in the indirect estimate of vocal fold vibration such as photoglottography or inverse filtering.

Measurements of fundamental frequency can be obtained from the electroglottograph as well as measures related to the opening, closing, or closed phases of vibration.

TECHNIQUES FOR THE STUDY OF THE ACOUSTICS OF PHONATION

Fundamental Frequency

Fundamental frequency reflects the vibrating rate of the vocal folds. It can be obtained in a number of ways from such devices as the electroglottograph, photoglottograph, high speed films, and direct measurements of the acoustic signal. Currently, there are a number of devices and computer programs that can extract fundamental frequency including the

Visipitch and the Computer Speech Laboratory (CSL from Kay Elemetrics, Inc., Pine Brook NJ), Dr. Speech (Tiger Eletronics, Seattle WA), CSpeech (Paul Milkenovic, Madison, WS), SpeechMaster (SpeechMaster, Sandy, UT), Sound Scope (GW Instruments), CSRE (AVAAZ Innovations, London, Ontario, Canada), and other computer programs. An example of an analysis of fundamental frequency in a simple sentence is shown in Figure 3–1. Many of these devices or programs can calculate perturbation in the normal voice signal such as jitter (frequency perturbation) and shimmer (amplitude perturbation), although they are somewhat limited in their use for analyzing disordered voices.

Vocal Intensity

The intensity of the acoustic signal can be measured with a variety of techniques including the devices and computer programs described above under Fundamental Frequency. An example of an analysis of vocal intensity in a simple sentence is shown in Figure 3–1. It is also possible to use a level recorder to obtain a graphic display of the intensity characteristics of a phonation. If absolute measurements of sound pressure levels are desired, it is necessary to calibrate these devices to produce accurate decibel (dB) readings.

Spectrum

Most elementary textbooks on basic acoustics state that the major acoustic correlate of quality is spectrum. An example of the spectrum of a sustained vowel is shown in Figure 3–2.

---

[1]These measurements are made when, supposedly, the vocal folds are closed. Without independent verification of vocal fold closing, we cannot be positive that the folds are completely closed. It is known that some normal subjects, particularly women, exhibit a small opening between the arytenoids often referred to as a posterior chink. If so, one would expect a small amount of airflow during the closed phase of the vibratory cycle.

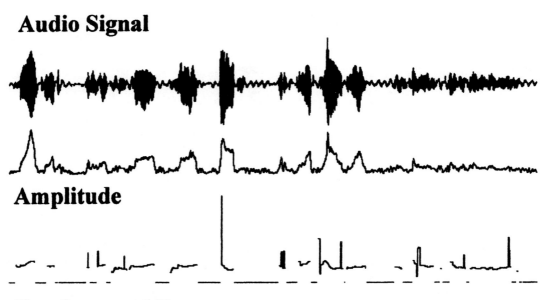

FIGURE 3-1. Example of a fundamental frequency and intensity analysis of a simple sentence as produced using CSpeech.

One problem with the analysis of spectrum, as is shown in Figure 3-2, is that it reflects the unique spectral characteristics of the sound produced. The spectrum obtained is not necessarily the voice quality of the person producing the sound. One way to obtain a spectrum characteristic of an individual's voice is to average the spectrum over many different kinds of speech sounds and reduce spectral effects of a specific sound in favor of the overall spectral characteristics of the speaker. This technique of Long Term Average Spectra, or LTAS, is an example of what is shown in Figure 3-3. The Kay Digital Sound Spectrogram and their computer program CSL can compute LTAS. Other programs would need some modifications to produce LTAS.

LTAS has been used with normal and abnormal voices and has been shown to be a good way to display the spectral characteristics of voice quality. Further information about LTAS analyses of nor-

mal and abnormal voice qualities will be presented in the following sections.

MALE/FEMALE DIFFERENCES OF VOICE QUALITY

Few listeners have difficulty recognizing the difference between a male and female voice. A major acoustic cue to male/female differences is the fundamental frequency of phonation. Male voices typically produce speaking fundamental frequencies between 100 and 130 Hz. Females typically produce fundamental frequencies between 180 and 220 Hz. Thus, there is about two thirds of an octave difference between male and female voices.

There are, however, other acoustic differences between male and female voices. Coleman (1971, 1973, 1976) demonstrated that differences between a male and female voice continued to exist even when fundamental frequency was identi-

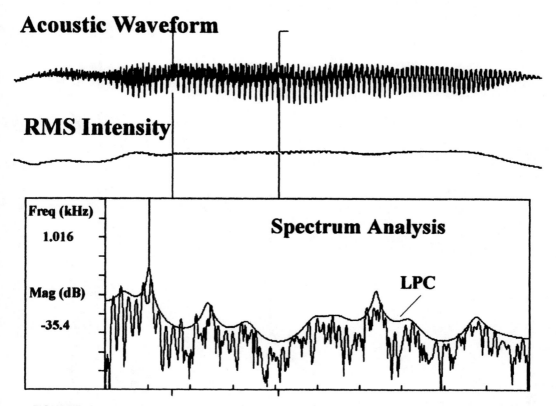

FIGURE 3–2. FFT and LPC spectrum analysis of the vowel /æ/ as produced by CSpeech.

cal. He attributed these differences to the relative sizes of the oral and pharyngeal cavities which would slightly alter the resonant frequencies of the vocal tract (Brown & Feinstein, 1977).

Physiological Differences Between Male and Female Voices

Physiologically, the larynx of the male voice is much larger than the female voice, accounting for the much lower fundamental frequency. The male thyroid cartilage is about 20% larger than that of the female. It also has been shown that the length of the membranous glottis (the part of the vocal folds that actually vibrates during phonation) is about 60% longer in males than in females. A schematic of these differences was presented by Titze (1989) and is shown in Figure 3–4.

Inverse Filtered Air flow

Gender differences have been found in measurements obtained from inverse flow glottograms produced by male and female subjects (Holmberg, Hillman, & Perkell, 1988). Figure 3–5 illustrates some of the differences. The top panel shows waveforms from the six male subjects, and the bottom panel from the six female subjects. Each subject produced phonations at soft, medium, and loud intensity levels. These differences are obvious when measurements of modulated and leakage airflow rates, closing quotient, speed quotient, glottal resistance and vocal efficiency are made.

In this study, the airflow modulated by the vibrating vocal folds is referred to as ac airflow rate. AC airflow rate differences between males and females are

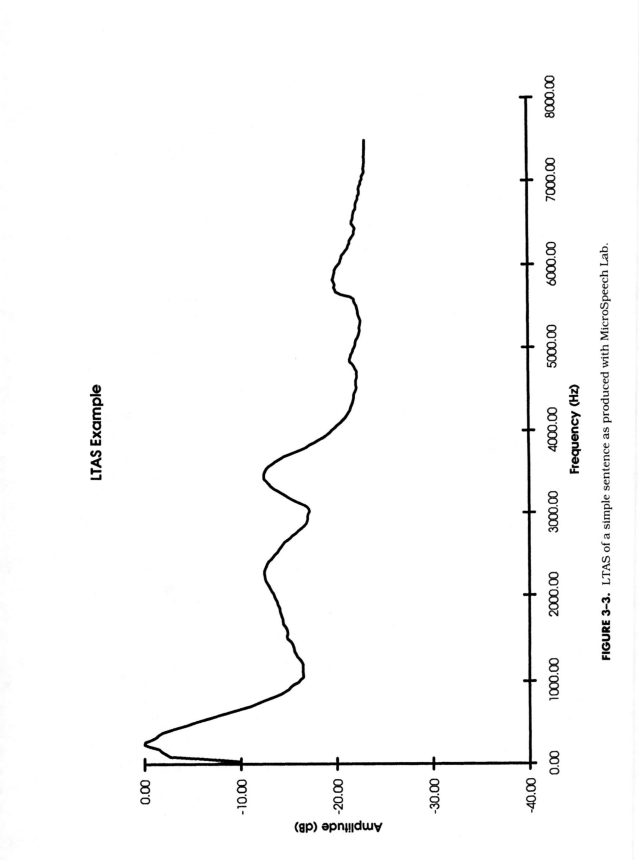

FIGURE 3-3. LTAS of a simple sentence as produced with MicroSpeech Lab.

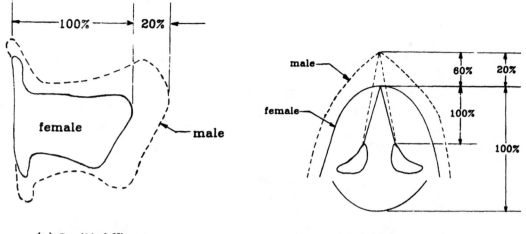

(a) Sagittal View **(b) Horizontal Section**

FIGURE 3–4. Male and female differences in the size of the thyroid cartilage *(left panel)* and membranous length of the vocal folds *(right panel)*. (From Physiologic and Acoustic Differences Between Male and Female Voices by I. Titze, 1989, p. 1699. *Journal of Acoustical Society of America, 85.* Reprinted with permission.)

shown in the lower panel of Figure 3–6. It is apparent that males have higher airflow rates than females, a finding reported by many other investigators (e.g., Hirano, 1981). The advantage of using flow glottograms is that the airflow modulated by the vocal folds can be separated from airflow that is escaping because of incomplete closure of the vocal folds. In the Holmberg study (Holmberg et al., 1988), this measure is labeled minimum airflow rate and is plotted in the lower panel of Figure 3–6. Minimum airflow rate may also be thought of as leakage airflow rate because it reflects the airflow when the vocal folds are presumably closed. Note that there is airflow leakage at all loudness levels. Males generally produce greater leakage flows, perhaps due to larger glottal openings. However, several studies (Biever & Bless, 1989; Rammage, Peppard, & Bless, 1992; Södersten & Lindestad, 1990; Södersten, Lindestad, & Hammarberg, 1991) have reported that females show a posterior glottal gap more often than males. The Holmberg et al.

(1988) data suggest that leakage flows are very large and further information is needed to assess the magnitude of leakage flows during speech.

Open Quotient

Open Quotient is a measure of the relative time the vocal folds are open during a cycle of vibration. One would expect that large open quotients would contribute to the magnitude of air flow rates. Average Open Quotients, as reported by Holmberg et al. (1988), are shown in the upper panel of Figure 3–7. Females produced larger open quotients than males, a result that may help to explain the perceptual impression that some females are more breathy than males. Interestingly, the larger open quotients do not appear to affect the magnitude of female ac airflow rates. However, they appear to affect the average airflow rates. This possible relationship was analyzed in the flow glottograms of 58 patients seen in the voice clinic at SUNY Health Science Center.

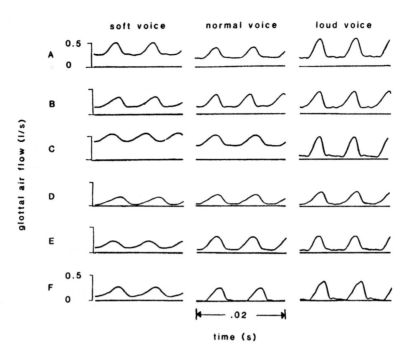

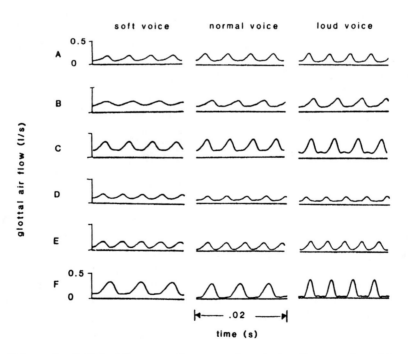

FIGURE 3–5. Schematic glottal airflow waveforms produced at soft, normal, and loud intensity levels by six males (upper panel) and six female (lower panel) normal speakers. (From "Glottal Airflow and Transglottal Air Pressure Measurements for Male And Female Speakers in Soft, Normal, and Loud Voice" by E. Holmberg, R. Hillman, and J. Perkell, 1988, pp. 517 and 519. *Journal of the Acoustical Society of America, 84*. Reprinted with permission.)

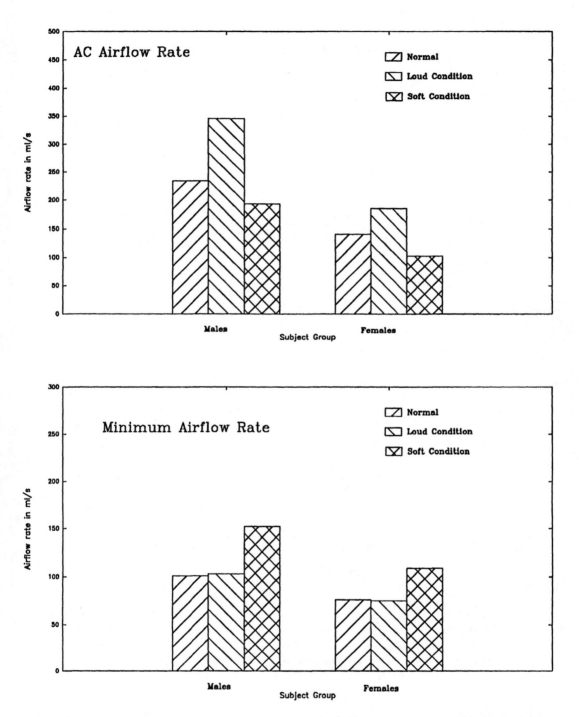

FIGURE 3–6. Mean AC airflow rates (upper panel) and Mean Minimum airflow rates (lower panel) for 25 males and 20 females producing a /pae/ syllable sequence at soft, normal, and loud intensity levels. (From data reported in "Glottal Airflow and Transglottal Air Pressure Measurements for Male and Female Speakers in Soft, Normal, and Loud Voice" by E. Holmberg, R. Hillman, and J. Perkell, 1988, pp. 517 and 519. *Journal of the Acoustical Society of America, 84.* Reprinted with permission.)

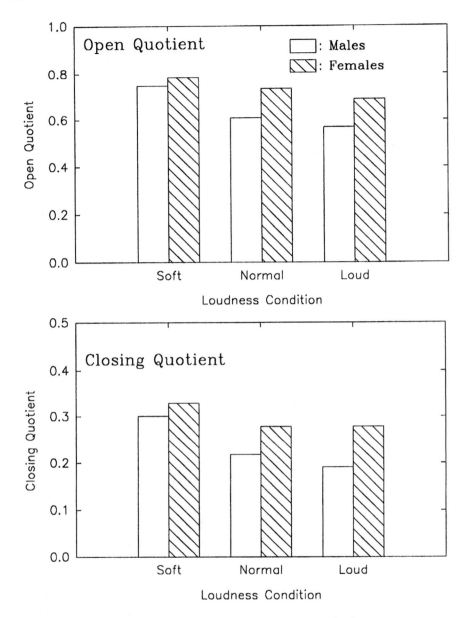

FIGURE 3–7. Mean Open Quotients *(upper panel)*, and Closing Quotients *(lower panel)* for 25 males and 20 females producing the syllable /pae/ at soft, normal, and loud intensity levels. (Based on data presented by Holmberg et al., 1988, *Journal of the Acoustical Society of America, 84.*)

One half of the patients had low open quotients (mean OQ = 51.87) and the other had high open quotients (mean = 66.14). Patients in each group were matched according to their peak airflow rates within ±1 ml/s. The low OQ group had significantly lower mean airflow rates (mean = 178.08 ml/s) than the high OQ group (mean = 284.13 ml/s; F = 30.70, p >.05). The relationship between

OQ and mean airflow rates are shown in Figure 3–8. A variety of factors may affect the magnitude of airflow rates in patients with phonatory disorders but it appears that variation of open quotient will affect mean flow rate but not peak airflow rates.

Closing Quotient

Closing Quotient was defined by Holmberg et al. (1988) as the time of the closing phase of the airflow waveform divided by the total time of the vibratory cycle. The measure is an indirect measurement of the speed of the closing of the vocal folds. The results are shown in the lower panel of Figure 3–7. The female group has a slightly larger closing quotient than males. This suggests that the speed of closure of the female speaker is slightly less than a male speaker. Slower closure speeds of the vocal folds may result in slightly less high-frequency energy in the acoustic waveform of female speakers.

Speed Quotient

Speed Quotient is defined as the speed of the opening phase of the vocal folds divided by the speed of the closing phase of the vocal folds. Opening and closing speeds may reflect the mechanical characteristics of the vocal folds and the aerodynamic properties of the airway. Speed of opening may be affected by the magnitude of the subglottal air pressures. Males appear to have slightly greater speed quotients than females (Figure 3–9). This could be due to slightly longer opening speeds or slightly shorter closing speeds. The data on closing quotient suggests that males have slightly faster closing speeds, thus the speed quotient data contributes some internal consistency about male/female differences with respect to speeds of opening and closing the vocal folds.

Glottal Resistance

Glottal resistance is a derived measure and is defined as the aerodynamic pressure divided by the airflow rate. It reflects the resistance of the vocal folds to vibration; resistance that may be due to differences of the mass and/or elasticity of the vocal folds and the degree of muscle activity. The glottal resistance measurements as reported by Holmberg et al. (1988), are shown in the upper panel of Figure 3–10. Females show greater glottal resistance at all loudness levels than males. These differences may be due to the higher pitch levels of the female subjects but most probably reflect a greater stiffness of the vocal folds to vibration.

Vocal Efficiency

Vocal efficiency is defined as the ratio of the sound energy and the aerodynamic energy. High ratios reflect much more efficient conversion of aerodynamic energy into sound energy. As shown in the lower panel of Figure 3–10, females have slightly greater vocal efficiencies at soft and medium loudness levels and a much greater efficiency at high intensity levels.

In Figure 3–11, some of the male/female flow glottogram differences are illustrated in a schematic way. These waveforms suggest spectral differences between males and females in addition to obvious differences of fundamental frequency.

Spectral Differences Between Male and Female Voices

Long term average spectrum (LTAS) has been used analyzing the spectral characteristics of normal (Löfqvist, 1986; Löfqvist & Mandersson, 1987; Pols, 1971; Pols, van der Kamp, & Plomp, 1969) and abnormal voice qualities (Hammarberg, 1987; Kitzing, 1986). The average LTAS of a sentence spoken by a group of 35 nor-

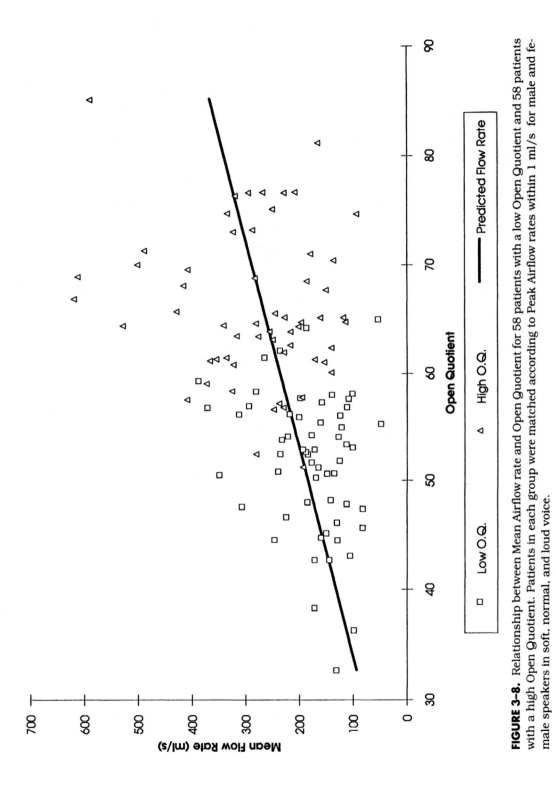

FIGURE 3-8. Relationship between Mean Airflow rate and Open Quotient for 58 patients with a low Open Quotient and 58 patients with a high Open Quotient. Patients in each group were matched according to Peak Airflow rates within 1 ml/s for male and female speakers in soft, normal, and loud voice.

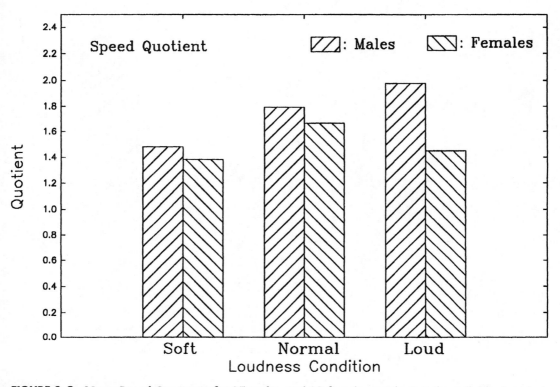

FIGURE 3–9. Mean Speed Quotients for 25 males and 20 females producing the syllable /pae/ at soft, normal, and loud intensity levels. (Based on data presented by Holmberg et al., 1988, pp. 517 and 519. *Journal of the Acoustical Society of America, 84.*)

mal speaking males and a group of 27 normal speaking females is presented in Figure 3–12. The major portion of the acoustic energy is between 200 and 5,000 Hz for both sexes. Females have lower low-frequency levels, probably due to their higher fundamental frequency.

Use of LTAS to Analyze Dysphonic Voices

Wendler, Doherty, and Hollien (1980) concluded that an LTAS analysis could differentiate degrees of hoarseness and that it could be used to classify patients into various hoarseness categories. Furthermore, they show how LTAS could be used to classify patients into different diagnos-

tic categories although with the small number of patients studied further research is needed.

Löfqvist (1986) analyzed normal and dysphonic voices using LTAS and derived two quantitative measurements: (a) the ratio of energy between 0 and 1 kHz and the energy between 1 and 5 kHz and (b) the energy level in the band from 5–8 kHz. He reported considerable variation in both of these measurements for normal voices recorded twice on the same day, suggesting that considerable variation may exist even for normal voices on these measures. He also failed to find a clear difference between a group of 37 normals and a group of 36 dysphonic voices. Löfqvist questioned the utility of LTAS measurements.

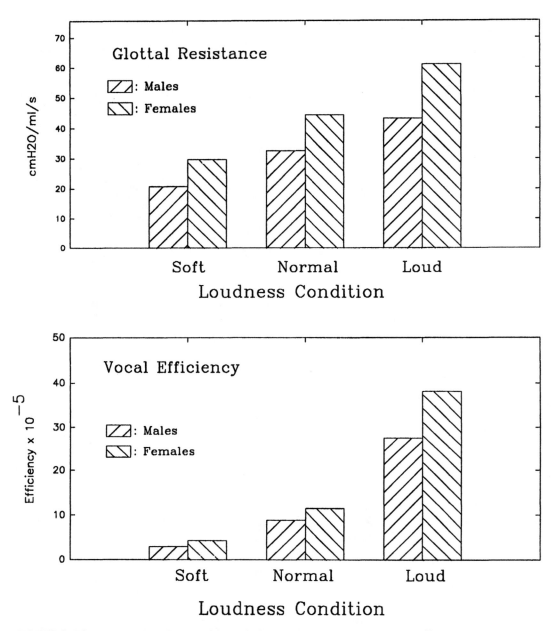

FIGURE 3-10. Mean Glottal Resistances *(upper panel)* and Mean Vocal Efficiencies *(lower panel)* for 25 males and 20 females producing the syllable /pae/ at soft, normal, and loud intensity levels. (Based on data presented by Holmberg et al., 1988, pp. 517 and 519. *Journal of the Acoustical Society of America, 84.*)

Use of LTAS to Analyze Normal and Abnormal Voice Qualities

Kitzing (1986) reported good results from an LTAS study of 10 normal speakers pro-

ducing examples of normal and abnormal voice qualities (leaky, strained, low intensity normal, moderate intensity normal voice). For example, there was a statistically significant difference between nor-

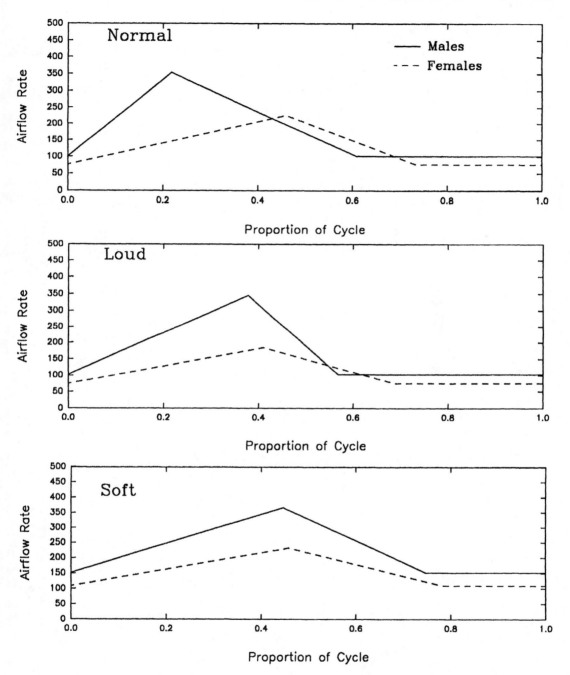

FIGURE 3–11. Schematic glottal airflow vs time waveforms produced by 25 males and 20 females producing the syllable /pae/ at soft, normal, and loud intensity levels. (Based on data presented by Holmberg et al., 1988, pp. 517 and 519. *Journal of the Acoustical Society of America, 84.*)

mal and leaky voices on the ratio of energy in the 0–1 KHz band to 1–5 kHz. There were statistically significant differences between all four voice qualities on the ratio of 0–1 kHz to 1–2 kHz energy. Thus, there appears to be some success in uti-

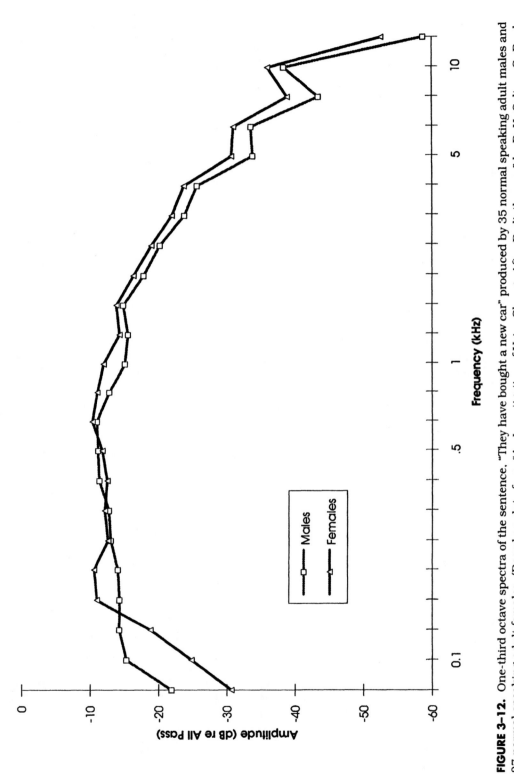

FIGURE 3–12. One-third octave spectra of the sentence, "They have bought a new car" produced by 35 normal speaking adult males and 27 normal speaking adult females. (Based on data from "An Investigation of Voice Change After Radiotherapy" by R. H. Colton, G. Reed, R. Sagerman, and C. Chung, 1982. Unpublished report to National Cancer Institute, Bethesda, MD.)

lizing LTAS measurements to distinguish among different voice qualities.

Sensitivity of LTAS in Distinguishing Vocal Differences Due to Emotional Stress, Disguising One's Voice, and Speaking Different Languages

LTAS appears to have merit in the classification of individual speakers. Hollien and Majewski (1977) studied the ability of LTAS spectral analysis to discriminate among speakers both within and across two languages (Polish and English) when a speaker spoke under emotional stress, and when a speaker attempted to disguise his voice. Fifty Polish and 50 American college-age speakers read a 2.5-minute passage. The passage was analyzed into 23 one-third octave bands, the data were normalized, and an n-dimensional Euclidean space was constructed. The Euclidean distances (a measure of dissimilarity) for the Polish speakers was smaller than for the American speakers. Thus, the technique appeared to be sensitive to language differences. The percent correct identification of the speakers was 96% for the Polish speakers and 94% for the American speakers. Lower correct identification scores were obtained when the passage was analyzed in a smaller number of one-third octave bands covering the frequency range from 315 to 3150 Hz (typical bandwidth of a telephone). When a group of 25 adult American speakers who spoke under emotional stress or tried to disguise their voices was analyzed with the same technique, the percent correct identification in the emotional stress condition was 92% but only 20% for the disguised voices (full bandwidth condition: 80 Hz–10 kHz). These authors concluded that LTAS can be used to correctly identify speakers although there are language differences; and under some condi-

tions of distortion (i.e., disguise), it is less useful for speaker recognition.

Use of LTAS Analysis in Discriminating Severity of Dypshonia

There is also evidence to conclude that LTAS analysis may be successful in discriminating among the severity of dysphonia. Wendler, Rauhut, and Kruger (1986) studied the LTAS characteristics of 162 male and 311 female patients and related these to perceptual severity ratings of hoarseness, roughness, and breathiness. The reading passage was analyzed using a discriminate analysis procedure to determine if LTAS data could be used to classify the patients according to severity. The average correct classification of the male patient group was 46.58%. Similar results were claimed for the female patient group although no data were reported. It appears that LTAS reflects something about the patient's degree of dysphonia although it may not be the same as found in the perceptual ratings of severity. Observer ratings of severity are not based solely on the spectrum characteristics of the voice but may include factors such as frequency level, loudness variation, phrasing, and other miscellaneous factors.

LTAS may be an important acoustic measurement for patients with voice problems. Hammarberg, Fritzell, and Schiratzki (1984) reported the LTAS characteristics of 16 patients who had received Teflon® injection for the treatment of vocal fold paralysis. Five quantitative measurements were made from the LTAS spectra. The only statistically significant difference between the pre- and post-treatment conditions occurred for the measurement of the SPL in the lowest frequency band analyzed (i.e., the 6th Bark[2]

---

[2]A Bark is a frequency band corresponding approximately to the critical bandwidth of the ear (Plomp, 1976).

band or about 200 Hz). Example pre- and post-treatment spectra for seven patients were shown and suggested spectral differences between the two conditions for most patients.

It is difficult to reach a definitive conclusion about the effectiveness of LTAS to discriminate among normal voices, discriminate normal voices from abnormal voices, and discriminate among abnormal voices. The data from the literature suggest that there is value in the LTAS, but the most productive method to extract the relevant data from LTAS analyses remains to be developed. It probably is not necessary to use the full frequency range of an LTAS analysis (usually from 20 Hz to 10k Hz). Therefore, some kind of summary measurements are needed. Many have been proposed; some are arbitrary, some are based on statistical or a priori reasons. No one measurement has proven to be the most effective most of the time.

ANALYSIS OF VIBRATORY FUNCTION

G. Paul Moore's most significant contribution to our knowledge about the human voice came from his series of articles with R. Timcke and H. von Leden (Timcke, von Leden, & Moore, 1958, 1959; von Leden, Moore, & Timcke, 1960) about vocal fold vibratory characteristics in normal and abnormal phonation as revealed from high speed films. He had, of course, reported on vibratory function in several previous articles and many since, but in these later articles considerable quantitative and qualitative information about vocal fold vibration was presented. In this section, a brief review of the findings from these studies will be presented, information that was augmented but not superseded by subsequent literature on vibratory function.

High Speed Film Measurements

The data reported in the three articles were derived from high speed films taken of the vocal folds of normal and pathological subjects producing a sustained vowel at different fundamental frequencies and intensity levels. In addition, the normal subjects produced examples of laughing, crying, coughing, vocal fry, head voice, and inhalation voicing. The area of opening between the vocal folds (glottis) was measured for each frame of a complete vibratory cycle. Usually there were 16–18 frames encompassing an entire cycle. These area measurements were plotted for each frame in the cycle. Because each frame represents a discrete time within the cycle, glottal area as a function of time is plotted.

Two additional measurements were made, Open Quotient (OQ) and Speed Quotient (SQ). OQ is defined as the time the vocal folds are open divided by the total time of the cycle. In a way, it is a reflection of the time during the vibratory cycle that the vocal folds are working, thus it is analogous to the engineering term of duty cycle. SQ is defined as the time the vocal folds take to open divided by the time they require to close. It has been speculated that the forces opening the vocal folds are different from the forces closing the vocal folds, although this may be true only with respect to the relative contribution of these forces because both myoelastic and aerodynamic forces are present throughout the entire vibratory cycle. SQ may be related to the spectral content of the vocal folds, although it is the pressure waveform that generates the acoustic disturbance in the vocal tract and not the area waveform; however, area and pressure waveforms are related.

Vibratory Characteristics of Normal Phonation

A variety of normal phonations were studied in the first two articles in the series (Timcke, von Leden, & Moore, 1958, 1959). Different subjects with no obvious pathology of the vocal folds were asked to produce a variety of phonatory tasks including phonation at different pitches (fundamental frequencies), loudness (intensities), registers (quality differences), laughing, inhalation voicing, and other examples of phonation one might encounter in normal subjects.

A plot of the area waveform from a normal subject is shown in Figure 3–13 (redrawn from the data presented by Timcke, von Leden, & Moore, 1958). Note that the opening phase occupies more than one-half of the total cycle; therefore, one would expect the OQ to exceed 0.5 (actual measurement of OQ was 0.69). The time it takes for the vocal folds to open is shorter than that required for the vocal folds to close; thus the SQ should be less than 1.0 (actual measurement = 0.58). Note the unusual bulge in the waveform

about one-third of the distance from the peak along the closing phase of the waveform. This bulge suggests a change in the rate of closing of the vocal folds and may reflect a different rate of closure by the upper and lower lips of the vocal folds.

Effects of Pitch Variation

The results of the measurement of OQ and SQ for phonations produced by four subjects at the same loudness level but at three different pitch levels are shown in Figure 3–14. From these data there does not appear to be any systematic variation of OQ or SQ as a function of fundamental frequency.

Effects of Loudness Variation

In Figure 3–15, the results of the measurement of OQ and SQ for phonations produced by four subjects at the same

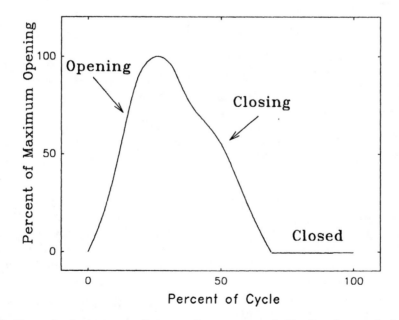

FIGURE 3–13. Example of an area-via-time waveform as presented by Timcke, von Leden, and Moore (1958). Time is expressed as percentage of the total cycle. (Reprinted with permission from *Archives of Otolaryngology, Head and Neck Surgery, 68*, 1–19. © 1958, American Medical Association.)

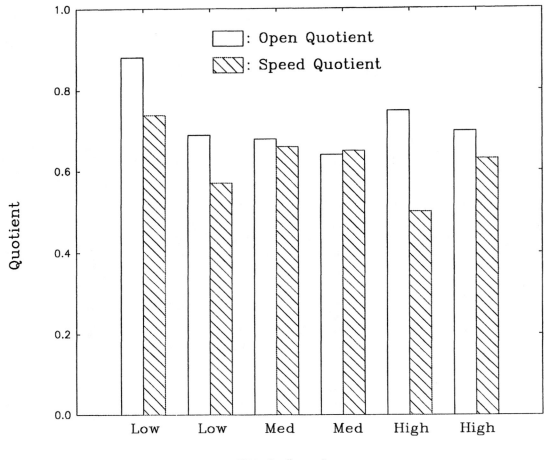

FIGURE 3–14. Open Quotients and Speed Quotients of phonations produced at three different pitch levels (low, medium, high) but at the same relative loudness level (weak) by four subjects. (Redrawn from data presented in Laryngeal Vibrations: Measurements of the Glottic Wave by R. Timcke, H. S. von Leden, and G. P. Moore, 1958, pp. 1–19. *Archives of Otolaryngology, Head and Neck Surgery, 68.* © 1958, American Medical Association. Reprinted with permission.)

pitch level but at three different loudness levels are shown. There is a tendency for OQ to decrease and SQ to increase as the intensity of the phonation increases. The authors noted that the width of glottal opening increased as the intensity increased. All three trends would be expected since with greater intensity, there are greater subglottal air pressures forcing the vocal folds to open and close at a faster rate. Furthermore, to generate the

increase of subglottal air pressure, the vocal folds must be abducted more forcefully, thus producing a shorter opening phase of the vibratory cycle. Greater air pressures would also force the vocal folds to open with greater lateral excursions.

Effects of Quality Variation

The OQ and SQ for one subject producing phonations in the chest and head regis-

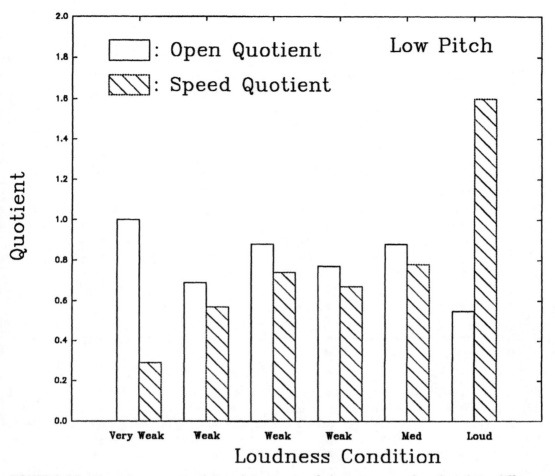

FIGURE 3–15. Open Quotients and Speed Quotients of phonations produced at three different loudness levels (weak, medium, and loud) but at the same relative pitch level (low) by four subjects. (Redrawn from data presented in Laryngeal Vibrations: Measurements of the Glottic Wave by R. Timcke, H. S. von Leden, and G. P. Moore. 1958, pp. 1–19. *Archives of Otolaryngology, Head and Neck Surgery, 68.* © 1958, American Medical Association. Reprinted with permission.)

ters but at the same intensity and frequency levels[3] are shown in Figure 3–16. The major difference between these two registers is quality (i.e., they sound different to a human ear). Note that the phonation produced in the head register had a much longer OQ than the phonations produced in the chest register. SQ between the two registers were very similar although slightly smaller in the head reg-

ister. Because these data are based on one subject, it would be difficult to reach any definitive conclusions about these aerodynamic differences between the two registers. However, the results of research following these articles have presented data supportive of the results of this pioneering work.

The nature of the qualitative differences between chest and head registers as

[3]According to the authors, the fundamental frequency of the two phonations was about 250 Hz.

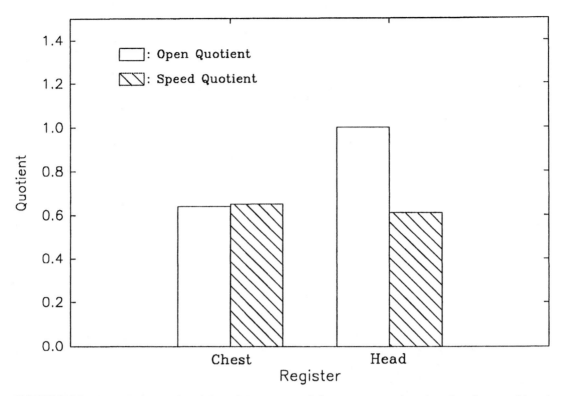

FIGURE 3–16. Open Quotients and Speed Quotients of phonations produced in the chest and head registers by a single subject at the same loudness level (weak) and pitch level (medium or about 250 Hz). (Redrawn from data presented in Laryngeal Vibrations: Measurements of the Glottic Wave by R. Timcke, H. S. von Leden, and G. P. Moore, 1958, pp. 1–19. *Archives of Otolaryngology, Head and Neck Surgery, 68.* © 1958, American Medical Association. Reprinted with permission.)

shown in high speed films is shown in Figure 3–17. The phonation produced in the head register has no closed phase. The closing phase is somewhat irregular, suggesting changes of velocity during this phase of vocal fold vibration. Although the SQs for both phonations are very similar, the actual speed of opening and closing is slower in the head register than for phonations produced in the chest register.

Vibratory Characteristics of Abnormal Phonation

In a later article (von Leden, Moore, & Timcke, 1960), Moore and his colleagues presented considerable high speed data from patients with a variety of voice disor-

ders. The quantitative results are shown in Figure 3–18. Considerable variation exists in both OQ and SQ for patients with different kinds of voice problems. Unilateral paralysis, edema, polyps, nodules, and a fixed arytenoid appeared to produce long Open Quotients, whereas a cyst and hematoma produced shorter Open Quotients. Speed Quotients differed among pathologies and between the two vocal folds. In general, the fold with the lesions produced the slower speeds.

Different pathologies produce drastic variation in the shape of the waveforms. There is greater irregularity in the period of the waveform and differences exist in the relative timing of each fold during vibration (producing a phase difference be-

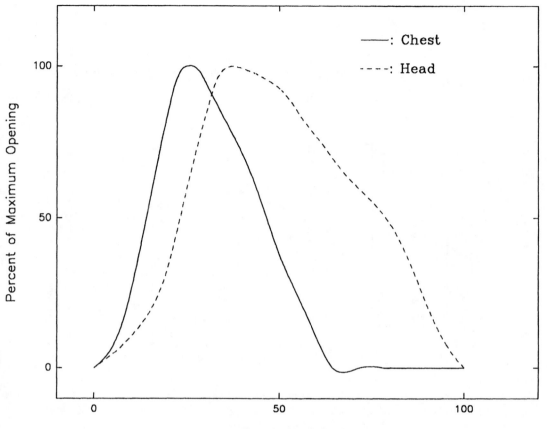

FIGURE 3–17. Example of area-via-time waveforms of phonations produced in the chest and head registers by a single subject at the same loudness level and pitch levels. (Redrawn from data presented in Laryngeal Vibrations: Measurements of the Glottic Wave by R. Timcke, H. von Leden, and P. Moore, 1958, pp. 1–19. Permission to reprint granted by *Archives of Otolaryngology, Head and Neck Surgery, 68.* © 1958, American Medical Association.)

tween the two folds). There is also variation in amplitude of vibration. A summary of the conclusions about the effects of pathology on vocal fold vibration, as reported in the original article, is presented in Table 3-1. All of these conclusions have been supported by the extensive work on vocal fold vibration in the pathological voice that has appeared in the literature since the publication of this landmark article in 1960.

Recent Work on Vibratory Function in Normal and Abnormal Voices

Equipment Development

Much of the early work with high speed filming of the vocal folds utilized a Fastex camera or similar devices. The basic camera facilities have changed little since then with the exception of the development of a high speed digital imaging de-

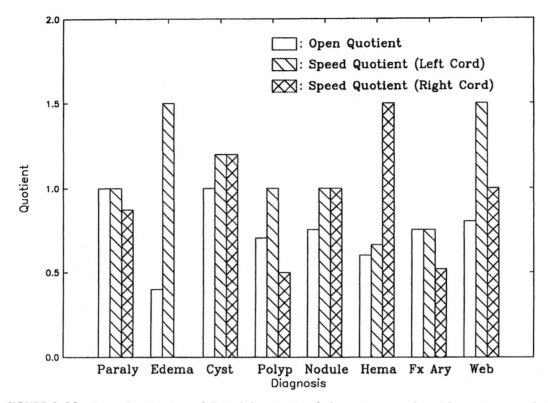

FIGURE 3–18. Open Quotients and Speed Quotients of phonations produced by patients with vocal pathologies. All were produced at about the same pitch and loudness levels. (Redrawn from data presented in Laryngeal Vibrations: Measurements of the Glottic Wave by H. von Leden, P. Moore, and R. Timcke, 1960, pp. 26–45. *Archives of Otolaryngology*, 71.)

vice as developed by researchers at the Research Institute of Logopedics and Phoniatrics in Tokyo, Japan (Hirose, 1988; Hirose, Kiritani, & Imagawa, 1987, 1988, 1991a, 1991b; Honda, Kiritani, Imagawa, Hirose, & Hashimoto, 1985; Imagawa, Kiritani, & Hirose, 1987; Imagawa, Kiritani, Honda, & Hirose, 1986; Kiritani, Imagawa, & Hirose, 1986, 1992).

The high speed digital device uses a standard 35 mm camera body and lens but the "film" has been replaced by a high speed, solid state image sensor. The image array is controlled by a computer which samples the image passing through the lens at rates up to 4,000 frames per second. Better image quality is obtained, however, when lower frame rates are used. The advantage

of the device is immediate visualization of the image and more convenient, less expensive digital storage. The latter simplifies the use of image analysis techniques to obtain measurements and expedite the collection of accurate data. Several reports have appeared in which some results of measurements made with the device have appeared (Hirose, Kiritani, & Imagawa, 1988, 1991a, 1991b; Kiritani, Imagawa, & Hirose, 1992).

Improvements in Illumination

Refinements in the illumination systems used with high speed cameras have also been reported. Metz and his colleagues (Metz, Whitehead, & Peterson, 1980) described a compact illuminating system

Table 3–1. Some conclusions about the effects of pathology on vocal fold vibration.

1. All vocal folds with benign lesions vibrate, even paralyzed vocal folds.

2. Normal vibratory pattern of a fold with a lesion is possible, especially if the lesion is small.

3. The vibratory pattern of the normal fold can be affected by the abnormal vocal fold.

4. Pronounced changes in the period of the vibratory cycle are possible in the presence of a lesion.

5. Pronounced changes in the amplitude of vibration are possible in the presence of a lesion.

6. There may be an asynchrony of vibration between the two folds producing a phase shift.

7. Phase shifts between the two folds may be constant or may vary throughout the vibratory cycle.

8. If phase shift continues throughout the closed phase, the vocal folds may execute a side-to-side motion.

9. One or both folds may cross the midline during vibration.

10. Unilateral, soft tumors tend to follow the movements of the normal vocal fold.

11. Most lesions will diminish the vibration of the fold on which they are located.

Source: Based on information in von Leden, H., Moore, P., & Timcke, R. (1960). Laryngeal vibrations: measurements of the glottic wave Part III: the pathologic larynx. *Archives of Otolaryngology, 71,* 26–45; Timcke, R., von Leden, H., & Moore, P. (1958). Laryngeal vibrations: measurements of the glottic wave. *Archives of Otolaryngology-Head and Neck Surgery, 68,* 1–19, Copyright 1958, American Medical Association.

that provides sufficient light for high speed filming, but requires much less space and produces a cooler light to minimize the possibility of heat damage to the vocal folds.

Measurement of High Speed Films

The measurement of high speed films is tedious and time consuming. Each picture frame from each vocal fold cycle (usually 15–20 frames) must be projected and held motionless while the desired measurements are made using a variety of devices including planimeters, rules, computer-controlled cursors, and similar measurement devices. An ever-present problem in all measurement schemes is the correct identification of appropriate landmarks on the image. Analysis of a single cycle of vibration may require an hour or more of measurement time. No wonder why so few of the available high speed films have been analyzed quantitatively![4]

There have been many attempts to simplify and expedite the measurement process. Most have used computers to assist in the measurement or to perform all measurements with little or no human intervention.

Procedures using computer-assisted measurement have usually projected the film, using a stop-frame motion picture projector, onto a screen or digitizing tablet. In some cases, the human operator controlled the location of light points or cursors and the computer was programmed to measure distances between these points (Tanabe, Kitajima, Gould, & Lambiase, 1975.) In other cases, the cursors were controlled via a computer which also made the measurements (Childers, Naik, Larar, Krishnamurthy, & Moore, 1983). In another scheme, the motion picture image was projected onto a digitizing tablet and the relevant landmarks on the image were marked with a pen, again

[4]It has been estimated that, of the many hours of high speed film that have been taken of the vocal folds, only about 8 minutes have been analyzed (Childers, Paige, & Moore, 1976).

connected to a computer that made the measurements (Hirano, Gould, Lambiase, & Kakita, 1980).

One early report (Childers et al., 1976) compared the results of hand measurements to automated measurements of the glottal area waveform. Two automated measurement schemes were evaluated: (1) a photocell method where a frame is projected onto a photocell that measures the light transmitted through the film, converted to digital values, and used to plot the glottal area, and (2) a television method where the film is projected onto a vidicon tube (TV camera) and special circuits where it is processed and displayed on a TV monitor. The special circuits provide what amounts to a contour of the glottal area. The results of these two procedures were compared to hand planimeter measurements (see Figure 3–19). The authors report a maximum absolute difference of 11% between the TV and planimeter and a 30% absolute difference between photocell and hand measurements. An additional problem with the photocell data was the lack of a true closed period which had to be estimated from the hand-measured data. Greater correspondence between the TV or photocell data and the hand measurements could be obtained with repeated automated processing, but this will add to the processing time.

Hildebrand (1976) used a sonic digitizer tablet scheme to make measurements from high speed films. The digitizer has sensitive microphones positioned at the periphery of the active tablet area. A special pen produces a brief impulse which is picked up by the microphones. Time of arrival of the impulse is used to determine distance anywhere in the active digitizing area. Hildebrand reported a close correspondence to hand and pen measurements of glottal area. In addition, reliability of the measurements with the pen was very high (>0.99).

The measurement schemes discussed above (except for the TV method of Childers et al.) all use the computer to aid in the calculation of distances that are entered by a human operator. There have been reports of methods where the measurement has been completely under control of the computer. Most of these techniques involve digitizing the original filmed image and then processing the digital image to extract the relevant data.

Booth and Childers (1979) described their system that produced reliable, automatic measurements of high speed films. High speed films were digitized and stored in a computer. A computer program was developed to identify the edges of the glottis. Glottal area was then computed and the next frame was loaded and analyzed. The authors report about a 13% difference between the area measured with a planimeter and the present system. They found that they could analyze about 1 frame per minute. They believed that some of this discrepancy was due to the coarse nature of the digital image because they only digitized the images into eight gray levels. Current digitizing techniques permit the acquisition of video images with considerably greater resolution (256 gray levels). The Booth-Childers technique may produce much better results with higher resolution images. At this point in time, no other investigators have used this technique to analyze high speed films.

Colton and his colleagues (Colton, Casper, Brewer, & Conture, 1989) presented the results of some preliminary efforts to apply standard image processing techniques to the analysis of high speed films using an inexpensive, personal computer. Images were projected via a step-motion projector and digitized. Image enhancement routines were tried to improve the glottal area boundaries. Edge detection schemes were then performed to identify the edges of the glottis. Once the

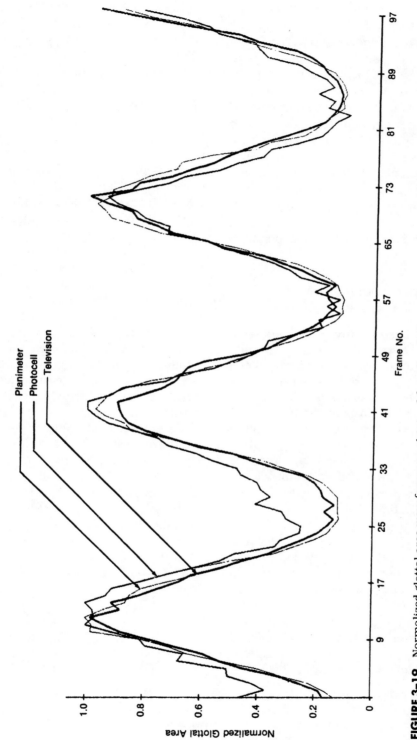
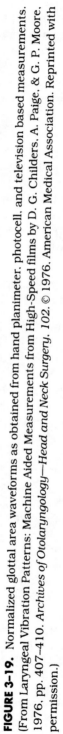

FIGURE 3–19. Normalized glottal area waveforms as obtained from hand planimeter. photocell. and television based measurements. (From Laryngeal Vibration Patterns: Machine Aided Measurements from High-Speed films by D. G. Childers. A. Paige. & G. P. Moore. 1976, pp. 407–410. *Archives of Otolaryngology—Head and Neck Surgery, 102.* © 1976. American Medical Association. Reprinted with permission.)

glottis was completely circumscribed,[5] the area of the glottis could be obtained.[6] The automated scheme compared favorably to hand measurement of glottal area, differing by about 1%. However, the technique still required considerable operator intervention to set the proper threshold values for the edge detector, fill in gaps in the edges, and fill the boundary with a uniform level to allow accurate area estimation. It is believed that image processing techniques exist or can be developed that will solve these problems and permit reliable, accurate measurement of vocal fold vibration using inexpensive, personal computers.

Some Recent Analyses of Normal Vibratory Patterns

There have been a number of reports in which the activity of normal vocal folds has been analyzed using high speed films. Some have used excised larynges where greater control can be exercised on the various structures in the larynx and better images of vibratory motion can often be obtained. Others have photographed actual voices and extracted data from the films obtained by hand or computer-assisted techniques as described below. In this section, a brief review of some of these reports will be presented.

Baer (1975, 1981a, 1981b) reported on his experiments with excised larynges in which he photographed the vocal folds in various simulated phonatory conditions. Of major interest were the patterns of vibratory motion which were interpreted in the framework of the body-cover model of the vocal folds (Baer, 1981a, 1981b; Hirano, 1974; Kakita, Hirano, &

Kawasaki, 1976a, 1976b; Kakita, Hirano, Kawasaki, & Matsushita, 1976). Other studies with excised larynges have also contributed to our knowledge about normal vibratory function (Matsushita, 1969; Matsushita, 1975; Titze, Jiang, & Hsiao, 1993; Yanagi & McCaffrey, 1992; Yumoto, Kadota, & Kurokawa, 1993).

Studies also have been reported in which human voices were photographed as they produced different phonatory maneuvers (Baer, Löfqvist, & McGarr, 1983; Brackett, 1947; Childers et al., 1983; Childers, Krishnamurthy, Naik, Larar, & Moore, 1983; Childers, Moore, Naik, Larar, & Krishnamurthy, 1983; Hildebrand, 1976; Hirano, Gould, Lambiase, & Kakita, 1980; Hirano, Kakita, Kawasaki, Gould, & Lambiase, 1981; Kiritani et al., 1986; Moore & Childers, 1984; Rubin & Hirt, 1960; Tanabe et al., 1975). Some of these studies have added further details to our knowledge about the vibratory characteristics of the vocal folds. Others have added new knowledge about vibratory function.

Rubin and Hirt (1960) reported a detailed analysis of the vibratory function when subjects produced phonation in falsetto voice. They carefully analyzed the chaotic motions of the vocal folds during the transition from normal to chest voice into falsetto (the so-called falsetto break). Once in falsetto, the vocal folds resumed a regular vibration but the folds barely touch each other. The authors postulated three mechanisms of falsetto based on their studies. In the first mechanism (open chink), the posterior portion of the glottis is always open and the vocal folds barely touch each other. In the second mechanism, the vocal folds close com-

---

[5]Considerable operator efforts were needed to ensure that there was a complete boundary around the glottis. This operator intervention slowed down the analysis considerably.

[6]Area was computed by simply counting the number of pixels (picture elements) circumscribed by the boundary. Because pixel size is fixed, absolute area can be determined by knowing how many pixels are presented in a known area.

pletely along their anteroposterior length but for a very brief period of time (the closed chink mechanism). In the third mechanism, there is progressive closure in a posterior-to-anterior direction as pitch is increased. This "damping" mechanism suggests that fundamental frequency is controlled by a systematic shortening of vocal fold length.

Hildebrand (1976) conducted a careful study of trained and untrained female speakers as they produced phonation at different fundamental frequencies and intensities. Measurements of Open Quo-

tient (OQ) and Speed Quotient (SQ) were made. The results are summarized in Figure 3–20. The average OQs rarely are less than 0.80 at any pitch or loudness condition and are much greater than those reported in the literature (see Figure 3–15). Perhaps, high OQs are a characteristic of female voices, or are due to the higher fundamental frequencies. At a low pitch level, OQ systematically decreased as intensity level was raised. This finding is consistent with previously reported empirical findings and supports the hypothesis that intensity is controlled by the

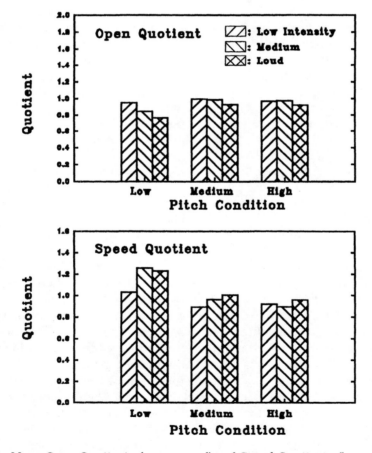

FIGURE 3–20. Mean Open Quotients *(upper panel)* and Speed Quotients *(lower panel)* for 10 female speakers. These data were obtained from high-speeed films of phonations produced at three pitch levels equally sampled throughout the subjects total pitch range and three intensity levels at each pitch level, again equally sampled through the subjects total intensity range for that pitch. (Data are from Hildebrand, 1976.)

closed time of the vocal folds. At the highest pitch level, the trend is not as systematic. The OQ at medium intensity level is greater than at low intensity level. Hildebrand reports a statistically significant difference of OQ between pitch and intensity levels. Any differences of OQ between the trained singers and the untrained speakers were not significant.

Speed Quotients show more variation as a function of intensity and pitch levels. There is an increase then a decrease of SQ as intensity was increased at the lowest pitch level but an increase of SQ as intensity was increased at the medium pitch level. At high pitch levels, there appears to be little systematic trend.

Speed Quotient is a ratio measurement and does not provide information about the actual speed of closure. At low fundamental frequencies, the actual velocity of the vocal folds may be slower than at high pitches. Furthermore, at high pitches, the speed of vocal fold opening or closing may be at its asymptote, suggesting that the upper limit of vocal fold velocity has been attained. This upper limit is probably due to the mass and other physical characteristics of the vocal folds. Attempts to further increase velocity of vocal fold vibration, for example, when a subject attempts to increase vocal intensity, result in little or no increase of velocity but may increase the variability of velocity of either or both folds. If true, this increased variability may manifest itself partly in variable SQ. Needless to say, these conjectures require experimental verification.

Hildebrand (1976) also presented some qualitative analyses of vocal fold vibration. First, about 65% of the films exhibited an opening in the posterior part of the vocal folds. This posterior gap, or chink, which may be a characteristic of female voices, has been also reported by Rammage et al. (1992). Second, many subjects showed an anterior-to-posterior

opening pattern as if the vocal folds were "zipping" open or closed. Both of these observations have been reported previously (Baisler, 1950; Moore, 1937, 1938; Timcke et al., 1958). Third, Hildebrand observed a slight phase difference between the two vocal folds in about 69% of the films. Therefore, it would appear that a slight difference in timing of each vocal fold is a normal characteristic of phonation in females.

Hirano et al. (1980) reported on an analysis of the phonatory behavior of single male speakers using high speed films. Plots of glottal width as a function of time were presented and show similarities in the details of motion as observed in glottal area plots. These authors introduced a new measure, speed index (SI), that they claimed was superior to SQ in providing a visual impression of the shape of the glottal waveform. Speed Index is defined as SQ − 1 divided by SQ + 1. Schematic, hypothetical, and highly improbable glottal area waveforms and their corresponding Speed Indexes are shown in Figure 3–21. A SI close to − 1 implies a very rapid opening phase and a rather slow (or much slower) closing phase. Equal opening and closing times would produce an SI of 0. Slow opening phases and very rapid closing phases will produce an SI close to 1. Note that the range of variation of SI is between − 1 and +1, whereas SQ ranges between 0 and some large positive number. Theoretically, waveform variations such as these, if mirrored in the acoustic pulse produced by the vocal folds, will produce differences in the spectrum of the glottal tone and, therefore, voice quality.

Hirano, Kakita, Kawasaki, Gould, and Lambiase (1981) analyzed the vibratory behavior of a male speaker and reported data on the propagation velocity of the mucosal wave. These measurements were based on the measurement of maximum lateral excursion of a vocal fold edge and demonstrated how the mucosal wave

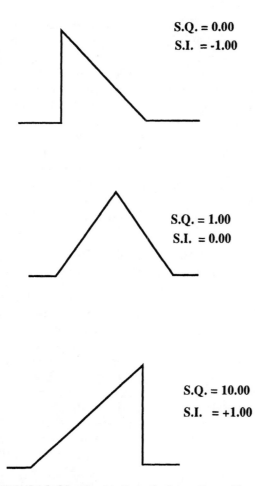

S.Q. = 0.00
S.I. = -1.00

S.Q. = 1.00
S.I. = 0.00

S.Q. = 10.00
S.I. = +1.00

FIGURE 3–21. Illustration of schematic and hypothetical glottal area waveforms and their corresponding Speed Quotients (SQ) and Speed Indexes (SI). (Based on data presented by Hirano, Gould, Lambiase, and Kakita, 1980.)

slowed as it approached the lateral boundary of the vocal fold. A velocity of 2.5 m/s was measured near the medial margin of the fold whereas it had slowed to 1.5 m/s near the lateral boundary. These are similar to propagation velocities measured from canine larynges as reported by Titze, Jiang, and Hsiao (1993) ranging from 0.5 m/s to 2.0 m/s. The presence of a mucosal wave and its lateral extent is an important feature observed in stroboscopy of normal and abnormal voice productions.

Quantification of its speed, either from high speed films or stroboscopic images, may be important in understanding the effect of pathology on vocal fold vibration.

Some Recent Analyses of Abnormal Vibratory Patterns

Since the classic studies by Moore and his colleagues concerning the physiology of vocal fold vibration in persons with vocal pathology, there have been a number of studies in which high speed films have been used to study the pathophysiology.

Vibratory behavior of patients with a unilateral paralysis of the vocal folds was described by von Leden and Moore (1961). They concluded that (1) both folds vibrate at the same fundamental frequency, (2) the healthy fold tends to exhibit greater amplitude of motion, (3) the paralyzed fold tends to precede the good fold but there are considerable phase differences, (4) the healthy fold tends to initiate vibration first, and (5) the paralyzed fold tends to cease vibration first. The authors claim that the paralyzed fold is at a slightly higher level than the good fold, creating a disturbance in air flow patterns which strike the paralyzed fold and may cause movement of the ventricular folds. The asymmetrical patterns of airflow and/or vocal fold configuration may explain the marked phase differences between the folds. The von Leden and Moore study is significant because it demonstrates how careful investigation of vocal fold vibration, even in pathology, can add significant information to our understanding of the pathophysiology of phonation.

Later studies by Hirano and his colleagues (Hirano, Matsushita & Kawasaki, 1974; Hirano, Gould, Lambiase, & Kakita, 1981) confirmed the importance of the investigation of vibration in pathology, this time for a unilateral polyp. Study of the motion of both folds in a patient revealed how the polyp moved during the vibratory cycle and how it affected the healthy fold when the two touched each other. Also measured from the high speed films was the velocity of the traveling or mucosal wave on the good fold of about 0.47 m/s. No such mucosal wave was observed on the fold with the polyp. There were differences of maximum amplitude between the two folds suggesting greater stiffness on the affected fold. Clinically, the mass of the polyp is often implicated as a possible cause for the abnormal vibrations and voice quality. However, for some patients, as was the case for the patient described in the Hirano study, stiffness changes may be the true underlying cause of the abnormal vibrations rather than mass differences.

Glottic closure patterns are also a significant feature of abnormal phonation. Moore, Cannon, and Wilson (1979) analyzed the high speed films of three female patients with nodules who produced phonation at different fundamental frequencies and intensities. They classified the glottal opening pattern at the most closed portion of the vocal folds into seven categories based on their measurement of glottal opening at nine points along the anteroposterior distance of the vocal folds. About 7% of the films showed a complete closure pattern. Sixty per cent showed a posterior opening of varying magnitude (their categories II, III, IV), whereas the remainder had an opening anterior to the nodule in addition to an opening posteriorly. The pattern of glottal closure would determine the shape of the acoustic pulse and therefore the quality of the voice. However, the precise effect of these closure patterns on the acoustic pulse has yet to be determined.

Another significant observation from Moore et al. (1979) was that the nodule of one subject was more easily seen or prominent during the closing phase of the vibratory cycle. This suggests that a nodule has its genesis on the lower lip of the vocal fold, since in normal vibration, the lower edge of the vocal folds leads the medial excursion of the vocal folds. Unknown is how prevalent this finding is among patients with nodules, especially when the nodule is small, soft, and in its formative stages.

A summary of the effects of a pathology on vocal fold vibration is presented in Table 3–1. All of the findings reported in this table are based on high speed film studies but also have been observed during stroboscopic examinations.

Stroboscopy: A Clinical Tool for the Analysis of Vibration

To understand the basic features and nuances of normal and abnormal voice, otolaryngologists, speech-language pathologists, and voice scientists need to analyze the vibratory characteristics of the vocal folds. Analysis of high speed films has added considerably to our knowledge about normal and abnormal vibration. However, the use of high speed films is difficult technically, and the technique has not been found acceptable for routine clinical use. Clinicians needed a technique that was reasonable in cost and could be used in the clinic with most patients. Such a technique is stroboscopy.

Although the basic technique of stroboscopy has been known for over a century, its acceptance and increased clinical use is much more recent, first in Europe, then Japan, and finally in the United States. In stroboscopy, the vibration of the vocal folds can be seen with the naked eye and recorded on ordinary video tape. But, the motion we see is an illusion. We miss many details of motion, details that may or may not be significant. On the other hand, we are able to visualize in real time the vibratory characteristics of the vocal folds, both in health and disease, which is more information than we can obtain from viewing the vocal folds

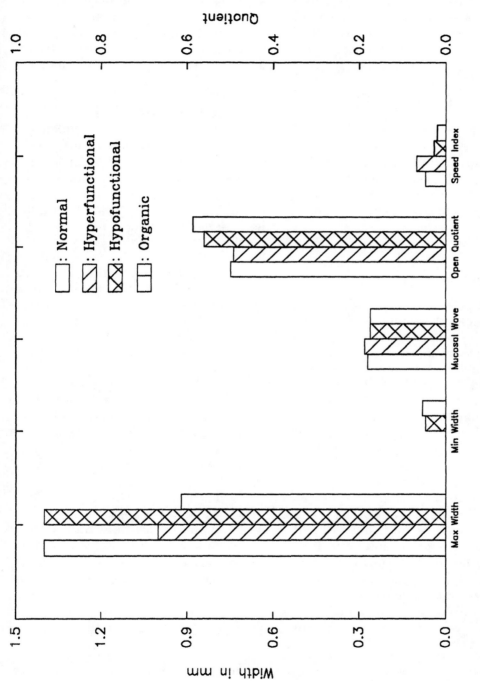

FIGURE 3–22. Average data for five measurements made on stroboscopic video recordings. Minimum and Maximum Glottal Width and Extent of Mucosal Wave are expressed in mm. Open Quotient and Speed index are dimensionless qualities. (Based on data presented by Wendler, Köppen, and Fischer, 1986.)

with the naked eye or by using regular, continuous light with an endoscope.

Much has been reported about the use of the stroboscope in a clinical setting and the value it has in the diagnosis and treatment of many voice problems (Alberti, 1978; Bless, Hirano, & Feder, 1987; Colton & Casper, 1996; Ford, Bless, & Lowery, 1990; Kallen, 1932; Kruse, 1989; Prytz, 1987; Remacle, Clerin, Dubois, Ryckaert, & Bertrand, 1986; Prytz, 1987; Sataloff, Spiegel, & Hawkshaw, 1991; Sessions et al., 1989; Woo, Colton, Casper, & Brewer, 1991, 1992). The following is a brief review of selected studies in which the stroboscope was used to quantify characteristics of vocal fold vibrations in humans.[7]

Quantification of Stroboscopic Images

Rasinger, Neuwirth-Riedi, and Kment (1986) described a digital and cursor-based video analysis system that they hoped to use to quantify videostroboscopic images. They demonstrated some simple image processing and measured the area of glottal opening. However, since this was primarily a preliminary report, little data were reported.

Wendler (Wendler, Köppen, & Fischer, 1986; Wendler & Köppen, 1988) presented the results of measurements of stroboscopic video recordings of 48 female subjects (14 with normal voices, 7 with hypofunctional voice difficulty, 13 with hyperfunctional voices, and 14 with organic voice disorders). He measured maximum and minimum glottal width, maximum extent of mucosal wave, Open Quotient, and Speed Index using a cursor-based video analysis system.[8] The re-

sults of this study appear in Figure 3–22. There were statistically significant differences among the four groups on the measures of maximum glottal width, minimum glottal width, OQ, and SI. In the hyperfunctional and organic groups, the vocal folds had small amplitudes of movement. Both normal and hyperfunctional speakers had no glottal opening at the most closed position of the vibratory cycle. Both the hyperfunctional and organic voice groups had incomplete closure. Lower OQs were evident for both the normal and hyperfunctional groups. Based on these measurements, Wendler classified the patients into the four original groups using a multivariate discriminate analysis statistical procedure. The results of the classification are shown in Figure 3–23. No group was perfectly reclassified using the quantitative measurements; however, the hyperfunctional and normal groups had the highest percentage of correct classification. Hypofunctional speakers exhibited the lowest correct classification percentage. Wendler concluded that, although the quantification of stroboscopic images may be an important research tool, there appears to be little need for such objective measurement clinically. He found the procedures time-consuming and felt they added little to our understanding of the nature of the clinical problem.

Although Wendler's conclusions about the clinical utility of objective stroboscopic measurements may be warranted based on his data, it is possible that the nature of the questions Wendler asked were not appropriate for the data collected. His goal was to use objective measurements to classify patients into one of four diagnostic categories. Diagnosis of voice prob-

---

[7]There have been studies in which the stroboscope has been used to quantify vocal fold behavior in an excised human or canine larynx (e.g., Moore, Berke, Hanson, & Ward, 1987). However, in the interest of brevity, these will not be reviewed here.

[8]A computer controlled cursor overlaid the video image appearing on a TV monitor. Measurements were made in mm.

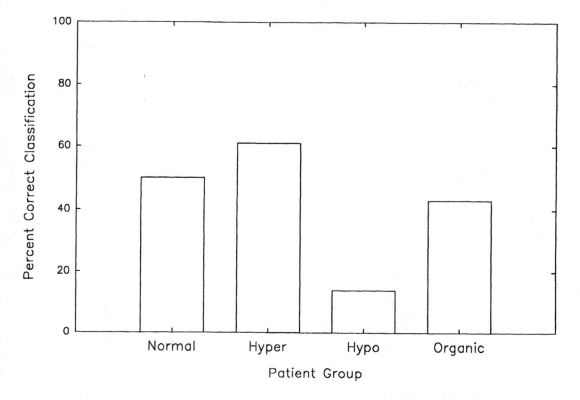

FIGURE 3–23. Percent correct classification of four patient groups: normal, hyperfunctional, hypofunctional, and organic based on a disriminate analysis of six measurements made on the stroboscopic video recordings. (Based on data presented by Wendler, Köppen, and Fischer, 1986.)

lems does not depend on a solitary piece of information, but is the result of careful consideration of patient and voice characteristics derived from a variety of sources. One wonders about the clinical reality of the three diagnostic groups studied by Wendler. It is possible (and indeed probable) that hypofunctional and organic voice patients share some common vibratory features. It is obvious from Wendler's data that hyperfunctional, hypofunctional, and normal voices share some common features; otherwise, they would not have been confused so frequently.[9] Addi-

tional varied objective measurements, as well as more careful definition of these diagnostic categories, probably are needed to correctly classify patients into diagnostic categories.

Another computer-based system for the analysis of stroboscopic video images was described by Watanabe, Shin, Matsuo, Oda, and Fukaura (1986). These authors used digital image processing techniques to subtract images from each other, thereby emphasizing the differences between them. Color intensity variation was employed to highlight the anatomical dif-

[9]Hyperfunctional voices were confused with normal voices about 29% of the time and with hypofunctional voices about 14% of the time. Hypofunctional voices were confused with normal voices about 21% of the time.

ferences. However, few quantitative data were presented.

Analysis of Stroboscopic Images and Other Measures of Vibratory Function

Anastaplo and Karnell (1988) and Karnell (1989) reported on a technique for the simultaneous recording of stroboscopic and electroglottographic data and demonstrated how it could be used to quantify the vocal fold vibratory waveform. Specifically, they investigated the relationship between the vocal fold opening, as viewed with a stroboscope, and features in the EGG waveform. They reported that the "knee"[10] of the EGG occurred at about the same moment in time as the vocal folds opened superiorly, although there was some variation in the exact time of appearance of the knee and opening of the vocal folds. These observations suggest that simultaneous recording of EGG and the videostroboscopic images can be useful in correlating the EGG signal to the movement patterns, thus permitting more precise descriptions of vibratory motion. Pedersen (1977) had reported earlier on the simultaneous use of stroboscopy and EGG in which the strobe images were used to identify or corroborate certain features of the EGG signal.

Using similar methodology, Karnell, Li, and Panje (1992) reported a quantitative study in which glottal length measurements were made from stroboscopic recordings of 24 subjects at three points on the EGG waveform: (a) the start of vocal fold closure; (b) at peak vocal fold closure, and (c) at the end of closure. The subjects were divided into four groups: six controls with normal voices; six pa-

tients who were found to exhibit normal voices; six patients with vocal fold nodules, and six patients who had polyps removed surgically. No statistically significant differences were found among the four groups at the point of maximum closure. Some statistically significant differences were found among the groups at either the start or end of closure or both points. Karnell and his colleagues concluded that vocal fold neoplasms do not necessarily reduce the amount of glottal closure.[11] They also made an important point about when to observe the effects of a neoplasm on vocal fold vibration by suggesting that clinicians pay attention to both the opening and closing phases of the vibratory cycle, rather than just the closed phase. Clinically, important information may be gained about the pathophysiology of vibration by careful examination of the entire vibratory cycle.

SUMMARY

Vocal fold physiology is a dynamic event resulting from the complex interaction of aerodynamic and myoelastic forces. There are important acoustic and physiological correlates that need careful study if one is to fully comprehend the dynamics of vocal fold vibration and the kind of acoustic disturbances it creates. Analysis of vocal fold vibration via high speed films, as pioneered by G. Paul Moore, has contributed greatly to this understanding in patients with and without vocal fold pathology. Other techniques, such as stroboscopy, EGG, and inverse filtering of the oral air flow waveform, also contribute to our understanding of the voice. The acoustic consequences of vocal fold vibra-

---

[10]The "knee" refers to a discontinuity in the opening phase of the EGG.
[11]Karnell et al. (1992) made measurements of glottal length and not glottal area. It is possible, as they recognize, that a neoplasm might result in an increased area of opening of the glottis when the vocal folds are maximally closed.

tion are varied and require careful study because the acoustic disturbance transmits to our ears, in a transformed manner, the effects of pathology or simple bodily functions. No clinician can be effective without a reasonably complete and current understanding of vocal fold physiology.

REFERENCES

Alberti, P. W. (1978). The diagnostic role of laryngeal stroboscopy. *Otolaryngology Clinics of North America, 11*, 347–354.

Anastaplo, S., & Karnell, M. P. (1988). Synchronized videostroboscopic and electroglottographic examination of glottal opening. *Journal of the Acoustical Society of America, 83*, 1883–1890.

Baer, T. (1975). *Investigation of phonation using excised larynges.* Unpublished doctoral dissertation, Massachusetts Institute of Technology, Cambridge, MA.

Baer, T. (1981a). Investigation of the phonatory mechanism. In C. L. Ludlow & M. Hart (Eds.), *Proceedings of the Conference on the Assessment of Vocal Pathology* (pp. 38–37). Rockville, MD: American Speech-Language-Hearing Association Reports #11.

Baer, T. (1981b). Observation of vocal fold vibration: measurement of excised larynges. In K. N. Stevens & M. Hirano (Eds.), *Vocal physiology* (pp. 119–133). Tokyo: University of Tokyo Press.

Baer, T., Löfqvist, A., & McGarr, N. (1983). Laryngeal vibrations: A comparison between high-speed filming and glottographic techniques. *Journal of the Acoustical Society of America, 73*, 1304–1308.

Baisler, P. (1950). *A study of intralaryngeal activity during production of voice in normal and falsetto registers.* Unpublished doctoral dissertation, Northwestern University, Evanston, IL.

Biever, D. M., & Bless, D. M. (1989) Vibratory characteristics of the vocal folds in young adult and geriatric women. *Journal of Voice, 3*, 120–131.

Bless, D. M., Hirano, M., & Feder, R. (1987). Videostroboscopic evaluation of the larynx. *Ear, Nose, and Throat Journal, 66*, 289–296.

Booth, J. R., & Childers, D. G. (1979). Automated analysis of ultra-high-speed laryngeal films. *IEEE Transactions in Biomedical Engineering, BME-26.*

Brackett, I. (1947). *An analysis of the vibratory action of the vocal folds during the production of tones at selected frequencies.* Unpublished doctoral dissertation, Northwestern University, Evanston, IL.

Brown, W. S., & Feinstein, S. H., (1977). Speaker sex identification utilizing a constant laryngeal source. *Folia Phoniatrica, 29*, 240–248.

Childers, D. G., Krishnamurthy, A. K., Naik, J. M., Larar, J. N., & Moore, G. P. (1983). Assessment of laryngeal function by simultaneous measurement of speech, electroglottography and ultra-high speed film. *Folia Phoniatrica, 35*, 116A.

Childers, D. G., Moore, G. P., Naik, J. M., Larar, J. N., & Krishnamurthy, A. K. (1983). Assessment of laryngeal function by simultaneous synchronized measurement of speech, electroglottography and high-speed film. In V. Lawrence (Ed.), *Transcripts of the Eleventh Symposium: Care of the Professional Voice: Part II. Medical/surgical sessions: Papers* (pp. 234–244). New York: The Voice Foundation.

Childers, D. G., Naik, J. M., Larar, J. N., Krishnamurthy, A. K., & Moore, G. P. (1983). Electroglottography, speech, and ultra-high speed cinematography. In I. R. Titze & R. C. Scherer (Eds.), *Vocal fold physiology: Biomechanics, acoustics and phonatory control* (pp. 202–220). Denver, CO: Denver Center for the Performing Arts.

Childers, D. G., Paige, A., & Moore, G. P. (1976). Laryngeal vibration patterns: Machine aided measurements from high-speed films. *Archives of Otolaryngology, 102*, 407–410.

Coleman, R. O. (1971). Male and female voice quality and its relationship to vowel formant frequencies. *Journal of Speech and Hearing Research, 14*, 565–577.

Coleman, R. O. (1973). Speaker identification in the absence of inter-subject differences in glottal source characteristics. *Journal of the Acoustical Society of America, 53*, 1741–1743.

Coleman, R. O. (1976). A comparison of the contributions of two voice quality characteristics to the perception of maleness and femaleness in the voice. *Journal of Speech and Hearing Research, 19*, 168–180.

Colton, R. H., Casper, J. K., Brewer, D. W., & Conture, E. G. (1989). Digital processing of laryngeal images: A preliminary report. *Journal of Voice, 3,* 132–142.

Colton, R. H., Reed, G., Sagerman, R., & Chung, C. (1982). *An investigation of voice change after radiotherapy.* Final Report National Cancer Institute. Bethesda, MD: National Institutes of Health. Bethesda, MD.

Ford, C. N., Bless D. M., & Lowery, J. D. (1990). Indirect laryngoscopic approach for injection of botulinum toxin in spasmodic dysphonia. *Otolaryngology—Head and Neck Surgery, 103,* 752–758.

Hammarberg, B. (1987). Pitch and quality characteristics of mutational voice disorders before and after therapy. *Folia Phoniatrica, 39,* 204–216.

Hammarberg, B., Fritzell, B., & Schiratzki, H. (1984). Teflon injection in 16 patients with paralytic dysphonia: Perceptual and acoustic evaluations. *Journal of Speech and Hearing Disorders, 49,* 72–82.

Hildebrand, B. H. (1976). *Vibratory patterns of the human vocal cords during variations in frequency and intensity.* Unpublished doctoral dissertation, University of Florida, Gainesville, FL.

Hirano, M. (1974). Morphological structure of the vocal cord as a vibrator and its variations. *Folia Phoniatrica, 26,* 89–94.

Hirano, M. (1981). *Clinical examination of voice.* Wein, Austria: Springer-Verlag.

Hirano, M., Gould, W. J., Lambiase, A., & Kakita, Y. (1980). Movements of selected points on a vocal fold during vibration. *Folia Phoniatrica, 32,* 39–50.

Hirano, M., Gould, W. J., Lambiase, A., & Kakita, Y. (1981). Vibratory behavior of the vocal folds in a case of a unilateral polyp. *Folia Phoniatrica, 33,* 275–284.

Hirano, M., Kakita, Y., Kawasaki, H., Gould, W. J., & Lambiase, A. (1981). Data from high-speed motion picture studies. In K. N. Stevens & M. Hirano (Eds.), *Vocal fold physiology* (pp. 85–91). Tokyo: University of Tokyo Press.

Hirano, M., Matsushita, H., & Kawasaki, H. (1974). Vibration of the vocal cords with unilateral polyp. An ultra-high speed cinematographic study. *Japanese Journal of Otolaryngology* (Tokyo), *77,* 593–610.

Hirose, H. (1988). High speed digital imaging of vocal fold vibration. *Acta Otolaryngologica* (Stockholm), *Suppl. 458,* 151–158.

Hirose, H., Kiritani, S., & Imagawa, H. (1987). High speed digital image analysis of laryngeal behavior in running speech. *Annual Bulletin RILP, 21.*

Hirose, H., Kiritani, S., & Imagawa, H. (1988). High speed digital image analysis of laryngeal behavior in running speech. In O. Fujimura (Ed.). *Vocal physiology: Voice production, mechanisms, and functions* (pp. 335–345). New York: Raven Press.

Hirose, H., Kiritani, S., & Imagawa, H. (1991a). High speed digital imaging of vocal fold vibration and its application for analysis of hoarseness. In J. A. Cooper (Ed.), Assessment of speech and voice production: *Research and clinical implications* (pp. 146–149). Bethesda, MD: U.S. Department of Health and Human Services.

Hirose, H., Kiritani, S., & Imagawa, H. (1991b). Clinical application of high-speed digital imaging of vocal fold vibration. In J. Gauffin & B. Hammarberg (Eds.), *Vocal fold physiology: Acoustic, perceptual, and physiological aspects of voice mechanisms* (pp. 213–216). San Diego, CA: Singular Publishing Group.

Hollien, H., & Majewski, W. (1977). Speaker identification by long-term spectra under normal and distorted speech conditions. *Journal of the Acoustical Society of America, 62,* 975–980.

Holmberg, E. S., Hillman, R. E., & Perkell, J. S. (1988). Glottal airflow and transglottal air pressure measurements for male and female speakers in soft, normal, and loud voice. *Journal of the Acoustical Society of America, 84,* 511–529.

Honda, K., Kiritani, S., Imagawa, H., Hirose, H. & Hashimoto, K. (1985). High speed digital recording of vocal fold vibration using a solid-state image sensor. *Annual Bulletin RILP, 19,* 47–54.

Imagawa, H., Kiritani, S., & Hirose, H. (1987). Further development in high-speed digital image recording system for assessment of vocal fold vibration. *Annual Bulletin RILP, 21,* 9–23.

Imagawa, H., Kiritani, S., Honda K., & Hirose, H. (1986). Improvements in the high-speed digital image recording system for observing vocal fold vibration. *Annual Bulletin RILP, 20,* 17–22.

Kakita, Y., Hirano, M., & Kawasaki, H. (1976a). Schematical presentation of vibration of the vocal cord as a layer-structured vibrator. *Nippon Jibiinkoka Gakkai Kaiho, 11,* 1333–1340.

Kakita, Y., Hirano, M., & Kawasaki, H. (1976b). Schematical presentation of vibration of pathological vocal cords. Japanese *Journal of Otolaryngology* (Tokyo), *79,* 1533–1548.

Kakita, Y., Hirano, M., Kawasaki, H., & Matsushita, H. (1976). Schematical presentation of vibration of the vocal cords as a layered-structured vibrator: Normal larynges. *Japanese Journal of Otolaryngology* (Tokyo), *79,* 1333–1340.

Kallen, L. A. (1932). Laryngostroboscopy in the practice of otolaryngology. *Archives of Otolaryngology, 16,* 791–807.

Karnell, M. (1989). Synchronized videostroboscopy and electroglottography. Journal of Voice, 3, 68–75.

Karnell, M. P., Li, L., & Panje, W. R. (1992). Glottal opening in patients with vocal fold tissue changes. *Journal of Voice, 5,* 239–246.

Kiritani, S., Imagawa, H., & Hirose, H. (1986). Simultaneous high-speed digital recording of vocal fold vibration, speech, and EEG. *Annual Bulletin RILP, 20,* 11–15.

Kiritani, S., Imagawa, H., & Hirose, H. (1992). High-speed digital imaging of vocal cord vibration at voice onset in consonants. *Annual Bulletin RILP, 26,* 29–37.

Kitzing, P. (1986). LTAS criteria pertinent to the measurement of voice quality. *Journal of Phonetics, 14,* 477–482.

Kruse, E. (1989). Differential diagnosis of functional voice disorders. *Folia Phoniatrica, 41,* 1–9.

Löfqvist, A. (1986). The long-time average spectrum as a tool in voice research. *Journal of Phonetics, 14,* 471–476.

Löfqvist, A., & Mandersson, B. (1987). Long-time average spectrum of speech and voice analysis. *Folia Phoniatrica, 39,* 221–229.

Matsushita, H. (1969). Vocal cord vibration of excised larynges: a study with ultra-high-speed cinematography. *Otologia* (Fukuoka), *15,* 127–142.

Matsushita, H. (1975). The vibratory mode of the vocal folds in the excised larynx. *Folia Phoniatrica, 27,* 7–18.

Metz, D. E., Whitehead, R. L., & Peterson, D. H. (1980). An optical illumination system for high speed laryngeal cinematography. *Journal of the Acoustical Society of America, 67,* 719–720.

Moore, G. P. (1937). Vocal fold movement during vocalization. *Speech Monographs, 4,* 44–55.

Moore, G. P. (1938). Motion picture studies of vocal folds and vocal attack. *Journal of Speech and Hearing Disorders, 1,* 235–238.

Moore, G. P., Berke, G. S., Hanson, D. G., & Ward, P. H. (1987). Videostroboscopy of the canine larynx: The effects of asymmetric laryngeal tension. *Laryngoscope, 9, 7,* 543–553.

Moore, G. P. , Cannon, K. A., & Wilson, L. I. (1979). Vocal fold vibration in the presence of vocal nodules. In V. Lawrence (Ed.), *Transcripts of the Eighth Symposium: Care of the Professional Voice: Part III. Medical/surgical therapy* (pp. 24–31). New York: The Voice Foundation.

Moore, G. P. & Childers, D. G. (1984). Glottal area (real size) related to voice production. In V. Lawrence (Ed.), *Transcripts of the Twelfth Symposium: Care of the Professional Voice* (pp. 92–96). New York: The Voice Foundation.

Pedersen, M. F. (1977). Electroglottography compared with synchronized stroboscopy in normal persons. *Folia Phoniatrica, 29,* 191–199.

Plomp, R. (1976). *Aspects of tone sensation.* New York: Academic Press.

Pols, L. (1971). Dimensional representation of speech spectra. *In Proceedings of the 7th International Congress on Acoustics* (pp. 281–284). Budapest, Hungary.

Pols, L. C. W., van der Kamp, L. J., & Plomp, R. (1969). Perceptual and physical space of vowel sounds. *Journal of the Acoustical Society of America, 46,* 458–467.

Prytz, S. (1987, September). Laryngeal videostroboscopy. *Ear, Nose, and Throat Journal Supplement, ENTechnology,* 34–41.

Rammage, L. A., Peppard, R. C., & Bless, D. M. (1992). Aerodynamic, laryngoscopic, and perceptual-acoustic characteristics of dysphonic females with posterior glottal chinks: A retrospective study. *Journal of Voice, 6,* 64–78.

Rasinger, G. A., Neuwirth-Riedi, K., & Kment, G. (1986). Erst ergebnisse digitaler videobildanalyseverfahren zur Auswertung von endoskopischen. *Laryngology Rhinology Otology, (Stuttgart) 65*, 333–335.

Remacle, M., Clerin, M., Dubois, P., Ryckaert, M., & Bertrand, B. (1986). Exploration of glottic function before and after injection of collagen for rehabilitation of the vocal cord. *Acta Otorhinolaryngology Belgium, 40*, 405–420.

Rubin, H. J., & Hirt, C. (1960). The falsetto: A high speed cinematographic study. *Laryngoscope, 70*, 1305–1324.

Sataloff, R. T., Spiegel, J. R., & Hawkshaw, M. J. (1991). Strobovideolaryngoscopy: Results and clinical value. *Annals of Otology, Rhinology and Laryngology, 100*, 725–727.

Sessions, R. B., Miller, S. D., Martin, G. F., Solomon, B. I., Harrison, L. B., & Stackpole, S. (1989). Videolaryngostroboscopic analysis of minimal glottic cancer. *Transactions American Laryngological Association, 110*, 56–59.

Södersten, M., & Lindestad, P. A., (1990). Glottal closure and perceived breathiness during phonation in normally speaking subjects. *Journal of Speech and Hearing Research, 33*, 601–611.

Södersten, M. , Lindestad, P. A., & Hammarberg, B. (1991). Vocal fold closure, perceived breathiness, and acoustic characteristics in young normal-speaking adults. In J. Gauffin & B. Hammarberg (Eds.), *Vocal fold physiology* (pp. 217–224). San Diego, CA: Singular Publishing Group.

Tanabe, M., Kitajima, K., Gould, W. J., & Lambiase, A. (1975). Analysis of high speed motion picture of the vocal folds. *Folia Phoniatrica, 27*, 77–87.

Timcke, R., von Leden, H. S., & Moore, G. P. (1958). Laryngeal vibrations: Measurements of the glottic wave. Part I: The normal vibratory cycle. *Archives of Otolaryngology, 68*, 1–19.

Timcke, R., von Leden, H. S., & Moore, G. P. (1959). Laryngeal vibrations: Measurements of the glottic wave. Part II: Physiologic variations. *Archives of Otolaryngology, 69*, 438–444.

Titze, I. (1989). Physiologic and acoustic differences between male and female voices. *Journal of the Acoustical Society of America, 85*, 1699–1707.

Titze, I. R., Jiang, J. J., & Hsiao, T. Y. (1993). Measurement of mucosal wave propagation and vertical phase difference in vocal fold vibration. *Annals of Otology, Rhinology and Laryngology, 102* , 58–63.

von Leden, H.S., & Moore, G. P. (1961). Vibratory patterns of the vocal cords in unilateral laryngeal paralysis. *Acta Otolaryngologica* (Stockholm), *53*, 493–506.

von Leden, H., Moore, P., & Timcke, R. (1960). Laryngeal vibrations: measurements of the glottic wave. Part III: The pathologic larynx. *Archives of Otolaryngology, 71*, 26–45.

Watanabe, H., Shin, T., Matsuo, K., Oda, M., & Fukaura, J. (1986). A new computer-analyzing system for clinical use with a strobovideo scope. *Archives of Otolaryngology Head Neck Surgery, 112*, 978–981.

Wendler, J., Doherty, E.T., & Hollien, H. (1980). Voice classification by means of long-term speech spectra. *Folia Phoniatrica, 32*, 51–60.

Wendler, J., & Köppen, K. (1988). Schwinungsmessunger der Stimmlippen: Zür klinischen relevantz der stroboskopie. *Folia Phoniatrica, 40*, 297–302.

Wendler, J., Köppen, K., & Fischer, S. (1986). The validity of stroboscopic data in terms of quantitative measures. In R. S. Hibi, D. Bless, & M. Hirano (Eds.), *Proceedings of International Conference on Voice* (pp. 36–43). Kurume, Japan: Kurume University.

Wendler, J., Rauhut, A., & Kruger, H. (1986). Classification of voice qualities. *Journal of Phonetics, 14*, 483–488.

Woo, P., Colton, R. H., Casper, J. K., & Brewer, D. W. (1991). Diagnostic value of stroboscopic examination in hoarse patients. *Journal of Voice, 5*, 231–238.

Woo, P., Colton, R. H., Casper, J. K., & Brewer, D. W. (1992). Analysis of spasmodic dysphonia by aerodynamic and laryngostroboscopic measurements. *Journal of Voice, 6*, 344–351.

Yanagi, E., & McCaffrey, T. V. (1992). Study of vibratory pattern of the vocal folds in the excised canine larynx. *Archives of Otolaryngology—Head and Neck Surgery, 118*, 30–36.

Yumoto, E., Kadota, Y., & Kurokawa, H. (1993). Tracheal view of vocal fold vibration in excised canine larynxes. *Archives of Otolaryngology—Head and Neck Surgery, 119*, 73–78.

LIFESPAN CHANGES IN THE LARYNX: AN ANATOMICAL PERSPECTIVE

JOEL C. KAHANE, Ph.D.

Changes in the human voice occur between infancy and old age and reflect a myriad of biological changes that influence the size, shape, and physical properties of the larynx. This chapter chronicles these changes in the larynx during infancy, childhood, adolescence, and adulthood, and their functional implications to voice production.

THE INFANT LARYNX

The infant larynx is not simply a miniature of the adult. Although clearly smaller (Figure 4–1), it differs from its adult counterpart in terms of its (a) position in the pharynx, (b) size and shape, and (c) structural maturity of its tissues.

During infancy, the larynx is located high in the neck (the lower border of the cricoid cartilage rests between the second and third cervical vertebra, C2–C3). It lies within a short, fairly horizontal pharyn-

geal cavity that offers little resistance to airflow. The epiglottis can contact the soft palate (Laitman & Crelin, 1976), affording an anatomical coupling of these structures. This arrangement enables the infant to breathe while it nurses. The laryngeal airway is protected by the epiglottis, which remains erect to divert the ingested contents into the pyriform sinuses while allowing air to pass from the nasopharynx into an unobstructed laryngeal cavity.

Cotton (1990) has pointed out that the infant's airway differs from the adult's. In the infant, the airway is funnel-shaped, narrowing through the vocal folds into the subglottal region (see Figure 4–1). In the adult, the funnel shape is lost and is replaced by a tubular configuration, resulting from growth of the cricoid cartilage that widens the subglottal area.

No significant sex differences exist in the infant larynx (Klock, 1968; Negus, 1929; Noback, 1925); consequently, it is not surprising that infant voices of both sexes are similar.

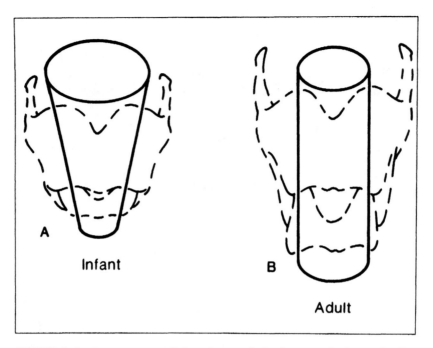

FIGURE 4-1. Comparison of the shape of the laryngeal airway in the infant and adult. (From Management and treatment of subglottic stenosis in infants and children by R. T. Cotton, 1990. In C. Bluestone & S. Stool, Eds., *Pediatric otolaryngology*. Philadelphia: W. B. Saunders. Reprinted with permission.)

Laryngeal Cartilages

The infant laryngeal cartilages are uniquely different from older counterparts because they are quite soft and pliable (Wilson, 1953). Similarly, great amounts of loose and highly vascular connective tissue (Ogrua & Mallen, 1977) make the infant larynx structurally more susceptible to becoming edematous than older individuals.

Abt (1923) and Bosma (1975) have noted that infant and adult larynges differ in shape and proximity to the hyoid bone (Figure 4-2). They observed that the shape of the infant larynx is more rounded than in the adult; this is particularly evident in the thyroid cartilage, which is broader and shorter in infants than adults. The infant larynx is also more compact than in the adult. Its cartilages assume a proportionally larger amount of the structure of the larynx (Figure 4-2), especially in the rima glottidis. Bosma suggests that the proportionally larger size of the arytenoid cartilages and their posterior cricoarytenoid ligaments stabilize the vocal folds posteriorly. The vocal processes in the infant assume a proportionally greater length of the rima glottidis (Figure 4-3) because the anterior dimension of the larynx is shorter. This structural reinforcement serves to accentuate the effects of the short vocal folds (3 to 5 mm, see Table 4-1) in producing a high fundamental frequency.

Vocal Folds

The length of the vocal folds, however, cannot entirely account for the fundamental frequency or vocal properties of the infant larynx. Clearly, the structure of the vocal

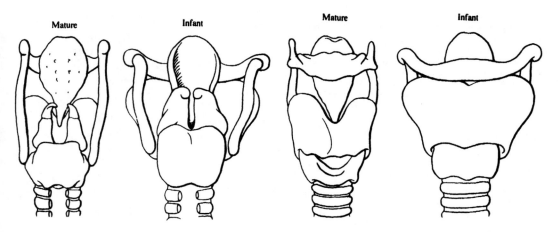

FIGURE 4–2. Posterior and anterior views of the infant and mature larynx. (Anatomic and physiologic development of the speech apparatus by J. Bosma, 1975, p. 476. In D. B. Tower (Ed.), *The Nervous System, Vol. 3, Human Communication and Its Disorders.* New York: Raven Press. Reprinted with permission.)

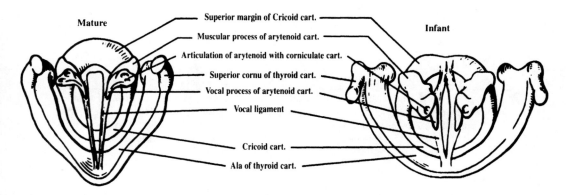

FIGURE 4–3. Superior view of the larynx showing laryngeal cartilages and vocal ligament in a mature male and infant. For demonstration purposes, these schematics are made dimensionally equivalent at the external diameter of the cricoid cartilage at midline. From Anatomic and physiologic development of the speech apparatus by J. Bosma, 1975, p. 477. In D. B. Tower (Ed.), *The nervous system, Vol. 3 Human Communication and Its Disorders.* New York: Raven Press. Reprinted with permission.)

folds is important. Hirano, Kurita, and Nakashima (1983) have shown that, in the infant, the connective tissue layers of the lamina propria of the vocal folds are not well defined, nor is a vocal ligament developed. Thus, not only is the infant vocal fold shorter and less massive muscularly than it is in older individuals, but it also lacks the physical properties of the mature structure. Additionally, although little is known about the neurological maturity of the infant larynx, morphological data from von Leden (1961) suggest that it is not fully developed until three years of age.

Table 4–1. Length of the membranous portion of the vocal fold from birth through adulthood.

Author	Sex	Age	Length of Membranous Portion of Vocal Folds (in mm)
Negus (1929)	F	3 days	3.00
	F	5 wk	4.00
	M	2 mo	5.00
	F	3 mo	4.50
	M	9 mo	5.50
	M	1 yr	4.00
	F	1 yr	5.50
	F	2.3 yr	5.00
	M	5 yr	7.50
	M	6.5 yr	8.00
	F	7 yr	6.60
	M	8.5 yr	7.00
Hirano et al. (1981a)	M	10	8.00
	M	10 (prepubertal)	10.41
Kahane* (1978)	F	12 (prepubertal)	10.38
	M	16 (pubertal)	16.93
	F	16 (pubertal)	13.89
Hirano et al. (1983)	M	20	15.18
Maue* (1971)	M	Adult	17.35
	F	Adult	12.88

*Length of the membranous portion of the vocal fold was derived from a measurement of total fold length which encompassed intercartilaginous and intermembranous portions of the rima glottidis. Of this measurement 60% was used to derive the length of the membranous portion of vocal folds. See text for details. Vocal fold length measurements from Kahane are based on 5 subjects each for prepubertal and pubertal groups and those from Maue are based on 20 men and 20 women.

Laryngeal Muscles

Although scant information is available on the morphology of the infant vocal fold, almost no information exists on the intrinsic muscles of the infant larynx. Kahane and Kahn (1984) examined the relationship among the weights of infant intrinsic laryngeal muscles as compared to their weight in adults. They dissected the intrinsic laryngeal muscles from nine infants. Infant laryngeal muscle weights ranged from 9.6 to 14% of their adult counterparts. No sex differences were found nor were there significant bilateral differences in respective pairs of muscles. The adductors, consisting of the lateral cricoarytenoid, thyroarytenoid, and interarytenoid muscles, represented the bulk of the intrinsic muscle mass, followed in order by the tensor, cricothyroid, and the abductor, posterior cricoarytenoid. The relationship among intrinsic muscle weights is shown in Figure 4–4. From a functional perspective, this is consistent with the principal activities of the infant that involve building up intrathoracic and intraabdominal pressures needed for de-

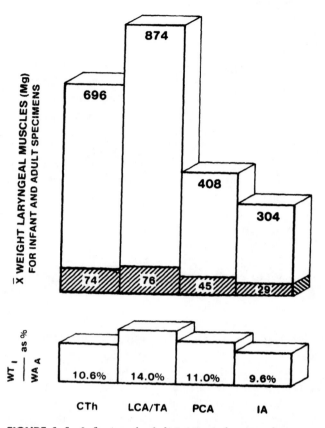

FIGURE 4–4. Infant and adult intrinsic muscles compared by mean weight (*upper graph*) and expressed as a percentage (*lower graph*). Adult values calculated from data from Bowden and Scheure (1960). (From Weight measurements of infant and adult intrinsic laryngeal muscles by J. C. Kahane & A. R. Kahn, 1984, *Folia Phoniatrica, 36*, p. 131. Reprinted with permission.)

velopment of upper body strength and erect posture, ambulation, and elimination of body wastes.

The importance of the cricothyroid in infancy is appreciated when it is compared with the adductors that, as Negus (1929) notes, function as a laryngeal sphincter. The weight of the cricothyroid muscle is 97% of the lateral cricothyroid-thyroarytenoid muscle mass. Thus, by weight, this is the most massive muscle in the infant larynx. Its developmental

status may be attributable to the need for the tensor of the vocal folds to be of adequate mass to regulate length, tension, and mass/unit area adjustments during infant reflexive vocalizations and vocal play. A significant feature of these activities involves experimenting with intonational variation which is mediated by cricothyroid muscle activity.

More discriminative analysis of the composition of infant laryngeal muscles is found in studies by Cooper and Petzinger

(1989) and Kersing (1983). These studies provide interesting information on the histochemistry of some infant laryngeal muscles, but unfortunately are based on very small samples (two to three specimens).

Cooper and Petzinger (1989) found that 50% of the intrinsic laryngeal muscles in the infant were immature and undifferentiated (type 2C). These types of fibers are present in 10–20% of other human muscles at birth (Colling-Saltsin, 1978; Farkas-Bargeton, Dibler, Aresnio-Nunes, Wehrle, & Rosenberg, 1977). Type 2C fibers are not normally found in mature muscle. Cooper and Petzinger found that, in their oldest specimen (9 months), type 2C fibers were present in only 9% of the muscle fibers. Thus, they suggest that the undifferentiated fibers differentiate into mature muscle fibers after birth, the specific interval not being determinable at this time.

Kersing (1983) reported similar findings in the thyroarytenoid muscle of two 8-week-old infants. Although data from these two studies must be interpreted cautiously, they suggest that, although basic biological mechanisms are operable in the neonate and infant larynx, the mechanism for more refined control needed during speech and voicing evolves over time. More work is needed to elucidate this point.

THE CHILD LARYNX

During childhood, the larynx is transported to lower positions in the pharynx. By age 5 years, the lower border of the cricoid cartilages is located at the middle of C5. This repositioning results from several factors: (a) vertical growth of the pharynx and cervical region, (b) changing angle of the base of the skull relative to the vertebral column, and (c) growth ("descent") of the posterior third of the tongue into the pharynx.

The combined effect of these events is to increase the distance between the tip of the epiglottis and the soft palate and change the shape of the oropharyngeal airway from a short, fairly linear pathway into a larger, more angulated one. This developmental pattern is illustrated in a series of radiographs (Figure 4–5) from Laitman and Crelin (1976). Note the close proximity of the soft palate and epiglottis and the short supralaryngeal airway in the 1- and 2-year-old child (Figure 4–5A & 4–5B). Sasaki, Levine, Laitman, and Crelin (1977) point out that, between 12 and 18 months, the soft palate and epiglottis interlock during swallowing, but remain separated during vocalization and crying. As the pharynx increases in length, these structures become more separated; and by age 5 years (Figure 4–5C), interlocking of the soft palate and epiglottis is no longer possible. The shape of the vocal tract begins to assume a more mature contour. By age 9 years, the shape of a child's vocal tract is comparable with the adult (Figure 4–5D), although it is smaller in size.

Growth of the larynx (Klock, 1968) and pharynx (King, 1952; Tanner, 1964) are correlated with growth in body height. Klock has shown that the larynx grows slowly but steadily in childhood with no sex differences appearing. Cartilages increase in size and firmness. He notes that there is a distinctive pattern to the growth of the larynx in childhood. The posterior dimension grows to a greater extent than the lateral and anterior dimensions, in that order. The laryngeal cavity also becomes significantly wider and deeper above the vocal folds than below them.

Childhood growth of the vocal folds can only be roughly estimated from data that is derived from a few sources (see Table 4–1). Based on these data, from ages 1 to 12 years, the vocal folds increase in length about 6.5 mm. Substantial internal changes also occur in the

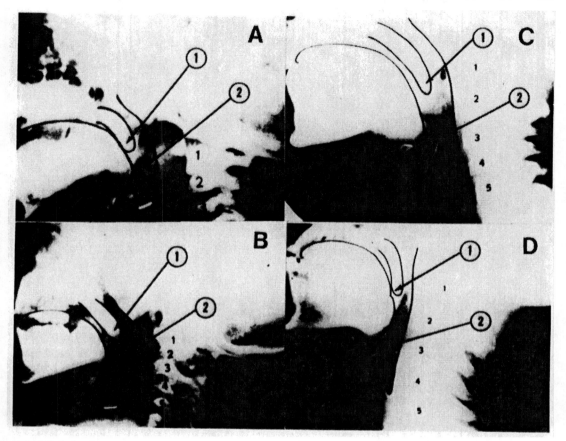

FIGURE 4–5. Radiographs from **A.** 1-year-old, **B.** 2-year-old, **C.** 5-year-old children and **D.** from an adult showing maximum descent of the larynx. Tongue, pharynx, larynx, and soft palate are outlined. 1: Soft palate; 2: Epiglottis. (From Postnatal development of the basicranium and vocal tract region in man in J. Laitman & E. S. Crelin, 1976, pp. 216–217. In J. F. Bosma (Ed.), *Symposium on development of the basicranium*. Washington, DC: Department of Health, Education and Welfare. Reprinted with permission.)

vocal folds during childhood. These have only recently been described by Hirano et al. (1981, 1983). They have shown that, even at age 4 years, the vocal folds (lamina propria) are poorly developed (Figure 4–6A). Throughout childhood, the fibrous connective tissues of the vocal folds increase in density and structural complexity. By age 10 years (Figure 4–6B), the vocal ligament and lamina propria, although still immature, are better developed. Hirano and associates show that these structures do not become mature until after puberty.

Wilson (1979), in his survey of the literature on fundamental frequency (F_0) in children, found that there is a substantial decrease in F_0 between ages 7 and 11 years. In girls, the reported F_0 was from 295 Hz (at age 7) to 265 Hz (at age 11), whereas in boys it was from 295 Hz (at age 7) to 235 Hz (at age 10). These decreases in F_0 undoubtedly result from a combination of factors, consisting of modest increases in length and mass of the muscle and connective tissues of the vocal fold. Biomechanical stability of the vocal folds appears to increase during

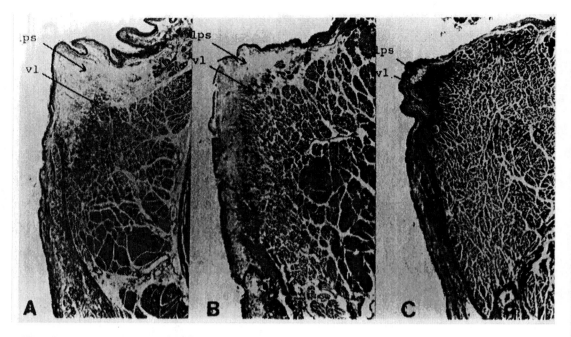

FIGURE 4–6. Coronal histological sections of the human vocal folds from a 4-year-old girl (A), 10-year-old girl (B), and 22-year-old woman. lps: superficial layer of the lamina propria; vl: vocal ligament. Structure of the vocal fold in normal disease states by M. Hirano, 1981, p. 15. In C. L. Ludlow and M. O. Hart (Eds.), *ASHA Reports, 11: Proceedings of the Conference on the Assessment of Vocal Pathology.* Rockville, MD: ASHA. Reprinted with permission.)

childhood, as suggested by the progressive decrease in variability of F_0 productions of older children compared with their younger counterparts (Eguchi & Hirsch, 1969).

THE ADOLESCENT LARYNX

During adolescence, the larynx is transformed into a mature organ. This takes place through markedly accelerated growth (Klock, 1968; Negus, 1929), which causes a short-lived (usually 3 to 6 months, but possibly up to 1 year) period of vocal change commonly referred to as vocal mutation or pubertal or adolescent voice change (Boone, 1983; Wilson, 1979). Because of the close relationship between the development of physical and vocal maturity, it is important to define adolescence

and puberty in terms of physiological differences and the time frames in which they occur. Such information will help to place vocal change precisely within the most appropriate developmental context. Timeras (1972) notes that "it is customary to view adolescence as beginning with the gradual appearance of secondary sex characteristics and ending with the cessation of somatic growth, generally occurring from 10 to 18 years of age in girls and 12 to 20 years of age in boys" (p. 318). She points out that puberty is that portion of adolescence when the capacity to procreate is attained. Puberty is associated with the dramatic increase in growth referred to as the adolescent growth spurt. It begins earlier in the female (10.5 to 13 years) than in the male (12.5 to 15 years). Timeras notes that it is easier to determine when puberty has occurred in girls because menarche is a clear physiological landmark of reproductive capacity, whereas there is no comparably reliable physiological sign in the male. She notes that "the transition from boyhood to adulthood is perhaps most dramatically seen in the voice change and appearance of facial hair rather than any single physiologic event" (p. 349). This is borne out in the voice science literature, as exemplified in the studies of Pedrey (1945) and Tossi, Postan, and Bianculli (1976).

It is well known that the larynx becomes positioned lower in the neck during adolescence. By the end of puberty, the inferior border of the cricoid cartilage lies at the lower border of C6. It continues to drop slightly to rest postpubertally between C6 and C7 in young adulthood. It remains at this level into old age. Until recently, little had been written about quantitative aspects of growth and development of the larynx during the circumpubertal period. Much of the information cited about pubertal changes in the larynx comes from the classic study by Negus (1929). Despite its usefulness, only a limited number of measurements were made, and sex differences were not always reported. This makes it difficult to obtain a complete picture of laryngeal development during the circumpubertal period.

Considerably more information on growth of the laryngeal cartilages and its soft tissue has come from more recent work reported by Kahane (1978, 1982a). He made numerous measurements of 20 human larynges consisting of five males and five females from the prepubertal period (mean ages, 10.7 and 12, respectively) and five males and five females from the pubertal period (mean ages, 15.8 and 16, respectively). The following discussion of pubertal laryngeal growth is based on these studies and will summarize trends rather than provide a detailed analysis of the specific measurements made. The interested reader should consult the references for such information.

Laryngeal Cartilage Changes During the Circumpubertal Period

The composite reconstructions of the thyroid cartilage in Figure 4–7 typify the morphological changes found in all the laryngeal cartilages at prepuberty and puberty. These illustrations should be interpreted as reflecting the overall pattern of maturation in the laryngeal cartilaginous skeleton during the circumpubertal period.

At prepuberty (Figures 4–7A, 4–7B), there is a high degree of morphological congruence between male and female laryngeal dimensions. The prepubertal female is developmentally more mature than the prepubertal male, as shown by the fact that prepubertal female dimensions (Figure 4–7C) are closer to pubertal counterparts than corresponding male dimensions (Figure 4–7D).

Significant growth takes place between prepuberty and puberty. It is greater in the male than in the female (compare prepubertal-to-pubertal differences in Figures 4–6C and 4–6D) owing to the fact that the female larynx requires less growth per unit time to reach maturity. This growth has been shown to be linearly related to growth in body height. By puberty (Fig. 4–7E), clear sexual dimorphism exists. The pubertal male laryngeal cartilages are significantly larger and heavier than their female counterparts. The thyroid eminence (Figure 4–6E) is clearly more pronounced in the male than in the female Figure 4–6F), although no significant mean differences were found between the angulation of the thyroid laminae. Similar findings were reported by Malinowski (1967) and others discussed by Zemlin (1981).

By puberty, adult size and form are established in the larynx in both males and females. A slight qualification is required, however, because significant postpubertal growth occurs in the anteropos-

A

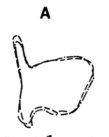

prepubertal ♂- prepubertal ♀

B

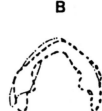

prepubertal♂- prepubertal ♀

C

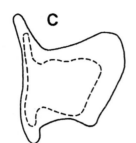

prepubertal - pubertal ♂

D

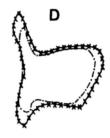

prepubertal - pubertal ♀

E

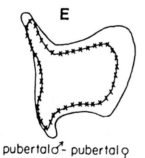

pubertal♂- pubertal ♀

F

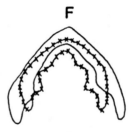

pubertal♂- pubertal ♀

FIGURE 4-7. Composite line drawings of lateral (A, C, D, and E) and superior (B and F) views of the thyroid cartilages depicting typical morphology at prepuberty and puberty (actual size). Tracings of individual cartilages were made from each specimen within each group and overlaid to produce a composite line drawing. Prepubertal male: ---; prepubertal female: - -; pubertal male: -; prepubertal female: -X-. (Reconfigured from A morphological study of the human prepubertal and pubertal larynx by J. C. Kahane, 1978. *American Journal of Anatomy, 151,* p. 13. Adapted with permission.)

terior dimension and anterior height of the male thyroid cartilage that enhances the prominence of the thyroid eminence beyond its size at puberty.

Vocal Fold Changes During the Circumpubertal Period

Growth of the vocal folds during puberty results from the action of sex hormones (Tanner, 1964; Timeras, 1972). A paucity of data is available on the size of the vocal folds in each sex at prepuberty and puberty (see Table 4–1). Negus (1949) reported that the female vocal folds at age 15 years were 12.5 to 17 mm, and they increased to 17 to 23 mm in the adult. No corresponding data were reported for males. Hirano et al. (1983) found that, in Japanese children at age 10, the length of the vocal folds measured 9 to 10 mm, whereas at age 20 they increased to 17.5 mm. Based on dissections of human cadaveric larynges of both sexes, Kahane (1982a) has provided specific information on vocal fold growth during the circumpubertal period. He measured the total length of the vocal folds (incorporating intermembranous and intercartilaginous portions of the rima glottidis) at prepuberty and puberty and compared them with adult data collected in a similar manner by Maue (1971).

The membranous length of the vocal folds was derived by taking 60% of the total vocal fold measurement. According to Aiken (1902) and Zemlin (1981), this corresponds to the membranous portion of the rima glottidis which consists of the vibrating (membranous) portion of the vocal folds. As such, the length of the membranous portion of the prepubertal vocal folds was 10.41 mm in the male and 10.38 mm in the female. By puberty, the vocal folds reach essentially adult size. In the pubertal male, they measured 16.93 mm and in the pubertal female, 13.89 mm. Thus, the male vocal folds underwent nearly twice as much growth as the female (6.52 mm and 3.51 mm, respectively) from prepuberty to puberty. These data compare favorably with those of Brod-

nitz (1971). He reported that the male vocal folds increased by 10 mm and the female by 3 to 4 mm from prepuberty to puberty.

Associated with increases in vocal fold length, Hirano (1981) has shown that maturation of the lamina propria and vocal ligament continues in adolescence and is not completed until after puberty (see the resulting mature morphology in Figure 4–6C).

Pubertal voice change is a physiological response and the by-product of several developmental factors:

1. A genetically predetermined difference in developmental maturity favors the female and causes the male larynx to grow to a greater extent than the female to reach its state of maturity. For example, the male vocal folds undergo twice as much growth as the female from prepuberty to puberty to reach adult size.

2. Pubertal growth of the larynx and growth in body height are closely related and influenced by similar hormonal mechanisms.

3. Maturation of the pubertal vocal folds involves changes in its geometry (length, width, and thickness) and its biomechanical properties. These changes, as reported by Brodnitz (1971), result in a change in fundamental frequency of one octave in the male and two to three notes in the female.

The pubertal and postpubertal voices resulting from physical changes in the preadolescent larynx have been studied empirically by a few investigators. Naidr, Zboril, and Seveik (1965); Cooksey (1977); and Cooksey, Beckett, and Wiseman (1984) have described voice changes in male singers, while Huff-Gackle (1987) and Gackle (1991) have described them in females.

THE ADULT LARYNX

Ramig and Ringel (1983) have stressed the importance of viewing age-related changes in vocal function as part of the process of physiological aging of the body's systems. Although chronological age is certainly a marker for evolution of the voice (i.e., changing fundamental frequency, increased variability of frequency and intensity output), physiologic changes in the respiratory, neuromuscular, and skeletal systems contribute significantly to the overall efficiency of voice production and to specific attributes or measures of laryngeal function. Thus, individuals of similar chronologic age, may have quite different voices because of differences in the robustness of their physical condition. These factors, along with intrinsic changes in the larynx, result in age-related changes in the voice.

Kahane (1982b) has referred to these age-related structural alterations in the larynx as "constitutional changes." These are nonpathological changes that occur gradually and involve changes in the microstructure and chemistry of laryngeal tissues. They may alter the biomechanical properties of some tissue, making them less responsive to muscular and aeromechanical forces to which they are exposed during voice production. It is reasonable to assume that, in older individuals, alterations in the physical properties of the larynx will interfere with the complex synergies required to obtain optimum levels of voice efficiency produced by younger voices.

Position and Proportions of the Adult Larynx

The dimensions of the adult larynx are established during puberty (Kahane, 1978), and no further linear growth in the cartilaginous skeleton or vocal folds occurs in the ensuing years of adulthood (Hicks, 1981). The larynx becomes repositioned to lower levels in the neck (as low as T2 to T3, according to Ferreri, 1959) because of losses of elasticity of the ligaments of the vertebral column and decreases in height of the vertebrae and interverterbral discs. Cartilages increase in weight during adulthood (Kahane, 1982a) as a result of calcification and ossification, but these intrinsic changes do not alter the size of the cartilages.

The adult larynx, however, does undergo significant age-related changes (Kahane, 1980b), some of which may result in evolutional changes in the voice. An excellent review of the acoustic aspects of vocal aging has been done by Kent and Burkard (1980).

Changes in Adult Laryngeal Cartilages

The hyaline cartilages of the adult larynx undergo significant changes throughout adulthood. Although once thought to calcify (Ardran, 1965; Negus, 1949), there is substantial evidence to show that they become ossified (Chamberlain & Young, 1935; Hately, Evison, & Samuel, 1965; Kahane, 1980b; Roncollo, 1949). That is to say, the cartilages change into bone as opposed to hardening due to the deposit of calcium salts. The elastic cartilages, consisting of the epiglottis, vocal processes, and apices of the arytenoid, do not ossify, but rather become calcified (Ardran, 1965; Kahane, 1980b; Malinowski, 1967). Each cartilage has its own pattern of ossification and the entire cartilage rarely is transformed into bone. Changes in the thyroid and cricoid cartilages begin earlier than in the arytenoid cartilages.

Figure 4–8 shows histologic sections, in the coronal plane, of the larynx through the region of the cricoarytenoid and cricothyroid joints. The typical effects of ossification are illustrated in 28-, 62-, and 72-year-old males. Note that, with

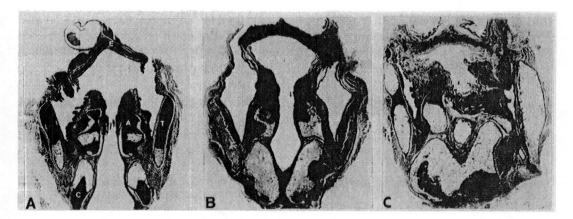

FIGURE 4–8. Coronal histological sections of the larynx at the level of the cricothyroid and cricoarytenoid joints to illustrate differences and patterns of cartilage changes in the adult male. 28-year-old male (A); 62-year-old male (B); 71-year-old male (C). a: arytenoid cartilage; e: epiglottis; t: thyroid cartilage; c: cricoid cartilage.

increasing age, the cartilages (dark areas) become replaced by bone (white areas). This process also occurs in females, proceeding in the same manner as in males, although starting later and usually not being as extensive.

The potential effects of these cartilage changes on voice production are not likely to be significant (Kahane, 1980b). The stiffening of the thyroid cartilages through ossification or calcification may limit the effects of lengthening and tensing the vocal folds that can be achieved by approximating the laminae of the thyroid cartilage (Zenker & Zenker, 1960). The contribution of this auxiliary pitch mechanism in normal vocal function has not been established, however.

Laryngeal Joints

The cricothyroid and cricoarytenoid joints of the larynx are important for changing the position of the laryngeal cartilages and altering soft tissue relationships. Of these joints, the cricoarytenoid is essential for airway protection, positioning of the vocal folds, and development of trans-

glottal impedance. Aging of the cricoarytenoid joint has been studied by Kahn and Kahane (1986), Kahane and Hammons (1987), and Kahane (1988). The basic architecture of the articular cartilage and the arrangement of collagen fibers in its matrix are well established in the infant (Kahn & Kahane, 1986) and consistent with those in the adult. This is also the case with the layering of the articular cartilage (Kahane & Hammons, 1987). Beginning in middle adulthood and continuing into late adulthood, changes occur in the articular cartilage of the joint. These vary in extent, but may consist of the following: thinning of the articular surface, appearance of surface irregularities, and breakdown and disordering of collagen fibers in the articular surface. These changes may result from additive effects of wear and tear as well as the normal aging of the constituent tissues. The synovial membrane undergoes atrophy, most evident in old age. This may result in reduction of lubrication and nourishment to the articular surfaces. These changes may affect function by (a) influencing the smoothness with which vocal fold adjustments (and positioning) may be made during voice and (b) affecting the degree of glottic closure (contributing to the formation of a glottal chink), and thus altering glottal resistance. This has been studied in males (Melcon, Hoit, & Hixon, 1989) and females (Hoit & Hixon, 1992), in whom glottal resistance appears to become less efficient with increasing age.

Vocal Fold Changes in Adulthood

The structure of the vocal fold is complex; it consists of epithelium, subepithelial connective tissue (the lamina propria) of which the vocal ligament is the most dense, and the thyroarytenoid muscle (see Hirano, 1974, for details). Laryngoscopic observations of aging human vocal folds are summarized in Table 4–2 (Kahane & Beckford, 1991). Our knowledge of how aging affects each of the vocal fold components is far from complete; however, available data point to several types of changes that may alter the biomechanical properties of the vocal folds and consequently voice quality.

The following discussion on aging of the vocal folds centers around changes for which empirical data are available. Much more information is needed.

Changes in Adult Laryngeal Epithelium and Mucous Glands

Several investigators (Eggston & Wolff, 1947; Hommerich, 1972) have reported that laryngeal epithelium thickens with increasing age, whereas others (Ryan, McDonald, & Devine, 1956) have found no age-dependent changes. Hirano et al. (1983) reported that laryngeal mucosa thickens up to age 20 but remains unchanged thereafter. Segre (1971) noted that in older persons laryngeal mucosa thins and appears yellowish in color. Persistent edema in the mucosa (Honjo & Isshiki, 1980) and submucosa (Hirano et al., 1983) have also been noted.

Noell (1962) noted that, with increasing age, the epithelium of the larynx becomes less firmly attached to its underlying lamina propria. This may decrease the structural support of the cover of the vocal folds and contribute to the increased frequency perturbation observed in older voices.

Detailed microscopic examination of the epithelium of the vocal folds has revealed it to be morphologically sophisticated. The epithelium on the vibrating surface of the vocal folds contains specialized surface adaptations, called microridges (Sperry & Wasserung, 1976; Tillmann, Pietzsch-Rohrschneifer, & Huenges, 1977). These cytoplasmic extensions raise above the cell surface and are thought to evenly spread and facilitate the retention of mucous secretions. This is important because it helps to prevent drying of the epithelium, thus reducing trauma from contact and aerodynamic forces, as well as maintain a healthy mucosal wave. Tillmann et al. report that the number of microridges decrease with increasing age. Thus, microscopic changes in the surface architecture of vocal fold epithelium can adversely affect voice production by affecting microdynamics of vocal fold vibration.

Associated epithelial changes may add irregularities to the contour of the leading edges of the vocal folds and, along with edematous changes, affect the compliance of the vocal folds. In addition, because the epithelium is so important to vocal fold vibratory activity (Hirano, 1974), alterations in it can have deleterious effects on vocal quality. Edema may contribute to the lowered fundamental frequency observed in older women by Honjo and Issiki (1980) and to the harshness and other acoustic distortions often attributed to older voices.

Some of these epithelial changes may be caused by atrophy of mucous glands in the laryngeal mucosa (Hommerich, 1972) and vestibular folds (Ferreri, 1959). Re-

Table 4–2. Laryngoscopic observations of aging human vocal folds. (From The Aging Larynx and Voice by J. C. Kahane & N. S. Beckford 1991, p. 167. In D. Ripick Ed., *Handbook of Geriatric Communication Disorders*. Copyright 1991 by Pro-Ed Publishers.)

Author	Epithelium	Bowing/Gap	Lamina Propria	Edema	Atrophy	Other
Behrendt and Strauch (1965)	Keratosis		Increase in collagenous and elastic fibers			Fatty degeneration of vocal folds
Segre (1971)	Yellow discoloration	Present	Decrease in elasticity			Vestibular fold atrophy
Honjo and Isshiki (1980)	Darkening of mucosa	Present 67% male 58% female	Sulcus vocalis	Present 56% male 74% female	Present 67% male 26% female	

duced lubrication of vocal fold epithelium resulting from diminished glandular activity may dry out these surfaces. This may make them more susceptible to injury or disease as well as affect their physical properties.

Laryngeal glands, mainly from the vestibular folds, lubricate epithelial surfaces and provide protection for them. Hommerich (1972) and Ruckes and Hohmann (1963) reported that mucous glands in the larynx degenerate or atrophy after age 70. This was not supported by Bak-Pedersen and Nielsen (1986), who found no significant difference in laryngeal glands based on age or sex.

Gracco and Kahane (1989) studied age-related changes in the vestibular folds of the human male larynx. They found that the glands of the vestibular fold underwent appreciable involution with age. These changes included fatty infiltration of the serous and mucous acini, fibrotic changes in the connective stroma of the gland, and alterations in the ratio of serous to mucous acini within the vestibular glands. Among the important effects of these vestibular gland changes is their impact on vocal fold hydration, which may contribute to dryness of the vocal fold epithelium. This may result in changes in surface topography at its leading edge, which may contribute to irregularities in vocal fold vibration such as have been reported by Honjo and Isshiki (1980), Wilcox and Horii (1980), Brown, Morris, and Michel (1989, 1990).

Connective Tissue Changes in the Adult Vocal Folds

A variety of age-related changes have been noted in the connective tissues of the larynx (Kahane, 1987); however, most interest has been directed toward changes in the lamina propria of the vocal folds. Sex differences have not been addressed. Kofler (1932) noted that elastic fibers in the

lamina propria atrophied in old age. This appears to be supported by Terracol and Azenar (1949) who found that the fiber density diminishes. Hirano et al. (1983) found that elastic fibers thinned with increasing age. Ferreri (1959) and Hommerich (1972) noted breakdown and disorganization of elastic fibers in older persons.

Similar changes have been reported by Kahane (1983a, 1983b) for the male vocal ligament. He found that histological changes in the adult vocal ligament became pronounced after age 50. These are well illustrated in Figure 4–9A, a coronal section of the vocal ligament which was obtained from the middle portion of the vocal fold from a 71-year-old man. It can be seen that elastic fibers become fragmented and straightened. There is an increase in the space between fiber bundles resulting in a decrease in density of the ligament. Based on preliminary studies, these changes have not been observed in women (Figure. 4–9B). It is evident that there is greater integrity of elastic and collagenous fibers, and a tighter weave of these fibers within the ligament. This histological appearance is qualitatively similar to that found in males younger than age 50. It appears therefore that connective tissue changes in the male vocal ligament increase with advancing age, whereas changes in the female are less extensive. The specific details of these sex differences need to be described in greater detail in future research. A similar pattern has been observed in the conus elasticus (Kahane, 1980). Changes in this fibroelastic tissue are important because of its intimate relationship to the thyroarytenoid muscle, and because of its contribution to the architecture and physical properties of the subglottal wall and the inferior and medial aspects of the vocal folds. Age-related changes in the conus elasticus, like those in the vocal ligament, appear to be greater in males than in females. They become established after age 50.

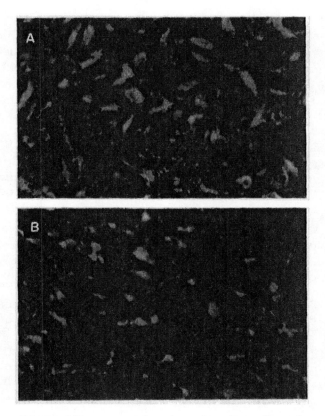

FIGURE 4-9. Coronal histological sections through the vocal ligaments of a 71-year-old man (A) and a 71-year-old woman (B) illustrating age-related differences. Galien-Elastic stain, original magnification 200X.

Structural changes in the aging vocal ligament and lamina propria may contribute to bowing of the vocal folds, and development of a persistent glottal chink, or other irregularities, in the margins of the adducted vocal folds. Changes like these could permit air to escape during voicing and introduce aperiodicity into the glottal signal.

The effects of the many connective tissue changes previously described on portions of the lamina propria, vocal ligament, and conus elasticus are likely to alter their mechanical properties. This has been shown to be the case for aging collagenous and elastic fibers elsewhere in the body (Hall, 1976). One major change in the physical properties of these tissues is that they become stiffer. The extent to which connective tissues of the larynx increase in stiffness with age is yet to be determined; however, the overall effect would be influenced by the extent of associated edema which also has been reported to increase with advancing age. Increased mass and compliance resulting from edema would reduce the effect of age-related increases in stiffness of the vocal fold connective tissues.

Lowering of fundamental frequency in older women (Honjo & Isshiki, 1980) may result because the edematous effects are greater than reversals in elastic tissue properties. The reverse may occur in men, as might be inferred from Hollien and Shipp (1972) who found that, in the male, fundamental frequency increased progressively after the sixth decade of life. This may be a result of stiffening of the vocal folds as well as loss of mass (this point is discussed in the following section).

Connective tissue changes also may affect the quality and regularity of vocal fold vibration. Wilcox and Horii (1980) found that older male voices contain greater amounts of vocal jitter (cycle-to-cycle variations in fundamental frequency) than younger counterparts. Such changes may add roughness to voice quality.

Changes in the Thyroarytenoid Muscle

Aging of the muscular portion of the vocal folds, the thyroarytenoid muscle, has been studied by only a few investigators. No information has been presented about sex differences. Ferreri (1959) and Hommerich (1972) found that the entire thyroarytenoid muscle atrophies. Leutert (1964) reported changes in only the vocalis portion.

The principal effects of the involution of the thyroarytenoid muscle appear to be: (a) decreased mass of the vocal folds and thereby, in the male, raised fundamental frequency (Brown, Morris, & Michel, 1990; Hollien & Shipp, 1972; Mysak, 1959) and (b) diminished neuromuscular control within the vocal folds that might cause sufficient destabilization of the aging vocal mechanism to result in strained vocal quality (Ptacek & Sander, 1966), laryngeal tension, and/or voice tremor (Ryan & Burk, 1974).

Intrinsic Laryngeal Muscle Changes in Adulthood

Despite limited research on the subject, there is ample evidence that laryngeal muscles undergo regressive changes with increasing age; however, there is not a consensus among investigators about the characteristics or extent of these muscle changes. No data have been reported on sex differences. It appears that all of the intrinsic muscles are affected to some extent.

Several investigators (Carnevalle-Ricci, 1937; Ferreri, 1959; Kofler, 1932) have reported that abductors and adductors are affected to equal extents. Bach, Lederer, and Dinolt (1941) reported that atrophy was greatest in lateral cricoarytenoid and thyroarytenoid muscles. Segre (1971) also noted that the cricothyroid muscle became hypertrophied as compensation for atrophy in the other intrinsic muscles.

Aging of the intrinsic muscles has been attributed to reduced blood supply resulting from narrowing of the arterial vessels (Ferreri, 1959; Hommerich, 1972; Leutert, 1964) or to impairment of the sympathetic nerves that supply these vessels (Bach et al., 1941). Malmgren and Ringwood (1988) reported that, in old recurrent laryngeal nerves, there was evidence of degeneration of neurons and evidence of attempts at regeneration. Neurohistological findings suggest that the regulatory mechanisms within the nerve involving ionic and oxidative processes may be adversely affected with aging.

These muscle changes may diminish vocal functioning in two ways. Weakness in the abductor muscles may result in less firm closure or inadequate approximation of the vocal folds which could add some breathiness to the voice. Muscle changes may also hamper development of optimum levels of muscle tonus and appropriate balance of muscle forces required for efficient voice production.

SUMMARY

Development and aging of the larynx are fertile areas for research. As the bodies of anatomical data begin to mount, it becomes imperative to develop acoustic and physiological studies to test the effects of the changes observed in laryngeal structure. Through these means, a more complete understanding of how the larynx works will emerge. As more information becomes available to both researchers and clinicians, our knowledge will increase and our clinical practice will surely improve.

REFERENCES

Abt, I. A. (1923). A summary of the anatomy of the infant and child. *Abt's Pediatrics* (Vol. 1, 10–35). Philadelphia: W. B. Saunders.

Aiken, W. A. (1902). The separate functions of different parts of the rima glottidis. *Journal of Anatomy and Physiology, 16*, 253–256.

Ardran, G. M. (1965). Calcification of the epiglottis. *British Journal of Radiology, 38*, 529–595.

Bach, A. C., Lederer, F. L., & Dinolt, R. (1941). Senile changes in the laryngeal musculature. *Archives of Otolaryngology, 34*, 47–56.

Bak-Pedersen, K., & Nielsen, K. O. (1986). Subepithelial mucous glands in the adult human larynx. *Acta Otolaryngologica, 102*, 341–352.

Behrendt, W., & Strauch, G. (1965). Die feinstruck des mechlichen Stimmbandes abhangig vom Lebensalter. *Archiv Ohein Nasen Keklkofheild, 184*, 510–520.

Boone, D. R. (1983). *The voice and voice therapy*. Englewood Cliffs, NJ: Prentice-Hall.

Bosma, J. (1975). Anatomic and physiologic development of the speech apparatus. In D. B. Tower (Ed.), *The nervous system: Vol. 3. Human communication and its disorders*. New York: Raven Press.

Bowden, R., & Scheure, J. (1960). Weights of abductor and adductor muscles of the human larynx. *Journal Laryngology and Otology, 74*, 971–980.

Brodnitz, F. S. (1971). *Vocal rehabilitation*. Rochester, MN: American Academy of Ophthalmology and Otolaryngology.

Brown, W. S., Jr., Morris, R. J., & Michel, J. F. (1989). Vocal jitter in young adult and aged female voices. *Journal of Voice, 3*, 113–119.

Brown, W. S., Jr., Morris, R. J., & Michel, J. F. (1990). Vocal jitter and speaking fundamental frequency characteristics in aged, female professional singers. *Journal of Voice, 4*(2), 135–141.

Carnevalle-Ricci, R. (1937). Osservazioni isopatologiche sulla laringe nella senescenza, *Archivo Italiano di Ootologia, Rinologia e Laringologia, 49*, 1.

Chamberlain, W. E., & Young, B. R. (1935). Ossification (so-called "calcification") of normal laryngeal cartilages mistakes for foreign bodies, *American Journal of Roetgenology, 33*, 441–450.

Colling-Saltsin, A. (1978). Enzyme histochemistry on skeletal muscle of the human fetus. *Journal of Neurological Sciences, 39*, 169–175.

Cooksey, J. M. (1977). The development of a continuing, eclectic theory for the training and cultivation of the junior high school male changing voice. Part II. Scientific and empirical findings: Some tentative solutions. *Choral Journal, 18*(3), 5–16.

Cooksey, J. M., Beckett, R. C., & Wiseman, R. (1984). A longitudinal investigation of selected vocal, physiological and acoustical factors associated with vocal maturation in the junior high school male adolescent. In E. M. Runfola (Ed.), *Proceedings: Research symposium on the male adolescent voice* (pp. 1–60). Buffalo: State University of New York at Buffalo

Cooper, D. S., & Petzinger, G. M. (1989, November). *Histochemical study of infant laryngeal muscles*. Paper presented at the Annual Conference of the American Speech-Language-Hearing Association, Atlanta, GA.

Cotton, R. T. (1990). Management and treatment of subglottic stenosis in infants and children. In C. Bluestone, & S. Stool, S. (Eds.), *Pediatric otolaryngology* (pp. 1194–1204). Philadelphia: W. B. Saunders.

Eggston, A. A., & Wolff, D. (1947). *Histopathology of the ear, nose, and throat*. Baltimore: Williams & Wilkins.

Eguchi, S., & Hirsch, I. J. (1969). Development of speech sounds in children. *Acta Otolaryngologica*, (Stockholm), *257* (Suppl.), 5–51.

Farkas-Bargeton, E., Dibler, M. F., Arsenio-Nunes, M. L., Wehrle, R., & Rosenberg, B. (1977). Etude de la maturation histochemique, quantitative et ultrastructurale du muscle foetal humain. *Journal of Neurological Sciences, 31,* 245–258.

Ferreri, G. (1959). Senescence of the larynx. *Italian General Review of Oto-Rhino-Laryngology, 1,* 640–709.

Gackle, L. (1991). The adolescent female voice: The characteristics of change and stages of development. *Choral Journal, 31*(2), 17–25.

Gracco, C., & Kahane, J. C. (1989). Age related changes in the vestibular folds of the human larynx: A histomorphometric study. *Journal of Voice, 3*(3), 204–212.

Hall, D. A. (1976). *The aging of connective tissues,* New York: Academic Press.

Hately, B. W., Evison, G., & Samuel, E. (1965). The pattern of ossification in the laryngeal cartilages: A radiological study. *British Journal of Radiology, 38,* 585–591.

Hicks, D. M. (1981). *A morphometric study of the aged human larynx.* Doctoral dissertation, Vanderbilt University, Nashville, TN.

Hirano, M. (1974). Morphological structure of the vocal cord as a vibrator and variations. *Folia Phoniatrica, 26,* 89–94.

Hirano, M. (1981). Structure of the vocal fold in normal disease states. In C. L. Ludlow & M. O. Hart (Eds.), *ASHA Reports, 11: Proceedings of the Conference on the Assessment of Vocal Pathology* (pp. 11–30). Rockville Pike, MD: ASHA.

Hirano, M., Kurita, S., & Nasashima, T. (1981). The structure of the vocal folds. In K. N. Stevens & M. Hirano (Eds.), *Vocal fold physiology* (pp. 33–44). Tokyo: University of Tokyo Press.

Hirano, M., Kurita, S., & Nasashima, T. (1983). Growth, development, and aging of the human vocal folds. In D. M. Bless, & J. H. Abbs (Eds.), Vocal physiology (pp. 11–43. San Diego: College-Hill Press.

Hoit, J. D., & Hixon, T. J. (1992). Age and laryngeal air resistance during vowel production in women. *Journal of Speech and Hearing Disorders, 15,* 55–159.

Hollien, H., & Shipp, T. (1972). Speaking fundamental frequency and chronological age in males. *Journal of Speech and Hearing Disorders, 15,* 55–59.

Hommerich, K. W. (1972). Der alternde Larynx: Morphologische Aspekte. *HNO, 20,* 115–120.

Honjo, I., & Isshiki, N. (1980). Laryngoscopic and voice characteristics of aged persons. *Archives of Otolaryngology, 106*(3), 140–150.

Huff-Gackle, M. L. (1987). *The effect of selected vocal techniques for breath management, resonation and vowel unification on tone production in junior high school female voice.* Unpublished doctoral dissertation, University of Miami, Miami, FL.

Kahane, J. C. (1978). A morphological study of the human prepubertal and pubertal larynx. *American Journal of Anatomy, 151,* 11–20.

Kahane, J. C. (1980). Age related histological changes in the human male and female laryngeal cartilages; Biological and functional implications. In V. Lawrence (Ed.), *Transcripts of the Ninth Symposium: Care of the Professional Voice, Part I* (pp. 11–20). New York: The Voice Foundation.

Kahane, J. C. (1982a). Growth and development of the human prepubertal and pubertal larynx. *Journal of Speech and Hearing Research, 25,* 446–455.

Kahane, J. C. (1983a). Age related changes in the elastic fibers of the adult male vocal ligament. In V. Lawrence (Ed.), *Transcripts of the Eleventh Symposium: Care of the Professional Voice* (pp. 116–122). New York: The Voice Foundation.

Kahane, J. C. (1982b). *Anatomical studies of postnatal changes in the human larynx: Insight into the voices of man.* Paper delivered at the Fiftieth Anniversary Symposium of the Brooklyn College Speech and Hearing Center, New York.

Kahane, J. C. (1983b). A survey of age related changes in the connective tissues of the adult human larynx. In D. M. Bless, & J. H. Abbs (Eds.), *Vocal physiology* (pp. 44–49). San Diego: College-Hill Press.

Kahane, J. C. (1987). Connective tissue changes in the larynx and their effects on voice. *Journal of Voice, 1*(1), 22–30.

Kahane, J. C. (1988). Age related changes in the human cricoarytenoid joint. In O. Fugimura (Ed), *Vocal physiology: Voice production, mechanisms and functions.* New York: Raven Press.

Kahane, J. C., & Beckford, N. S. (1991). The aging larynx and voice. In D. Ripich (Ed.), *Handbook of geriatric communication and disorders* (pp. 165–186). Austin, TX: Pro-Ed.

Kahane, J. C., & Hammons, J. (1987). Developmental changes in the articular cartilage of the human cricoarytenoid joint. In T.

Baer, C. Sasaki, & K. Harris, (Eds.), *Laryngeal function in phonation and respiration* (pp. 14–28). San Diego: College-Hill Press.

Kahane, J. C., & Kahn, A. R. (1984). Weight measurements of infant and adult intrinsic laryngeal muscles. *Folia Phoniatrica, 36,* 129–133.

Kahn, A. R., & Kahane, J. C. (1986). India ink pinprick assessment of age related changes in the cricoarytenoid joint (CAJ) articular surfaces. *Journal of Speech and Hearing Research, 29,* 536–543.

Kent, R. D., & Burkard, R. (1980). Acoustic correlates of speech production. In D. S. Beasley & G. A. Davis (Eds.), *Aging communication and disorders* (Chap. 3). New York: Grune & Stratton.

Kersing, W. (1983). *De Stembandmusculatur. En hostologische en histochemische Studie.* Dissertation. University of Utrecht.

King, E. W. (1952). A roentgenographic study of pharyngeal growth. *Angle Orthodontist, 22,* 23–37.

Klock, L. E., Jr. (1968). *The growth and development of the human larynx from birth to adolescence.* Master's thesis, University of Washington School of Medicine, Seattle.

Kofler, K. (1932). Die Altersueranderungen in Larynx. *Monatschrift fuer Ohrenheil-kunde und Laryngo-Rinogogie* (Wein), *66,* 1468.

Laitman, J., & Crelin, E. S. (1976). Postnatal development of the basicranium and vocal tract region in man. In J. F. Bosma (Ed.), *Symposium on development of the basicranium* (Chap. 13). Washington, DC: Department of Health, Education and Welfare.

Leutert, G. (1964). Uber die histologische Biomorphose der meschlichen Stimmlippen. *Morphologisches Jakrfach, 106,* 11–72.

Malinowski, A. (1967). The shape, dimensions and process of calcification of the cartilaginous framework in relation to age and sex in the Polish population. *Warszawa Folia Morphologica, 26,* 118–128.

Malmgren, L. T., & Ringwood, M. A. (1988). Aging of the recurrent laryngeal nerve: An ultrastructural morphometric study. In O. Fugimura (Ed.), *Vocal physiology: Voice production, mechanisms and functions.* New York: Raven Press.

Maue, W. M. (1971). *Cartilages, ligaments and articulations of the adult human larynx.*

Doctoral dissertation, University of Pittsburgh.

Melcon, M., Hoit, J., & Hixon, T. (1989). Age and laryngeal airway resistance during vowel production. *Journal of Speech and Hearing Disorders, 54,* 282–286.

Mysak, E. D. (1959). Pitch and duration characteristics of older males. *Journal of Speech and Hearing Research, 2,* 46–54.

Naidr, J., Zboril, M., & Seveik, K. (1965). Die pubertalan veranderungen der stimme bei jugen im verlauf von 5 jahren. *Folia Phoniatrica, 17,* 1–18.

Negus, V. E. (1929). *The mechanism of the larynx.* St. Louis: C. V. Mosby.

Negus, V. E. (1949). *The comparative anatomy and physiology of the larynx.* London: W. Heinemann Medical Books.

Noback, G. J. (1925). The lineal growth of the respiratory system during fetal and neonatal life expressed by graphic analyses and empirical formulae. *American Journal of Anatomy, 36,* 235–268.

Noell, G. (1962). On the problem of age related changes in laryngeal mucosa. *Archiv fur Klinische und Experimentelle Ohren-Nasen-und Kehlkopfheilkunde, 179,* 361–365.

Ogura, J. H., & Mallen, R. W. (1977). Developmental anatomy of the larynx. In J. J. Ballenger (Ed.), *Diseases of the nose, throat and ear* (12th ed., pp. 325–329). Philadelphia: Lea & Febiger.

Pedrey, C. P. (1945). A study of voice change in boys between the ages of eleven and sixteen. *Speech Monographs, 12,* 30–36.

Ptacek, P., & Sander, E. (1966). Age recognition from voice. *Journal of Speech and Hearing Research, 9,* 353–360.

Ramig, L., & Ringel, R. L. (1983). Effects of physiological aging on selected acoustic characteristics of voice. *Journal of Speech and Hearing Research, 26,* 22–30.

Roncollo, P. (1949). Researchers about ossification and conformation of the thyroid cartilage in men. *Acta Otolaryngologica, 103,* 169–171.

Ruckes, J., & Hohmann, M. (1963). On the topography and presence of fatty tissue in the human superior vocal cord in relation to age, weight, and disease. *Anatomischer Anzeiger, 112,* 405–425.

Ryan, R. F., McDonald, J. R., & Devine, K. D. (1956). Change in laryngeal epithelium: Relation to age, sex and certain other factora, *Mayo Clinic Proceedings, 31,* 47–52.

Ryan, W. J., & Burk, K. W. (1974). Perceptual and acoustic correlates of aging in the speech of males. *Journal of Communication Disorders, 7,* 181–192.

Sasaki, C. T., Levine, P. A., Laitman, J. J., & Crelin, E. S. (1977). Postnatal descent of the epiglottis in man. *Archives of Otolaryngology, 103,* 169–171.

Segre, R. (1971). Senscence of the voice. *Eye, Ear, Nose and Throat Monthly, 50,* 62–68.

Sperry, D. G., & Wasserung, R. J. (1976). A proposed function for microridges on epithelial surfaces. *Anatomical Record, 185,* 253–257.

Tanner, J. M. (1964). *Growth at adolescence* (2nd ed.). Oxford: Blackwell Scientific.

Terracol, J., & Azenar, R. (1949). *La senescence de la voix.* Paris: Societe Francoise. Phoniatrie.

Tillmann, B., Pietzsch-Rohrschneifer, I., & Huenges, H. L. (1977). The human vocal fold surface. *Cell and Tissue Research, 185,* 279–283.

Timeras, P. S. (1972). *Developmental physiology and aging.* New York: Macmillan.

Tossi, O., Postan, D., & Bianculli, C. (1976). Longitudinal study of children's voices at puberty. *Proceedings XVI International Logopedics and Phoniatrics* (pp. 486–490). Buenos Aires, Argentina: Casa Ares.

von Leden, H. (1961). The mechanism of phonation: A search for a rational theory. *Archives of Otolaryngology, 74,* 72–87.

Wilcox, K. A., & Horii, Y. (1980). Age and changes in vocal jitter. *Journal of Gerontology, 35,* 194–198.

Wilson, K. D. (1979). *Voice disorders in children,* Baltimore: Williams & Wilkins.

Wilson, T. G. (1953). Some observations on the anatomy of the infantile larynx. *Acta Otolaryngologica, 43,* 95–99.

Zemlin, W. R. (1981). *Speech and hearing science* (3rd ed.). Englewood Cliffs, NJ: Prentice–Hall.

Zenker, W., & Zenker, A. (1960). Ueber die Regelung der Stimmilippenspannung durch von aussen eingreifende Menchanismen. *Folia Phoniatrica, 12,* 1–36.

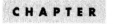

THE VOICE CARE TEAM

GAYLE E. WOODSON, M.D., F.R.C.S.

Voice disorders can result from a variety of causes. Even subtle derangements of the physical properties of the vocal folds can result in severe voice impairment. Such problems range from mild edema to large tumors. Furthermore, the human voice is a complex physiologic phenomenon, involving the coordination of breathing, phonation, and resonance, and can, therefore, be disrupted by a variety of neurologic diseases. Systemic diseases, as well as iatrogenic responses to pharmacotherapy, may also affect the voice. In fact, it is not at all uncommon to identify more than one organic factor contributing to vocal difficulty in a given patient. It is also true that vocal output is dependent not only on the organic substrate, but also on the functional and emotional response of the patient.

Given the complex pathophysiology of voice disorders, it is clear that management is best accomplished by the joint efforts of a multidisciplinary team. In the United States, the core elements of such a team are the otolaryngologist and the speech-language pathologist, each with special training or experience in the care of the voice. Each contributes special expertise in diagnosis and management, and optimal treatment of the vast majority of patients with voice disorders cannot be achieved without the collaborative efforts of both. Other specialists are important to patient care, including singing teachers, vocal coaches, psychiatrists or psychologists, neurologists, and internists (see Figure 5–1). The speech scientist can also make significant contributions to voice care, and in the future, as the validity of objective vocal function tests is established, this member of the team will become increasingly important.

Patients with voice problems may initially be referred to an otolaryngologist or to a speech-language pathologist by their primary physician or family doctor. In the case of children, it is often the school nurse who makes the referral. The high degree of collaboration required in the management of voice patients is best accomplished when the surgeon and speech-language pathologist evaluate the patient together. Continued management of the patient also requires frequent consultation. In an ideal situation, the two will practice in the same office space, with equipment for objective vocal assessment readily available. If circumstances preclude this, both parties should strive to keep the lines of communication as open as possible.

THE VOICE CARE TEAM

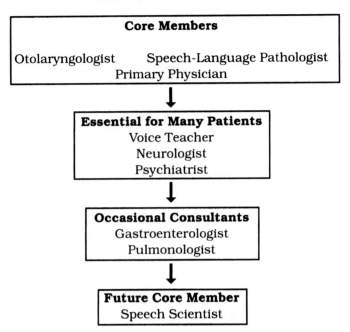

FIGURE 5–1. The voice care team.

THE ROLE OF THE OTOLARYNGOLOGIST AND THE SPEECH-LANGUAGE PATHOLOGIST

Otolaryngology

A history and physical examination by an otolaryngologist are essential. Systemic diseases, previous surgery or trauma, current medications, and co-existing problems such as gastroesophageal reflux, asthma, or sinusitis are all potential contributing factors to vocal dysfunction, so the history must be thorough. The patient's primary care physician is an excellent source of reliable information and should be included in management decisions. Specific details of the vocal symptoms, such as the circumstances surrounding the onset and exacerbating factors, can provide valuable clues to the etiology. Moreover, case history informa-

tion obtained by the laryngologist provides a framework for differential diagnosis and evaluation by the speech-language pathologist and other members of the voice care team.

The neck and upper airway must be carefully inspected. If videoendoscopy or stroboscopy is required for this evaluation, it should be personally performed by the physician. Many speech-language pathologists are quite competent in recording images of the glottis, as well as in interpreting the mucosal wave, and assessing glottic closure. However, the surgeon cannot abdicate the responsibility for physically inspecting the larynx and pharynx. In contemporary practice, endoscopy is an extension of the physical examination.

Speech-Language Pathology

Speech-language pathologists can detect faulty vocal habits, specify the type of vocal abnormality, and, in many cases, identify the mechanism of dysfunction. As an example, a patient with a unilateral vocal fold paralysis may achieve adequate glottic closure by compensatory function, yet still have a dysphonia due to vocal hyperfunction. In such a patient, a medialization procedure is not likely to improve the voice. It is also true that, in some cases, an organic lesion of the vocal fold is a "red herring." That is to say, a patient with a functional voice problem may have an identifiable defect which does not actually contribute to the vocal dysfunction. For example, a small polyp or varicosity on the superior surface of the vocal fold may not impede the mucosal wave. In such a patient, surgery would not improve the voice, and could possibly result in disastrous scarring. Although stroboscopy frequently is helpful in making a determination, a trial period of voice therapy is the definitive criterion. The speech-language pathologist uses information obtained from visual examination as well as from physiologic acoustic measures to initiate a plan of treatment. While the otolaryngologist makes the primary examination of the larynx to identify disease, the speech-language pathologist utilizes information from the visual records to identify faulty patterns of vocal fold opening and closing.

Voice therapy should be a part of the management of virtually every patient with a voice disorder. It is always essential to ensure the best possible vocal outcome from laryngeal surgery. Even when a patient has a lesion that is clearly anatomic and of organic etiology, evaluation and treatment by a speech-language pathologist with expertise in voice care can greatly enhance the outcome. In some patients, vocal patterns may have been modified as an adaptation to the lesion. For example, patients with vocal fold lesions may resort to false vocal fold phonation or may use anterior-posterior glottic compression. Patients with laryngeal paralysis frequently achieve phonation by using the falsetto or loft register. Such adaptations will generally persist for some time after surgery, perhaps indefinitely, unless they are specifically addressed in voice therapy. In some cases, particularly individuals with vocal nodules or contact granulomas, faulty vocal habits caused or contributed to the problem. Without correction of vocal technique, the lesions are not likely to resolve and, if surgically removed, will often recur. In all cases of phonosurgery, the procedure alters glottic function, temporarily or permanently, subtly or drastically. Voice therapy is required to help the patient adjust to the new anatomy and to obtain the optimal vocal result. A hand surgeon would not dream of operating on a patient without the perioperative support of a physical and/or occupational therapist. The vocal mechanism is just as complex as the hand, if not more so, and optimal function demands precision among the team members.

The voice therapist must attempt to use the objective measures of vocal function and the information in the video recordings to guide treatment. By using a treatment approach based on objective baseline measures, the therapist will maximize the treatment methods despite the fact that the changes take place without direct physical manipulation of the vocal folds.

Vocal Pedagogy

The otolaryngologist and speech-language pathologist should develop and maintain an effective working relationship with singing teachers and vocal coaches in the community. Teachers are essential in the management of actors, singers, and other patients with heavy public speaking demands. Certainly, if a patient has a teacher or coach, that person plays an integral part in management of the problem and is a defacto member of the team. When performers who are untrained, or who do not currently have a teacher, experience problems, it is important to be able to refer them with confidence to a skilled teacher who will be able to interact with the team. In an ideal situation, a voice teacher participates in the voice clinic to either directly manage the patient's care or facilitate communication with the patient's own teacher.

Many singers and actors who develop problems are referred by their teachers for evaluation. In such cases, the teacher functions in the same role as the referring physician, providing insight into the genesis of the problem and sharing in the responsibility for management. Vocal problems in a well-trained singer are much more likely to result from a medical problem or from misuse or strain during conversational speech than from technical problems in singing. This is true even when the presenting complaint is related to performance problems. This is partially because conversational speech is less taxing, but is also due to the fact that the performer is usually less concerned about and, thereby less critical of, his or her conversational voice. Moreover, the conversational voice is the most often used voice and the one to which the performer generally does not pay attention. In these patients, the primary thrust of management is to treat the underlying medical problem and/or retrain the speaking voice, eliminate abusive situations, and prescribe adequate voice rest. But, during resolution of the problem, it is usually necessary to modify, reduce, or eliminate practice or performance schedules, especially those in large, empty rehearsal halls. Judicious teaching and vocal exercises during this period are essential for maintaining skills and keeping the patient "in shape." Similarly, when the time is right to resume a normal performance schedule, the transition should be supervised by the voice care team.

Sometimes a well-trained singer or speaker may experience difficulty when the performance schedule becomes too demanding or when a specific program places new demands on the voice. For example, an increased range, a strenuous vocal quality, or a performance over loud background noise can be taxing. The voice teacher can help to assess the situation and suggest steps to alleviate the problem, such as changes in the performance or modification of the rehearsal or performance environment. The schedule can be made less taxing, as well. In some cases, the patient may need help in adapting to the new demands.

Even patients who are not performers can benefit substantially from interaction with a voice teacher. Patients can frequently relate to a teacher on a more personal and practical level than to a physician or speech-language pathologist. The teacher is probably less likely to use technical language. Patients who are ambivalent toward health care professionals may relate quite well to a teacher or coach. For example, a patient with a conversion (hysterical) aphonia may be coaxed into phonation in the context of singing behavior. This can serve as a starting point to generalize phonation into conversation. The artistic viewpoint of the teacher is a substantial asset in communicating with patients.

THE ROLE OF OTHER PHYSICIANS

Other physicians are frequently involved in the comprehensive management of patients, including internists, neurologists, and psychiatrists. The patients may be referred from these practitioners, but more often, it is necessary to identify a collaborating physician. It is important for the voice care team to cultivate relationships with referring physicians, as they are usually unfamiliar with voice disorders. However, a consultant physician who gains experience in treating patients with voice disorders becomes a valuable resource. Depending on the demographics of a particular patient population, specific physicians may be recruited as permanent members of the team.

Neurology

If a neurologic problem is suspected as a possible cause of the vocal problem, the patient should be referred for evaluation by a neurologist, preferably one who has both interest and experience in evaluating vocal problems. A complete neurologic examination is performed to rule out the presence of focal neurologic signs, and to look for signs of generalized neuropathology. The neurologist also may assist with electromyographic testing. When a focal neurologic lesion is detected, further tests are required to determine whether or not the patient has a serious disease, such as a tumor, or a demyelinating disorder, which needs treatment. In some cases, such as vocal tremor or myasthenia gravis, medication may be useful in diminishing symptoms. Sometimes a neurologic problem is diagnosed for which there is no effective therapy. Even in these cases, knowledge of the etiology is extremely helpful because it spares the patient of the burden of being considered neurotic or hysterical. It may also spare the patient from unnecessary therapy, surgery, or both. If a practice has a high volume of neurolaryngologic problems, such as laryngeal paralysis or spasmodic dysphonia, it is very helpful to have a neurologist on the voice care team.

Psychiatry or Psychology

The voice has been described as the mirror of the soul. It can convey strong emo-tional content without words. It is not surprising, therefore, that the voice is profoundly affected by emotional and psychiatric problems. Conversely, a vocal disorder constitutes a severe emotional handicap, because the patient is repeatedly frustrated in his attempts to communicate thoughts and feelings. For these reasons, psychiatric input may be needed in the care of any patient with a voice disorder, whether organic, functional, or psychogenic.

In the absence of anatomic alteration of the larynx, the differential diagnosis of a voice disorder has always included psychogenic dysphonia. The most cogent example of this is hysterical aphonia. However, in recent years, it has become clear that neurologic disease must also be considered. It is frequently very difficult to determine whether laryngeal dysfunction is neurogenic or psychosomatic. For example, in spasmodic dysphonia, symptoms can be inconsistent, fluctuating over time, and often becoming worse with emotional stress. Moreover, focal dystonias (of which spasmodic dysphonia is one), are usually task-specific, so that physical signs of dysfunction may become manifest only during certain vocal activities (e.g., in spontaneous speech but not laughter). Psychological testing alone is of limited value because a neurologic voice disorder can produce anxiety and depression, resulting in abnormal test results. Thus, a psychiatric consultation is often necessary.

Many patients react negatively to the suggestion of psychiatric consultation. It is helpful to stress to such patients that the consultation is being requested to explore the possibility of psychological overlay, and that they have not, in fact, been labeled as "crazy." The patients may also appreciate the fact that a psychiatrist may help in coping with the frustration of the vocal handicap. Psychiatric input can be much more acceptable to the patient if it is presented as a fairly routine component of voice evaluation.

It is certainly not difficult to make a case for including a psychiatrist or psychologist as a regular member of the voice care team. Not only is it important to detect possible psychogenic factors in some patients, but all patients with voice disorders experience some degree of emotional distress, and perhaps even severe depression. The psychiatrist is invited to consult in voice disorders under the assumption that the voice problem may have led to depression or anxiety associated with speaking. Furthermore, emotional distress can be implicated in the pathogenesis of many functional disorders. In some practices, the volume of psychological problems could be sufficient to justify the inclusion of a psychiatrist or psychologist on the staff of the Voice Clinic. At a minimum, the voice care team should identify at least one psychiatrist who is willing to become familiar with the ramifications of voice disorders and serve as a resource.

Gastroenterology

Gastroesophageal reflux is a very common cause of hoarseness. The signs and symptoms of this are usually easy to elicit clinically. Moreover, management of mild to moderate reflux is well within the capabilities of most otolaryngologists. However, in obscure or recalcitrant cases, a gastroenterology consultation is indicated for pH monitoring studies or management of medication. Some patients may require fundoplication to achieve control of this problem. It is essential for the voice care team to monitor vocal function in the presence of gastroesophageal reflux and to offer voice care assistance during and after control of reflux.

Pulmonary

Pulmonary disorders such as asthma and emphysema can adversely affect vocal function due to impaired breath support.

However, such patients do not, as a rule, present with a chief complaint of a voice problem. More often, patients who are marginally compensating for some vocal difficulty are unable to cope in the face of diminishing pulmonary reserve. Also, inhalant steroids, frequently used in the treatment of these disorders, can cause laryngeal irritation and swelling. In such a situation, the physician managing the pulmonary problem must be contacted and informed that alternate medical management is indicated, if available.

THE ROLE OF THE SPEECH SCIENTIST

In recent years, there has been a continuing and broad-based effort to develop objective measures of vocal function, analogous to the audiometric evaluation of hearing. The use of these techniques has become more widespread, but the validity of such measures in clinical practice has not been definitively established. Furthermore, the utility of these measures in patient management must be demonstrated before vocal function testing can be considered as an absolute requirement for voice care in general. However, at a minimum, voice care centers engaged in research should be using acoustic and/or aerodynamic measures of vocal function to assess patients and document treatment results. Speech-language pathologists are increasingly developing sufficient expertise to administer and analyze these tests. However, with increasing technical complexity, it is not difficult to imagine that a speech scientist may be included as a core member of the Voice Care Team.

CLINICAL ISSUES AND RESEARCH PROSPECTIVES

At present, most otolaryngologists who care for patients with voice disorders have been self-taught from the literature, conferences, and clinical experience. Some have unofficially spent time with mentors in the field. Most otolaryngology training programs include little or no training in the area of voice care. In contrast the European system has, for many years, included, in addition to laryngeal surgeons, the specialty of Phoniatrics, or medical care of the voice. Only recently have specific voice fellowships requiring completion of an otolaryngology residency begun to appear in the United States. Similarly, training in speech-language pathology usually includes little or no exposure to voice care. This is a trend which fortunately is gradually reversing. The care of voice disorders in this country could be greatly improved by the evolution and standardization of training, either within existing residencies or training programs or as fellowships.

SUMMARY

Voice disorders result from a variety of causes and are very often multifactorial. No single individual possesses all the skills and insights necessary to evaluate and manage these problems. Optimal care of voice patients requires the concerted efforts of a variety of professionals from diverse disciplines. Each professional brings important knowledge and experience from training, but each must also learn and develop from their experiences in caring for these patients, as well as from the interactions with other members of the team. With further advances in technology and standardization, the management of voice disorders is likely to become more complex, yet more precise. The status of voice care in the United States could be greatly enhanced by the development of adequate training in voice care under the disciplines of both otolaryngology and speech-language pathology.

CHAPTER 6

DIAGNOSIS AND MEASUREMENT: ASSESSING THE "WHs" OF VOICE FUNCTION

DIANE M. BLESS, Ph.D.
DOUGLAS M. HICKS, Ph.D.

There has been a considerable increase in knowledge about all aspects of voice disorders since G. Paul Moore published his classic book entitled *Organic Voice Disorders* (1971) 25 years ago. His book provided the framework upon which subsequent gains in knowledge, clinical assessment batteries, and physiological treatment programs could be based. In the last quarter of a century, objective quantitative and qualitative methods for assessment of organ system status have become increasingly important in all specialties of clinical medicine, and assessment of voice is no exception. For voice, decades of clinical efforts have returned few new practical benefits for assessment. There are no universally accepted, much less standardized, clinical methods for evaluation of the human voice. The only agreed on test procedure is a carefully taken case history by a clinician knowledgeable about anatomy, physiology, voice production, and the psychopathophysiology of laryngeal disease. Thus, although the knowledge of voice has increased at astronomical rates, the clinical application to assessment has been sporadic, and the single most important ingredient in successful assessment continues to be a knowledgeable clinician (Bless & Baken, 1992; Stemple, 1993).

The assessment of voice disorders today is a complex and demanding endeavor. The individual patient often poses a changing sequence of different problems, each demanding separate attention. Increased knowledge of interactions between body and mind, of diseases, of vocal demands, increase in longevity and needs to communicate, changes in health care delivery and in technology have co-conspired the clinician's task more difficult was 25 years ago when Moore wrote his classic text. There was a time when referrals to specialists for specialized testing and recommendations for treatment could be made without blazing paper trails to get HMO approval; a time when voice production was less critical to most employment opportunities; a time when quality of life into one's octogenarian years did not have so many demands for oral communication.

There are at least five basic steps in assessing voice: interviewing, observing, describing voice, comparing observations to standards and normal values, and integrating information to determine a treatment plan or to evaluate its effectiveness. Most often it is necessary to use a variety of subjective and objective measures to accomplish these steps. Assessment is prerequisite to determination of the effectiveness of any method of laryngeal treatment. A plethora of assessment methods exist, including laryngeal imaging, acoustic, aerodynamic, movement, and neurophysiologic direct and indirect measures of the laryngeal structure and its function. The specific measures selected for evaluating treatment depend on the laryngeal pathology and its clinical symptomatology. Interpretation of results are contingent on a number of factors including age, gender, and individual variability of the patient being tested. The purpose of this chapter is to present an overview of principles and practices of clinical assessment of voice.

Organic voice problems are multifarious and cannot be viewed solely as a lesion reflected in the acoustic or perceptual end-product of vocal fold vibration. Organic voice disorders are biological, psychological, and sociocultural. Dysphonias can be debilitating and impair the quality of life. Despite the down side of voice problems (expense of health care, loss of time on the job, inability to social-ize, talk on the telephone, or carry out job responsibilities), for some patients secondary gains accrue from having a dysphonia. The increased attention from friends or would-be friends is rewarding. Others enjoy financial gain from unemployment insurance. Still others find the perceived physical voice problem is more acceptable than admitting to emotional pain. Thus, any discussion of assessment of organic voice disorders must consider the psychological as well.

Dubovsky (1985) and Blumenfield and Thompson (1985) suggest that every psychological illness has a physical component, and every physical disease has a psychological component. The more we learn about neurobiology, the more we recognize how chaos in one part of the body affects biochemical changes, and may increase anxiety and tensions or cause problems or illness elsewhere. To iterate the obvious, as clinicians we must recognize the difficulty in separating what's what or be in danger of making some erroneous decisions. The same symptoms typically associated with anxiety could similarly be listed for voice problems related to reflux, asthma, or cardiac problems. Similarly, the problems associated with depression could also signal problems with general health.

In *Anatomy of an Illness as Perceived by the Patient* (1979), Norman Cousins writes, "Attempts to treat psychological problems as though they were completely free of physical problems, and to treat bodily diseases as though mind were not involved must be considered archaic" (p. 109). To avoid being engaged in archaic folly, we must consider the whole person and spend as much time taking a careful history as we do in listening to the voice, or in obtaining laboratory measurements in our attempt to describe and explain organic dysphonias.

To describe the multidimensional nature of voice, clinicians need a precise system of measurement that includes the patient's impression of his or her voice, and how it impacts on daily living. Examples of such tools are shown in Figures 6–1 and 6–2.

Unlike the precision provided by the metric system for describing dimensions of cells, tissues, and organs, there is no single system used to describe the multidimensional nature of voice. The underlying caution of this chapter is that "one cannot look at an isolated phenomenon without running the risk of misinterpreting results" (Titze, 1991). Therefore, the authors would like to state at the onset that any single measure presented here should be considered as only one part of the battery of tests of vocal function, and should not be done to the exclusion of other measures. It is not enough to know what the patient thinks about his or her voice, what the clinician hears, or the otolaryngologist sees. Moreover, not all tests described here are appropriate for all persons with voice disorders. Thus, the challenge for the voice clinician is to determine what minimal testing can be done to describe the disorder presented by the patient and to determine the appropriate treatment, or monitor change resulting from treatment.

As an example, one need look no further than the faces and body shapes of people around him or her to see the uniqueness of human beings. The same kind of variability seen in the face and other parts of the body holds for the larynx and its measurements. Thus, not every detail of observation accurately describes all people or all larynges. In some individuals, a particular cartilage may be misshapen, missing, or out of place compared to the cadaver image represented in most texts. The functional consequences of these anatomical variations are unknown, but the need to recognize variations in structure, and probable function, in the normal population is clear. It is only through recognition of

normal variability that one can truly understand a diseased structure and how it may relate to abnormal function.

Diagnosis is defined in the *Random House Dictionary of the English Language* (1967; p. 397) as, "the process of determining by examination the nature and circumstances of a diseased condition." The speech-language pathologist's role in determining the nature and circumstance of the diseased condition is the focus of this chapter and "process of determining by examination" the basis of the aforementioned principles. Yet, the speech-language pathologist is only one of several members of the voice care team involved in the diagnostic process, and no discussion of diagnosis would be complete without mention of the interdisciplinary nature of this effort. Over the past couple of decades, this interdisciplinary approach has been fundamental in increasing knowledge about assessment and treatment of dysphonias. On most teams, the speech-language pathologist evaluates laryngeal dysfunction and vocal performance problems; conducts perceptual, acoustic, aerodynamic and movement assessment; clarifies contributing and causal factors; establishes a thorough vocal/lifestyle history; and, based on measures of vocal function and case history information, provides conclusions, a prognosis, and recommendations for the patient. The otolarygologist on the team provides the official medical diagnosis and clearance for treatment, describes and labels the pathologic condition, and suggests medical/surgical implications. The vocal pedagogist assesses vocal technique and suggests ways the technique might contribute to the vocal problem. Other physicians may play a role in addressing other relevant body symptoms such as pulmonary or gastrointestinal problems. The patient's needs dictate who needs to participate in the team evaluation. Local interests, circum-

VOICE DISABILITY INDEX

Name _____Date_____

INSTRUCTIONS: First, mark on the line where appropriate. Then circle corresponding number.

Work

Because of my voice problems, my work is impaired

1	2	3	4	5	6	7
Not at all		Mildly		Moderately		Markedly Very Severely

Social Life/Leisure Activities

Because of my voice problems, my social life/leisure time is impaired

1	2	3	4	5	6	7
Not at all		Mildly		Moderately		Markedly Very Severely

Family Life/Home Responsibilities

Because of my voice problems, my family life/home responsibilities are impaired

1	2	3	4	5	6	7
Not at all		Mildly		Moderately		Markedly Very Severely

FIGURE 6–1. A Vocal Disability Index adapted by Koschkee (1993) from Disability Scale Psychiatry Clinic, UW Hospital and Clinics, Madison, Wisconsin.

VOICE PROFILE

Read each statement and then circle the number which best indicates how you presently feel about your voice.

1 = Almost Never   2 = Sometimes   3 = Often   4 = Almost Always

1. I have to alter daily activities because of my voice.   1 2 3 4

2. My voice interferes with communication.   1 2 3 4

3. My voice is distracting to others.   1 2 3 4

4. It is difficult for others to hear me in noisy environments   1 2 3 4

5. My voice gets tired during the day.   1 2 3 4

6. It takes a lot of energy to produce voice.

7. I miss work because of my voice.   1 2 3 4

8. I think about my voice problem.   1 2 3 4

9. My voice sounds worse than other speakers.   1 2 3 4

10. People make comments about my voice.   1 2 3 4

11. On a scale of 1 to 7, where 1 = normal, 4 = moderate impairment, and 7 = severe impairment, circle the number that best describes how bad your voice is.

1	2	3	4	5	6	7
Normal			Moderate			Severe

FIGURE 6-2. A Voice Profile inventory designed to help measure the impact of dysphonia (Koschkee & Rammage, in press).

stances, expertise, and regulations help determine the specific roles each member plays. The role of each team member is explained more thoroughly in Chapter 5, The Voice Care Team.

HISTORICAL DEVELOPMENT OF ASSESSMENT

Historically, the origins of assessment of vocal function can be traced to physicians, scientists, teachers of singing, and voice laboratories of the 19th century (Bless & Baken, 1992; von Leden, 1991). During the latter quarter of the 19th century, scientists and clinicians reported clinical application of instruments, including apparati for stroboscopic and aerodynamic observations. Clinical applications of acoustic analysis came much later; it was not until the development of the sound spectrograph in the 1940s that it was used with any regularity. In the early development of assessment tools, researchers and clinicians were limited in the range of activity by the design and capabilities of the equipment. In the early part of the 20th century, persons evaluating voice were working under very primitive conditions. Equipment was generally expensive, large, cumbersome, and tedious to calibrate. Analysis and recording procedures were time-consuming and labor intensive, and some equipment (such as the stroboscope) did not provide a hard copy. It was not until the advent of the personal computer and inexpensive high quality recording systems (audio, video, FM, digital) that acoustic and physiological assessment of voice became a clinical reality. With improved equipment, clinicians were able to make permanent recordings of measurable laryngeal events, measure and observe movement, and make detailed analysis of both gross and fine measures of aerodynamic and acoustic events. Advances in technology resulted in an explosion of reports on various measures of normal speakers and speakers with voice disorders. During the last two decades several thousand articles have been published on various facets of voice production and its assessment. Despite these advances and reports, the application has been limited by gaps in knowledge about tests and test practices, about normal and disordered speakers' performances, multiparameter testing, and pathophysiology of laryngeal disease.

Since its inception in the 19th century, assessment of vocal function—like the general definition of assessment—has evolved to mean deriving a description of voice production or voice profile that allows clinicians to make inferences about the functioning of the underlying anatomical and physiological condition of the larynx. Voice profiling ranges from a simple description of voice obtained from auditory perceptual judgments to a more comprehensive voice profile describing the aerodynamic, acoustic, and movement characteristics, and the patient's perspective of the impact of the dysphonia on his or her life. Voice profile characteristics are dependent on several factors including the method of assessment and the manner in which the individual with a vocal dysphonia responds. Unless the method of collection and the manner of response are well controlled, the results may be neither reproducible nor interpretable. Fortunately, these two influential factors can be controlled by rigidly adhering to a protocol; unfortunately, standardized protocols are nearly nonexistent making inter- and intra-institutional comparisons nearly impossible. Unreliable profiles are useless and add little to the information gained from the case history.

There are two general categories of application of vocal function tests: diagnosis and monitoring treatment effects. First, vocal function assessment is used as part of a diagnostic evaluation. In this application, the clinician compares the values and observations obtained from the patient to normal responses. For example, an airflow that is abnormally high suggests a pathologic condition and suggests incomplete closure of the glottis. Yet, airflow does not differentiate disease. Rather, it helps describe how the larynx functions in conjunction with the task as shown in Table 6–1.

Table 6–1. Summary of selected measures of vocal function, as they differentiate disease, are influenced by variables of gender, age, and practice on the example pathologies of nodules, paralysis, sulcus vocalis, and cancer.

Vocal Function Measure	Differentiate Disease	Influencing Variables				Severity	Nodules/Polyps			Other Diseases
		Gender	Age	Practice	Singing		Degree of Glottal Gap	Compared to Normal	Monitor Changes	
MPT	No	Yes	Yes	Yes	Yes	Decreased	Inversely Related	Overlap	Yes	Overlap
Airflow MFRm	No	Yes	Yes	No	Yes	Decreased	Positively Related	Overlap	Yes	Overlap
Airflow MFRc	No	Yes	Yes	No	Yes	Decreased	Positively Related	Overlap	Yes	Overlap
(PQ)	No	Yes	Yes			Decreased	Positively Related	Overlap	Yes	Overlap
Relip between: MPT, MFRm, MFRc, and PQ	No									
P(sub) and GE	No	No	Yes	Yes	Yes					Not Determined
Habitual F$_0$, LPT, HPT and F$_0$ Range	Yes	Yes	Yes	Yes	Yes	Inversely Related	Inversely Related	Decreased	Yes	Overlap
SPL and SPL Range	No	Yes	Yes	No	No	Inversely Related	Inversely Related	Overlap	Yes	Overlap
Stroboscopy	Yes									
Perceptual Evaluation of Hoarseness	No					Positively Related				
Acoustic Analyses	No	Yes							Yes	Overlap
EMG	Yes									

(continued)

Table 6-1. *(continued)*

Vocal Function Measure	Paralysis				Sulcus Vocalis				Cancer			
	Severity	Degree of Glottal Gap	Compared to Normal	Monitor Changes	Severity	Degree of Glottal Gap	Compared to Normal	Monitor Changes	Severity	Degree of Glottal Gap	Compared to Normal	Monitor Changes
MPT	Inversely Related	Inversely Related	Decreased	Yes	Decreased							
Airflow MFRm	Conversely Related	Positively Related	Increased	Yes	Decreased							
Airflow MFRc		Positively Related	Increased	Yes	Decreased						Increased	
(PQ)	Decreased	Positively Related			Decreased	Positively Related						
Relip between: MPT, MFRm, MFRc, and PQ												
P(sub) and GE												
Habitual PO, LPT, HPT and FO Range		None Noted	Decreased	Yes		Inversely Related	Decreased			Inversely Related	Decreased	
SPL and SPL Range	Inversely Related			Yes	Inversely Related	Inversely Related			Inversely Related			
Stroboscopy												
Perceptual Evaluation of Hoarseness	Positively Related	Positively Related			Positively Related							
Acoustic Analyses				Yes								Yes
EMG												

The second use of vocal function testing is to document change resulting from treatment. This is currently one of its best applications (Hirano, 1981, 1989). Within certain limits, vocal function testing can provide information about such things as improved movement of the structure, improved closure, and improved coordination. Baseline measures are compared to measures obtained following treatment. The values then can document the effectiveness of treatment and provide a measurement of success of treatment that typically use either a checklist with absolute measures of change recorded (see Figure 6–3) or a graph of values obtained over several sessions on a treatment response form (Figure 6–4).

Both forms of comparison use specific measures recorded at another time. Some clinicians have attempted to take the values a step further, and compare post-treatment values to normative data reported in the literature. This practice is questionable because of limitations in the values reported to date in the literature, and test conditions have not been standardized. Sample sizes are small and do not reflect lifespan changes in age, and profiles of speakers with specific vocal dysphonias are limited to a few pathologies or test measures.

A further impediment to routine vocal assessment is that there are few accepted guidelines that recommend when tests of vocal function should be administered (Bless & Baken, 1992). In most settings, tests of vocal function are done when either an otolaryngologist or speech-language pathologist believes they are indicated. This may be an acceptable practice with well-trained clinicians, but this practice does nothing to ensure equal quality of service in all facilities. Widespread similarity of quality of service could be facilitated by indication guidelines as suggested by the American Speech-Language-Hearing Association's

Special Interest Group in Voice (SIDS III, 1995) and the National Center for Voice Recommendations for Acoustic Assessment (Titze, 1996). SIDS III guidelines suggest stroboscopic assessment is recommended in the following cases:

■ when voice production sounds abnormal;
■ when the patient complains of voice problems even though they are not perceived by the examining clinician;
■ when the patient complains of vocal fatigue;
■ when the larynx appears abnormal even though the voice is perceived to be normal;
■ when the results have potential to expedite rehabilitation decisions;
■ when the results could confirm accuracy of a diagnostic impression in cases of conflicting data;
■ when results are needed to monitor the effectiveness of treatment and need to change or augment status quo.

Testing also may be recommended when treatment is being initiated which is likely to reduce the size of the lesion or modify vocal fold closure or movement patterns. These suggestions apply equally well to voice assessment in general, although some procedures may be better able to address specific rationales than others.

Conversely, testing of vocal function is not indicated if the test does not answer a question about the presence of disease, the site or size of the lesion, the degree of vocal dysfunction, the patient's vocal ability without surgical intervention, or if equally reliable information can be obtained by another simpler procedure without discomfort or expense to the patient.

Currently there is not agreement as to what specific measures (frequency, intensity, airflow, air pressure, stroboscopy, perceptual perturbation, EGG, inverse filter, EMG, glottal efficiency, adduction quotient) are the most sensitive or specif-

MEASUREMENT OF SUCCESS OF TREATMENT

ELIMINATION OF
  DISORDER _____

BEHAVIORAL
  Normal voice _____
  Improved quality _____
  Pitch improved _____
  Loudness improved _____
  Tension reduced _____

PERCEPTUAL
  Auditory
    voice improved on any
    parameter _____
  Visual
    vibration improved on
    any parameter _____
  Effort level reduced _____
  Patient accepts voice _____

AERODYNAMIC
  Decreased airflor _____
  Increased airflow _____
  Change in R_G _____
  Increase in V _____
  Increased control _____

ACOUSTIC
  Frequency range increased _____
  Habitual frequency age-sex appropriate _____
  Intensity range increased _____
  Habitual intensity situation appropriate _____
  Jitter decreased _____
  Shimmer decreased _____
  SNR increased _____

VOICE EDUCATION
  Know how to best use voice _____
  Know voice limitations _____
  Know how to avoid voice problems _____

FIGURE 6–3. A checklist of objective and subjective measures of vocal function used to measure success of treatment.

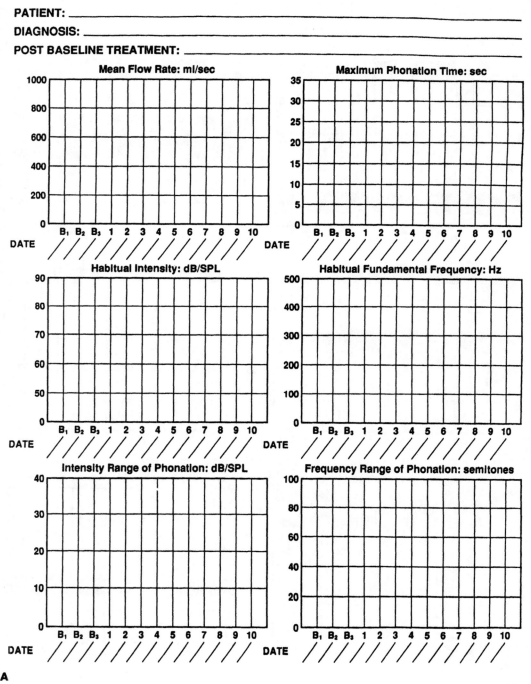

FIGURE 6–4. A. A treatment response form used to chart mean flow, phonation time, intensity, frequency, and range of phonation across three baseline measures (B1–3) and ten therapy (T1–10) sessions (From Koschkee and Rammage, in press).

Typical Values for Adult Females

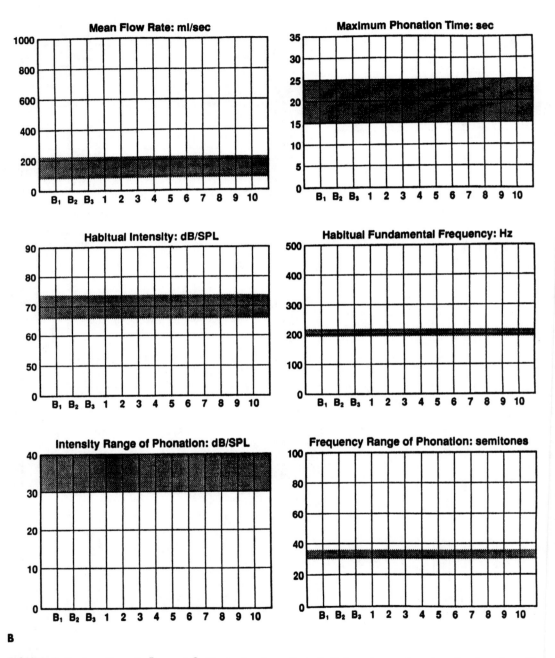

B

FIGURE 6–4. *(continued)* **B.** and **C.** Typical values for adult females and males displayed on the treatment response form (From Koschkee and Swift, 1993).

Typical Values for Adult Males

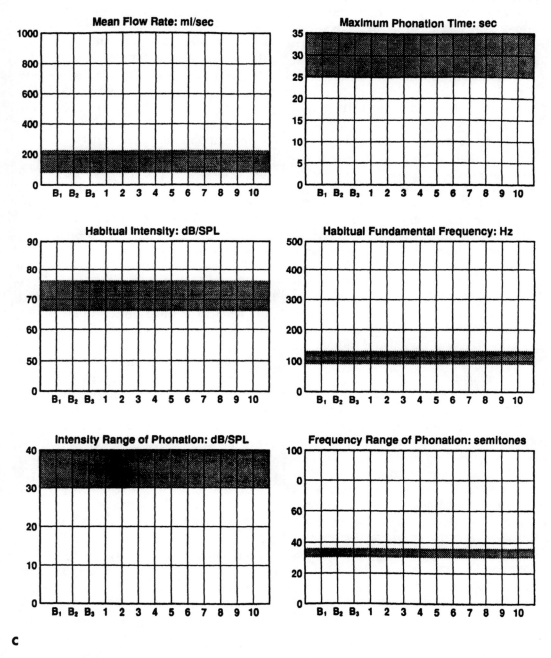

C

FIGURE 6–4. *(continued)*

ic to laryngeal disease or dysfunction. This is due in part to differing reasons for obtaining measures, different disciplines completing the test procedures, and different levels of experience and comfort with various available apparati. In the absence of guidelines, definitions, or standards, it is up to individual clinicians to decide on the measures used, once again underscoring the important role of the clinician.

Recent advances in recording and computer technology have propelled many laboratory techniques into the mainstream of clinical voice assessment. As information is gained about the histological structure (Gray, Hammond, & Hanson, 1995; Gray, Titze, & Lusk, 1987; Gray, Hammond, Zhou, & Hammond [in press]) and healing properties of the vocal folds, and as instrumentation is updated and experience expanded, specialized areas of application continue to be proposed. The acid test of their applicability is clinical relevance (i.e., does the yielded information improve treatment?). Thus, it is not only the assessment and equipment, but also the clinical usefulness and appropriate applications that are in question. The question of clinical applicability cannot always be answered directly because the science of voice testing is not static. Experience obtained in the past two decades with aerodynamic, acoustic and movement assessment, coupled with technical aspects of development of computer programs, foreshadows the upcoming decade as one in which a clinical explosion of information and answers can be expected. To be ready for this explosion, clinicians need to grapple with the issues related to the who, how, when, what, where, and why one clinically assesses voice production.

WHO SHOULD BE CLINICALLY ASSESSED?

Aside from the guidelines and recommendations previously stated, there are other factors to consider when determining who should be tested. Within the populations of persons with organic voice disorders, singers constitute a special group; they do not demonstrate the same aging effects seen in untrained speakers (Brown, Hicks, & Howell, 1993, Morris, Brown, Hicks, & Howell, 1995), and they exhibit greater ranges than nontrained singers, frequently even when a pathology is present (Peppard & Bless, 1991). This means that clinicians need to use different measurement standards for singers.

Patients with organic voice disorders rarely have a single factor as the cause or maintenance of their difficulty. When testing to describe vocal function, clinicians may need to adjust protocols to accommodate other health problems. Patients with temporo-mandibular joint dysfunction will not be able to keep their mouths open for extended periods of testing with rigid endoscopy. Persons with arthritis may have difficulty sitting for long periods and be unable to move their head in all directions. A careful case history taken prior to testing, combined with common clinical sense, will guide the wise clinician in determining who needs testing modifications different than the standard protocol (see Appendix 6-A for examples and Sataloff [1991] for a definitive discussion.)

WHEN SHOULD TESTING TAKE PLACE?

When to test is not always under the direct control of the examining clinician. Schedules of the clinic, patient, and other team members and availability of equipment often dictate when a person is seen. Within scheduling confines, clinicians need to be mindful of the time variables that influence phonation. This is particularly important in assessment of patients with seasonal allergies, esophageal reflux, and vocal fatigue. Patients with reflux are likely to be worse in the morning. Patients with allergies are likely to be worse when suffering from allergic reactions in the spring or fall and may be asymptomatic at other times. To ignore time of testing may obscure the symptoms, or in other cases of repeated testing, may demonstrate pseudo changes—differences that merely reflect a contrast in testing a person once at his best, asymptomatic time and another at his worst.

Laryngeal fatigue presents a particularly difficult scheduling dilemma for cost-conscious clinicians who want to understand the nature of the dysphonia presented. Laryngeal fatigue is a common, and often the sole, complaint of dysphonic patients (Koufman & Blalock, 1988; Stemple, Stanley, & Lee, 1995). Colton and Casper (1990) suggest vocal fatigue is characterized by restricted phonation range, reduced variability of fundamental frequency, increased flow rate, and the closed phase of the vibratory cycle is inadequate as viewed from stroboscopy. Stemple et al. (1995) added the observation of the presence of an anterior glottic gap and intermittent dysphonia. The question of when to test patients with vocal fatigue complaints has led many clinicians to test these patients twice. After completing the standard assessment battery, patients are given prolonged voice tasks, such as loud reading, and then administered a second set of vocal function tests. The prolonged voice task often demonstrates patient complaints not observed in the initial testing. This double testing is both time-consuming and costly, but it may be the only way to determine the nature of the dysphonia. The voice care team has a tough decision to make as to when this extended testing is necessary to make the best management decision in a cost-effective manner. It is also noteworthy that many individuals, particularly those with trained voices, have the ability to increase their voicing effort to overcome fatigue. In so doing,

they may negate the more subtle perceptual, aerodynamic and acoustic events (Stemple et al., 1995).

HOW TO ASSESS VOCAL FUNCTION

Because there are no standards of acceptable testing of vocal function, the "how" of testing is determined by individual clinicians and institutions. The method of testing that is chosen can be totally perceptual or involve a variety of instrumental recording procedures. Regardless of whether the testing of vocal function involves the ear or elaborate instrumentation, there are principles of calibration, test technique, data interpretation, reliability of measures, hygiene, and examiner training that are fundamental to valid outcomes.

Test Environment

There are at least two levels of concern for test environment: patient comfort and recording conditions. For patient comfort, rooms should be spacious enough to comfortably accommodate wheelchairs and family members who accompany the patient. The room should be free from outside distractions and insure that patient privacy is protected.

Equally important to the patient's comfort is the creation of an environment that will facilitate natural voice production and repeatable results. Without spending a considerable amount of money, it is impossible to exclude all extraneous sound from the test environment. However, it may not be desirable to have an artificially quiet environment. The sound level in a "quiet" room is seldom less than 30dBA scale, more often being closer to 40–50 dBA scale. With background noise, individuals will elevate their voices to a level at which they can be easily heard. This can appreciably influence voice assessment in at least two ways: (a) it can cause the patient to elevate laryngeal tension to speak louder and consequently change the measured vocal dimensions and (b) it can result in noise being recorded along with the voice signals and thereby change parameters of interest such as signal-to-noise level and perturbation measures. The source of background noise can come from air conditioning units, adjacent rooms, overhead paging, recording equipment, telephones, and other such environmental noises. Minimal standards need to be set so that measures obtained from different institutions, and within the same institution from recordings made at different times, are comparable.

Calibration

Far too often clinicians are left with the erroneous impression that the only thing needing calibration is electronic equipment. In fact, equal attention should be paid to calibration of the ear and eye for perceptual observations. Perceptual observations will only be as good as the training the observer has, and are subject to bias from the internal referents of the judge.

More obvious is the need to calibrate equipment. Clinicians need to monitor equipment output as part of routine maintenance. Much of the maintenance has to do with verifying timing and frequency characteristics. The sound level output, airflow, air pressure, and other measures of phonation function analyzers can change with time, which means that a test apparatus requires regularly scheduled calibration. Whether this means daily, weekly, or monthly calibration depends on the stability of the equipment.

Calibration cannot be ignored because uncalibrated equipment or ears can result in considerable measurement error and subsequently misinterpretation of the significance of the pathology. The old adage "garbage in, garbage out" is most apt in considering testing without calibration. Without calibration, the num-

bers are meaningless; with poor calibration, the numbers obtained must be regarded with skepticism.

Review of Test Techniques

Suggestions for test protocols, or a kind of "game plan," are needed to ensure minimum standards. It is important to stress that any standard protocol must be flexible to enable the insightful clinician to capture as much information as possible about the vocal system of the individual. At the same time, the procedure is somewhat determined by knowledge of the vocal mechanism and the information needed to characterize the disorder and determine the best treatment. The plan is determined by the nature of the primary information being sought, roughly grouped as descriptive or diagnostic. For example, if the purpose of the test is to obtain baseline measures to determine if surgery is indicated, the protocol is likely to be quite different than when the purpose is to monitor treatment results. In the first instance, the protocol is likely to be more comprehensive to provide an overall protocol of what the patient does and is capable of doing with his or her voice; whereas in the latter instance the protocol may be circumscribed around parameters predicted to change as a function of the treatment administered.

Recent studies of exercise physiology suggests that testing should include measures of range of motion, flexibility, endurance, and strength (Saxon & Schneider, 1995). Saxon and Schneider also suggest testing should be interpreted relative to distribution of fiber types in the laryngeal muscles.

Interpretation of Data

Because the clinician must be prepared to share test results with colleagues in a variety of disciplines, interpretation of test results should be relevant to the patient's overall diagnosis and rehabilitative program. The report should compare the results to predicted responses from normal speakers, with care taken to point out the critical limits of the technique. Clinicians must also be mindful of differences specific to pieces of instrumentation (Karnell, Scherer, & Fisher, 1991). The wise speech-language pathologist will also avoid any attempt to diagnose the abnormality. This is a medical decision to be made by an otolaryngologist, since any reasonable variation may be caused by one of several laryngeal and respiratory conditions.

The test report should provide some information about test conditions because there is no standard protocol, and test environment, test instructions, and patient compliance are variables known to play a role in test outcome. Clinicians wishing to replicate the tests need to have specific knowledge of the test conditions, including the tasks, the type of instrumentation (when used), phonatory conditions (e.g., level of loudness and pitch, type of phonation), test-retest reliability of the measure, whether the patient understood the tasks and appeared to be performing maximally, and the bases for defining abnormal. Clinicians wishing to interpret the results need similar information. Sharing knowledge in this manner is necessary for replication until some of these variables are specified in a commonly accepted protocol.

Assessment made when physical constraints are placed on the vocal mechanism or when something is physically connected to the airway is not necessarily the same as assessment obtained in a normal unencumbered position. These factors must be considered in the context of the test environment. Masks and mouthpieces may reduce auditory feedback of voice production, increase back pressures, and extend the length of the vocal tract. All of these environmental forces have an effect on voice production and must be taken into account when interpreting the test results.

Reproducibility

For any single measure (pitch/frequency, loudness/intensity, time, airflow, pressure, videostroboscopy, or laryngeal quality judgment), little is known about the test-retest variation. It is necessary to know test-retest variation so that the degree of deviation that is significant can be specified, provided the instrument's calibration and the test environment have been taken into account. Because of the many variables involved, changes of any magnitude have to be interpreted with caution.

Examiner

Although many organizations have specified qualifications necessary to practice laryngology, speech-language pathology, and phoniatry, they have not specified the qualifications necessary to examine voice. While these may seem to be self-evident, they are not. Some clinicians do not have well trained ears, others do not know how to run instrumentation and/or interpret results of data gathered, and still others have little information about normal phonation and/or laryngeal disease. In many cases, the practices of individuals in these three professions are not limited to voice disorders, and voice disorders may be rare or a very small part of their practice. Persons who rarely see voice disorders, even when well trained, may not have adequately developed skills. The ideal examiner has the skills necessary to identify and describe a voice disorder within a framework that would provide a psychophysiological basis for interpretation that would result in the most efficacious quality of service to patients.

Ideally, everyone assessing patients with voice disorders would have extensive knowledge about laryngeal disease, normal production for speaking and singing, laboratory instrumentation, knowledge of singing, behavioral treatment, and medical and surgical management. This is not always possible, and with teamwork, some tradeoffs can be made without compromising patient care. For example, the average laryngologist need not be required to have a detailed knowledge of laboratory techniques or be able to make detailed interpretation of the laboratory results, unless he or she wishes to carry out the testing. In those instances, he or she would be advised to learn under the supervision of a speech-language pathologist rather than by trial-and-error. If, on the other hand, all laryngologists understood the advantages and disadvantages of the main types of vocal function tests (movement, aerodynamic, acoustic, perceptual, and videostroboscopic), the appropriate test could be requested for each patient in whom a vocal dysphonia is present. Similarly, speech-language pathologists need not necessarily know everything about the pathophysiology of every laryngeal disease, but they do need to have sufficient knowledge to interpret the vocal function test results and recognize when there is a mismatch between the diagnosed disease and the test results.

Attempting to define the kind of lesion with any single test of vocal function is a serious abuse of the tests, and in most cases unnecessary because laryngologists can determine this from indirect mirror examinations. In addition, interpretation of vocal function without any other collaborative data, whether subjective or objective, is an unwarranted gamble. Seldom are all tests in agreement (Colton & Casper, 1990; Hirano, 1981, 1989; Karnell & Finnegan, 1994; Sataloff, 1991; Scherer, 1988, 1990, 1991; Stemple, 1993; Titze, 1989). Interpreting results must be based on the functional framework provided by documentation from perceptual, physiological, and acoustical procedures; retest; and other critical clinical information including the patient's history.

Use of "WH questions" helps guide clinicians in making relevant interpreta-

tions (Hicks, 1990). The "WH" questions provided below are intended to highlight some questions that should be addressed before vocal function measures can be put to best use:

1. Why is the test being done? Is it to describe the severity of the voice disorder, to determine the site of lesion, to monitor effectiveness of treatment, or some other purpose?
2. What additional data (radiologic, neurologic, psychological) are necessary for interpretation of the data?
3. What use will be made of the test outcome (will the patient be followed medically or in a voice therapy treatment program)?

WHAT SPECIFIC TESTS SHOULD BE USED?

The Case History

Voice testing begins with what you can see and hear, which means taking a careful case history and listening to the voice of the patient. Assessments often are completely subjective and depend entirely on the experience of the examining clinician. Sometimes, the subjective assessment triumvirate—indirect mirror examination, case history, and simply listening to the voice—provides a sufficient basis on which to make a management decision. At other times, these triumvirate are inadequate. Good diagnosis in all fields often hinges on asking the right questions and listening carefully to the answers (Sataloff, 1991, 1995). Recently, expanded comprehensive histories that recognize the complexity of phonation and the role that any body system may have in voice disorders force clinicians to think about voice in nontraditional manners. This is interpreted to mean that the medical history, voice usage, family history, history of the voice problem, work history, psychological history (including current stressors), and the impact of the voice disorder on the patient's life must be investigated to determine the origins of the voice complaint and the best treatment (see Figure 6–1 and appendixes).

Whether clinicians use history questionnaires, face-to-face interviews, or a combination of the two, *no assessment is complete without a thorough case history.* Information from the case history helps determine the assessment methods, diagnosis, prognosis, and treatment plan (Billings & Stoecky, 1989; Coulehan & Block, 1992). Model case history forms have been published by Sataloff (1991) and Colton and Casper (1990). These forms are organized around factors thought to cause or maintain vocal dysphonias. The complexity of voice problems necessitates that clinicians think about how the body and mind interact to produce voice disorders. Koschkee (in press) has provided a list of the major topical divisions of the case history and the factors that should provoke clinicians into making wise interpretations (see Appendix 6-A). This case history guideline, coupled with a chart of neurologic voice signs developed by Aronson (1990a, 1990b), should go a long way in guiding clinicians in obtaining comprehensive case histories.

Perception

Perceptual judgments of voice are a routine part of voice assessment, and they begin with the first encounter with the patient. Clinicians make judgments of the patient's pitch, loudness, and quality in a variety of situations that include comparisons of sustained versus connected speech, neutral versus emotionally loaded contexts, and tasks of maximum range. Clinicians' perceptions are matched with case history information to clarify factors that might affect production such as voice training and the presence or absence of trigger events (e.g., noisy environments, talking on the telephone, or speaking for extended periods of time).

For many, the ear is considered the gold standard, but like all equipment, to be of any value, the ear must be calibrated. Without continual training, clinicians who rarely see voice disorders may have a difficult time making valid perceptual judgments. To make reliable qualitative judgments, clinicians need to keep their ears keenly trained and be aware of factors known to affect perception such as expectation bias, recency effects, experience with wide range of dysphonias, case history bias, and clinician training. Moreover, clinicians need to be mindful that they may be fooled by the complex nature of the signal. For example, clinicians perceive persons with nodules to have a lower pitch, but physical measures of fundamental frequency demonstrate that this is not always the case.

Auditory perceptual judgments are aided by scales for grading the parameters of interest. The scales most commonly used are magnitude estimation, equal-appearing-intervals, and visual analogues. Most equal-appearing-interval scales employ seven equal-appearing steps, either between polar pairs, such as high and low pitch, or on a single judgment parameter compared to normal, such as breathiness. A scale of one to seven is commonly used to allow a sufficient margin of change to be demonstrated with treatment; judges tend to avoid the end points (1 and 7), leaving a span of 5 for rating; psychophysical research demonstrates seven digits are readily handled by most listeners. During the last decade, there has been increased use of the visual analogue because it provides a more discrete rating scale. Ramo's (1996) adaptation is displayed in Figure 6–5.

The perceptual parameter of interest varies with the population being assessed and the clinician doing the assessment

Generally, one wants to have some composite of perceptual information that speaks to the severity of the disorder, the quality, pitch, and loudness of the voice and takes into account signs of fatigue, level of effort, and consistency of vocal deviations. The single most important judgment is whether or not deviant perceptual parameters can be modified with facilitating techniques. This requires careful listening while administering probe therapies (Boone, 1983) and putting the patient through a variety of vocal gymnastics and laryngeal reposturing maneuvers.

As stated earlier in this chapter, there is not a one-to-one relation between perceptual judgments and quantitative measures. For seminal work in this area see Titze (1994). Judgments of breathiness relate not only to airflow but also to glottal configuration and conditions of the side walls. Harshness is related primarily to perturbation but is also affected by pharyngeal constrictions, phase symmetry, surface moisture, and breath support. Hoarseness relates primarily to tissue stiffness but also is affected by muscle balance, laryngeal posturing, and breath support. Pitch relates to the size of the structure, tension, and shape changes to the vocal fold cover applied by the cricothyroid contraction and extrinsic laryngeal muscles. Finally, loudness relates to the amplitude of vibration which is affected by muscle and tissue characteristics as well as respiratory driving force.

Movement

Rhythmic interruptions of the air column transduce the DC energy supplied by the lungs into the AC energy called sound. Vocal fold oscillations, or movement, provide the source of these interruptions, making movement measurements an essential component of describing vocal function.

In order for clinicians to determine what the patient does with his larynx, as well as what he is capable of doing, movement is recorded at a variety of pitch and loudness levels during laryngeal vocal fold diadochokinesia, and during nonphonatory respiratory activities such as whistling and laryngeal gymnastic maneuvers. This provides the clinician with information on whether movement appears normal by watching for increasing length with increases in pitch, increases in mucosal wave and amplitude with increases in loudness, and decreases in amplitude with increases in pitch. Movement may be assessed by a variety of techniques including high-speed photography, videostroboscopy, electroglottography (EGG), inverse filtered waveform, and acoustic analysis of periodicity of the waveform.

High-speed photography, one of the most valuable techniques for providing detailed information about vocal fold movement, will not be discussed here because it is not clinically practical. High-speed photography equipment is expensive and bulky, and the recorded images must be developed, so the results may not be known for several days. Also, the voice sample collected during high-speed photography is limited to a few seconds of sustained vowels. The movement techniques discussed below are less expensive, provide indirect measures of vocal fold oscillations in a variety of phonatory contexts, and easily can be used clinically to provide immediate knowledge of vocal function.

Videostroboscopy

Videostroboscopy became the "in" voice investigation in the latter part of the 1980s, with every voice clinic aspiring to have its own equipment, and it continues to be a vital part of voice assessment

Auditory-Perceptual Rating Form

Name:_____   Clinician: _____

MR. # _____   Date of Eval:_____

D.O.B.:_____   Audio Tape #: _____

Gender: _____   Diagnosis:_____

LOUDNESS

Strong   _____ Weak

Monoloudness   _____ Excess Loudness Variation

PITCH

Excessively Low pitch   _____ Excessively High pitch

Unsteady/Tremorous   _____ Monotone

QUALITY

Hyperfunction/tone   _____ Hypofunction/Lax

Clear   _____ Breathy

Rough   _____ Smooth

Muffled/Dampened   _____ Resonant

Hypernasal   _____ Hyponasal

Hard Glottal Attack   _____ Breathy Attack

Shrill   _____ Creaky Voice/Glottal Fry

TEMPO

Staccato   _____ Smooth Flowing

Rapid Rate   _____ Slow Rate

OTHER

25 yrs. old   _____ 75 yrs. old

Normal   _____ Abnormal

FIGURE 6–5. Auditory-Perceptual Rating Form adapted after Gelpher by Ramos (1996).

(Bless & Baken, 1992; Hirano & Bless, 1993; Sataloff, Spiegel, Carroll, Schiebell, Darby, & Rulnick, 1988; and Woo, Colton, Casper, & Brewer, 1991). Initially this would appear to be a laudable aim because there are undoubtedly many circumstances where stroboscopy can be of considerable benefit. As with any newly applied technique, however, its potential value tends to be overestimated, and its limitations and drawbacks are fully appreciated only when a clinician has extensive personal experience with the technique. This is not to undervalue stroboscopy's contribution to assessment of voice disorders. Sataloff et al. (1988) and Woo et al. (1991) have shown that stroboscopy changed diagnosis or treatment in approximately 30% of their cases.

Phonovideolaryngostroboscopy (PVLS) is a long word that describes a technique which enables clinicians to visualize the superior surface of the vocal folds during a variety of phonatory and breathing maneuvers. It allows clinicians to determine the vibratory characteristics of the vocal folds. PVLS exploits the observational limits of the eye which can differentiate no more than five distinct images per second. The stroboscopic pulsed light source illuminates sequential aspects of movements of glottal vibrations or cycles. The illuminated segments are recorded and played back at the video recording rate of approximately 33 frames/second. The observer's eye fuses these rapidly presented images into what is perceived as a complete picture of cycle-to-cycle vibration; thus, the name "apparent motion."

Judgments made from observing this apparent motion are based on knowledge of the histological structure of the vocal folds, and its two-layered mechanical equivalents of the generally pliable cover (epithelium and superficial layer of the lamina propria) and body (thyro-arytenoid muscle) with the intermediate and deep layers of the lamina propria serving as the transition or tie be-

tween the body and cover (Hirano, 1981). During normal pitch/normal loudness productions the cover is loose and the body is stiff. In cases of paralysis, the body is loose and behaves like the cover. In the case of vocal fold lesions, the cover at the site of the lesion becomes relatively stiff and behaves more like the body.

PVLS is one of the most practical clinical assessment techniques available to today's clinician. The image of apparent motion allows clinicians to determine the functional significance of laryngeal disease and/or inappropriate laryngeal posturing. It also can document small changes in the vibratory structure or patterns of vibration resulting from treatment. A hard copy of the video image can also be placed in patient folders for future reference as shown in Figure 6–6.

PVLS is not an objective test of laryngeal movement patterns. It is true that the vocal folds are visualized during a variety of tasks. As such, it is extensively used in describing function. Although it may be possible to obtain objective measures at some time in the future, at present, PVLS is limited by a number of factors including the frame rate of the video recorder system. What the stroboscope produces are apparent images of the larynx which someone has to interpret. It is here that the method stops being objective and becomes subjective, with any small asymmetry or change in vibration being interpretable as an abnormality. Correspondingly, interpreting the image is only for the experienced who have tested many different types of normal and abnormal speakers of different sexes and ages (Hirano & Bless, 1993).

Recently, the application of learning principles to interactive computer training (Poburka & Bless, 1995) has resulted in reliability of judgments of beginning clinicians matching those of their more experienced counterparts. The training programs capitalize on modern technolo-

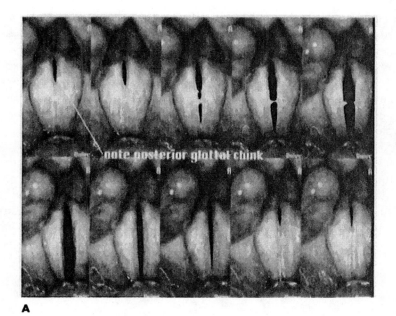

FIGURE 6-6. Video prints obtained from stroboscopy. **A.** Sequential frames captured with videostroboscopy demonstrating the opening and closing patterns and a posterior glottal chink. **B.** An enlargement of one of the frames so that the EGG signal on the bottom of the image can be better visualized.

gy to teach clinicians what the parameters mean and to provide them live rating experiences from video images while getting immediate auditory feedback of errors of judgment (Figure 6–7).

Figure 6–8 illustrates a typical PVLS rating form. The top half of the figure relates to movement patterns observed under the stroboscopic light, and the bottom half is used for recording other observations such as supraglottic hyperfunction.

Glottic closure pattern, phase closure, phase symmetry, regularity of vibration, and amplitude of movement are generally accepted as the best parameters to describe vocal function. These parameters are rated during normal pitch/normal loudness conditions and related to variations in loudness and pitch. Simultaneous recordings of frequency and intensity provide additional explanation of the dysphonia and help ensure clinicians can match conditions when making comparative recordings.

Electroglottography (EGG)

EGG is a popular method of measuring laryngeal movement. It is clinically appealing because it is quick, inexpensive,

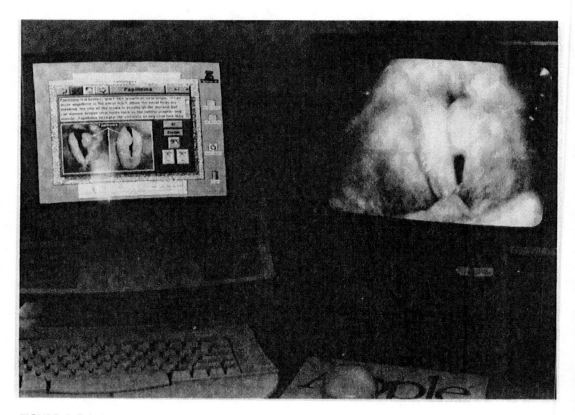

FIGURE 6–7. Photographs illustrating the multimedia computer-aided instruction (CAI) program developed to train visual perceptual judgments of stroboscopic images of the larynx. The left side of the figure illustrates the didactic information and feedback screen; the right side displays the video images to be judged by the person being trained with the CAI.

University of Wisconsin
STROBOSCOPIC ASSESSMENT OF VOICE

GLOTTIC CLOSURE: Complete | Posterior | Irregular | Spindle | Anterior | Hourglass | Incomplete

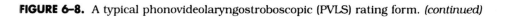

SUPRAGLOTTIC ACTIVITY	(0) None	(1) slight compres. of ventricular folds	(2)	(3)	(4)	(5) Dysphonia plica Ventricularis- VFolds not visible
VERTICAL LEVEL OF VF APPROX IMATION	(0) Glottic Plane	(1)	(2)	(3)	(4)	(5) OFF Plane
VOCAL FOLD EDGE LEFT	(0) Smooth Straight	(1)	(2)	(3)	(4)	(5) Rough Irregular
RIGHT	(0)	(1)	(2)	(3)	(4)	(5)
AMPLITUDE LEFT	(0) Normal	(1) Slightly Decreased	(2) Moderately Decreased	(3) Severely Decreased	(4) Barely Perceptable	(5) No Visible Movement
RIGHT	(0)	(1)	(2)	(3)	(4)	(5)
MUCOSAL WAVE LEFT	(0) Normal	(1) Slightly Decreased	(2) Moderately Decreased	(3) Severely Decreased	(4) Barely Perceptable	(5) ABSENT
RIGHT	(0)	(1)	(2)	(3)	(4)	(5)
NON-VIBRATING PORTION LEFT	(0) None	(1) 20%	(2) 40%	(3) 60%	(4) 80%	(5) 100%
RIGHT	(0)	(1)	(2)	(3)	(4)	(5)

PHASE CLOSURE: (−5) (−4) (−3) (−2) (−1) (0) (1) (2) (3) (4) (5)
Open Phase Predominates (Whisper dysphonia) — Normal — Closed Phase Predominates (Glottal fry-extreme hyper adduction)

PHASE SYMMETRY	(0) regular	(1) irregular during end or begin tasks	(2) irregular during extremes pitch or loud	(3) irregular during 50% +	(4) generally irregular 75% +	(5) always irregular
REGULARITY	(0)	(1)	(2)	(3)	(4)	(5)

NAME _____
HOSPITAL ID # _____
DATE _____
COMPLAINT _____
_____
_____
_____
_____
_____
Abuse _____
_____
Allergies _____
Arthritis _____
Aspiration _____
Esophageal reflux _____
Neurological _____
Psychological _____
Thyroid _____
Other health problems _____
_____
STROBE COMMENTS AND INTERPRETATIONS _____
_____
_____
_____
_____
_____
_____
AERODYNAMICS _____
Flow _____ Volume _____
Pressure _____
ACOUSTICS _____
Frequency _____ Intensity _____
PERCEPTUAL QUALITY _____
Pitch _____ Loudness _____
Stridor _____ GRBAS _____
Breaks Pitch/Phonation _____
RECOMMENDATIONS _____
_____
_____
_____

STROBOSCOPIC ASSESSMENT OF VOICE
University of Wisconsin-Madison

PARAMETER							COMMENTS
Overall Strobe Quality	1 Poor	2 Fair	3 Good	4 Excellent			
Supraglottic Activity (latero-medial)	0 None	1 Slight Compression of Ventricular Folds	2	3	4	5 Dysphonia Plicae Ventricularis	
(antero-posterior)	0 None	1 Slight Advancement of Petiole	2	3	4	5 Complete Obscuration of TVF	
Vocal Fold Edge Right	0	1	2	3	4	5	
(Smoothness) Left	0 Smooth	1	2	3	4	5 Rough	

FIGURE 6-8. A typical phonovideolaryngostroboscopic (PVLS) rating form. *(continued)*

143

FIGURE 6-8. *(continued)*

	Right	0	1	2	3	4	5	
	Left	0	1	2	3	4	5	
(Straightness)		Straight					Irregular	
Predominant Glottic Closure	Complete	Posterior	Irregular	Spindle	Anterior	Incomplete	Consistency Y N	
Vertical Level	0	1	2	3	4	5		
	Glottic Plane					Off Plane		
Amplitude ● NPNL	Right	0%	19%	39%	59%	79%	100%	
	Left	0%	19%	39%	59%	79%	100%	
Mucosal Wave ● NPNL	Right	0%	19%	39%	59%	79%	100%	
	Left	0%	19%	39%	59%	79%	100%	
Non-vibrating Portion	Right	None	20%	40%	60%	80%	100%	
	Left	None	20%	40%	60%	80%	100%	
Phase Closure ● NPNL	Open	100%	80%	60%	40%	20%	0%	
	Closed	0%	20%	40%	60%	80%	100%	
Phase Symmetry ●NPNL		0%	20%	40%	60%	80%	100%	
% of time		Assymmetrical					Symmetrical	
Phase Regularity ● NPNL		0%	20%	40%	60%	80%	100%	Which method did you use for your rating? :
% of time		Irregular					Regular	___Stop Phase ___Running Phase

Other observations:

	Presence and Location		Presence and Location
1. Hyperemia/ Erythema	_____	7. Mucus	_____
2. Hematoma/ Capillary Ectasia	_____	8. Web	_____
3. Edema	_____	9. Paresis of Vocal Fold	_____
4. Stiffness	_____	10. Paralysis of Vocal Fold	_____
5. Thinning of Epithelium	_____	11. Sulcus Vocalis	_____
6. Thickening of Vocal Fold	_____	12. Other	_____

Overall Rating of the Larynx:

Please place a mark along the line to indicate how you would describe this subject's larynx.

Which influenced
your decision ?
(in %, should add
to 100%):

___Structure
___Movement   Normal Larynx   Profoundly Abnormal
                                                                        Larynx

noninvasive, and easy to perform. EGG measures provide an indirect measure of vocal fold closure patterns that reflects the degree of contact between tissues in the neck. This sophisticated equipment uses a pair of electrodes positioned on either side of the thyroid cartilage. A high-frequency electric current is passed between electrodes using the neck/laryngeal tissue as a conductor. Changes in conductance are reflected in changes in voltage. As the vocal folds contract, voltage increases; it decreases as they abduct, resulting in a glottal waveform. Frequent users of EGG are strong advocates of this technique, suggesting that specific shapes and patterns have diagnostic significance. Opponents argue additional work is needed to classify abnormal movement patterns because current applications of EGG demonstrate its inability to differentiate subtle dysphonias from normal voice or pathologic laryngeal conditions from normal accumulations. To fully exploit its potential, clinicians need to understand the underlying theoretical bases and be able to discern abnormal movement patterns that actually reflect disorder rather than artifact. Unfortunately, many speech-language pathologists and laryngologists do not have the theoretical background and training to allow them to be competent users of this tool and do not recognize that factors such as placement of the electrodes and the type of speech sample elicited have profound effects on the resultant signal recorded. As a result, many EGG units and clinically recorded data lie dormant because nobody has the expertise to use and interpret the data. Baken (1992) provides an impressive review of important issues of which clinicians should be aware.

Inverse Filter

Inverse filter techniques provide an estimate of the waveform produced by the vocal folds. It can be performed on either the acoustic sound pressure waveform or the airflow waveform (Rothenberg, 1973). The signal from a sustained sound is passed through filters set to provide the inverse effect of the vocal tract. In effect, this eliminates the resonant characteristics leaving a glottal volume velocity waveform representation of the voice source. The waveform is similar to that obtained from EGG. However, unlike the EGG waveform, the inverse filter signal is not affected by mucus and electrode placement, although it is affected by the recording conditions (the microphone and filter used) and may be more representative of the examiner's ability to tweak the signal into looking like the glottal signal than it is representative of reality.

Aerodynamics

Aerodynamics refer to the average air pressures, airflows, and air volumes that are produced as part of the peripheral mechanics of the respiratory, laryngeal, and supralaryngeal airways. As such, clinical measures of airflow, air pressure, and air volume are thought to reflect laryngeal valving efficiency and respiratory support (Bless, 1988; Hirano, 1981). These indirect measures of voice production change as a function of respiratory support and should be used to supplement acoustic, glottal kinematic, and other measures of vocal function. Aerodynamics is related to acoustics through the fluid mechanics of air motion (Allen, 1982). Quantitative aerodynamic measures for voice tend to follow a dichotomy between gross and fine characteristics, as do acoustic measures (Scherer, 1990). Measures of gross characteristics are taken over a few hundred milliseconds or more; fine measures of aerodynamic characteristics deal with short-term calculations on the order of tens of milliseconds or less and often deal with aspects of pressures and flows within individual phonatory cycles.

The major purposes for measuring laryngeal aerodynamics are to differentiate between respiratory and laryngeal problems, monitor change of the voice, and evaluate degrees of dysphonia. According to Hirano (1981), the most "popular" measures have been the mean airflow rate and the maximum phonation time, which appear to show significant change between pre- and post-treatment of vocal fold paralysis and polyps. Hirano also points out that glottal acoustic efficiency appears to be significantly reduced in a number of patient groups following treatment.

It is not the purpose of this chapter to compare and contrast the myriad of techniques (strain gauges, pneumotachographs, magnetometers, hot wire aneomometry, spirometers, u-tube manometers, or plethesmographs) available for aerodynamic assessment. The reader is referred to Baken (1987) and Scherer (1990) for beautifully written comparisons of advantages and disadvantages of these techniques. It is important to point out that different groups have adopted different techniques to measure airflow rate, vital capacity, and air volume with apparently equal satisfaction. Familiarity with, and availability of, a particular technique appears to outweigh the disadvantages inherent in each technique.

Pressure

Intraoral pressure measures made by the airway interruption technique or end-oral pressure provide indirect measures of subglottal pressure (Löfquist, Carlborg, & Kitzing, 1982; Scherer, 1990; Schulte, 1992). It has been repeatedly stated that subglottal pressure decreases with age and is similar for male and female speakers (Bless, 1988, 1991). It also has been shown that subglottal pressure can be used in combination with other measures to provide an index of glottal efficiency

(Schutte, 1980). Subglottal pressure and glottal efficiency change with hyperfunctional and hypofunctional voice disorders. No information concerning the critical values for normal speakers is available. Information concerning predicted values for speakers with different pathologies is deficient. Lack of standards in this area makes clinical interpretation of results of questionable value.

In the past 23 years, estimation of subglottal pressure has developed increasing clinical relevance (Löfquist et al., 1982; Rothenberg, 1973; Scherer, 1988; Shipp, 1973; Smitheran & Hixon, 1981; Verdolini, Titze, & Pruker, 1990). In this procedure, a CVC string such as /pip/ is repeated at a rate of 1.5 syllables/second during a single exhalation. The theory underlying this technique is that, when the lips close for the bilabial consonant, the glottis opens in order to produce the voiceless consonant and there is equilibration of pressure throughout the vocal tract. The estimate of subglottal pressure is taken from a measure of the oral pressure during the consonant closure, and avoids the necessity of taking a direct measure from a subglottal puncture. Recently, this indirect measure has been used to obtain subglottal pressure threshold measures (Titze, 1988; Verdolini, Titze, & Druker, 1995). Subglottal pressure threshold, defined as the pressure where the vocal folds just begin to oscillate, appears to have clinical relevance. Lower threshold pressures correspond to less expiratory work, or effort, to phonate thus allowing phonation, speaking, or singing to feel easier. Conversely, higher threshold pressures are caused by such things as scarring and increased tissue viscosity, making initiation of vocal fold oscillation more effortful.

Subglottal pressure plays a significant role in changing fundamental frequencies and intonation control. At the lower frequencies, as the subglottal pressure increases, the lateral extension of the vocal folds in each of the vibratory cycles is increased, which increases the effective length and tension of the vocal folds (Titze, 1989), thereby changing pitch.

Airflow

Airflow provides an indirect measure of a speaker's ability to valve efficiently. Airflow rate in normal speakers covers a large range and, when used alone, often is not a clinically sensitive measure because clinically relevant differences can be buried in the variability. Critical values for normal speakers have been established and the same values appear to be accepted internationally. Hirano (1981) suggests a critical range between 40–200 cc/sec. The magnitude or change necessary to be considered clinically significant, or that can be expected to be readily noticed by the patient, has not been reported. Nor have standards for acceptable or typical test-retest variations been reported. Clinical experience indicates that persons at the high and low end of the critical ranges should be regarded with suspicion for marginal or excessive closure. The mean flow rate appears to be relatively high in many cases of recurrent laryngeal nerve paralysis and large tumors (Hirano, 1981, 1989) and low in cases of hyperfunction without large glottal gaps from obstructive lesions. The mean flow rate can be used in following treatment of the larynx if significant changes are anticipated in glottal competency. The primary value of mean flow rate, however, is probably in conjunction with subglottal pressure in measures of glottal resistance and subglottal aerodynamic power (Scherer, 1988). Glottal resistance (subglottal pressure divided by airflow), rather than flow rate alone, is more informative regarding glottal competence, and subglottal power (subglottal pressure times airflow) specifies the power

that can be used and dissipated by the larynx and upper airway during speech.

Measures of airflow and glottal flow resistance may not correspond well to clinical voice quality judgments. The detection of phonatory changes and accurate mapping to diagnostic categories and voice qualities may require finer analysis. Measures of subtle voice change, smaller measurement error, and a strong connection to phonatory theory are required.

What is the relationship between these measures of average airflows and average air pressure and clinical needs? In his pivotal paper on aerodynamic assessment, Scherer (1990) suggests that, like other measures of vocal function, changes of pressures and flows can be examined over time for a patient undergoing phonatory change or for post-treatment checks. For example, phonosurgery often changes the adductory nature of the larynx, and relatively large changes in airflows and air pressures and derived measures of glottal resistances and subglottal power may occur. Also, for example, regaining steadiness of the voice following BOTOX® treatment in patients with spasmodic dysphonia can be monitored by using the patient's average airflow during sustained vowels. Unfortunately these useful examples do not represent standard protocol in most clinics.

Maximum phonation times are used by many clinicians to indirectly determine if the presenting dysphonia is respiratory or laryngeal. This crude measure has the advantage of requiring no more equipment than a watch. Clinicians attempting to get the "maximum" production will find the task frustrating as practice improves the scores and the task can be both tiring and time-consuming. Accepting an adequate production or comparing /s/ and /z/ productions seems to be a more clinically practical method of obtaining the same information (Eckel & Boone, 1981).

One factor critical to these maximum performance tasks is the ability of the tester to motivate the subject to give maximum effort. Part of the motivation comes from instructions which are all too frequently ignored as a critical variable in the outcome of the measurements. Instructions that specifically ask patients to inhale and exhale maximally and encourage them to keep going near the end of their phonation yield longer and more reliable productions.

Acoustics

Perhaps the most widely studied of all voice measures is acoustics. Acoustics includes the measures of frequency, intensity, and time. Summaries of the plethora of acoustic study results may be found in Baken (1987) and Colton and Casper (1990).

Unlike most other areas of voice assessment, standards have been suggested for clinical recording of acoustic signals (National Center for Voice and Speech, 1995). Table 6–2 shows the entire set of test utterances recommended for clinical recording and analysis of the acoustic signal.

The Voice Range Profile (VRP)—frequency-intensity profile or phonetogram—is a recording of frequency versus intensity (Figure 6–9). It circumscribes the maximum range a person can produce and as such can be used to establish the boundaries for further testing.

Low, medium and high pitch are defined as a percentage of the fundamental frequency range (e.g., 10%, 50%, and 80%), and soft, medium, and loud as a percentage of intensity range. Strategic vowels are elicited at specific locations within the range to determine stability. A series of pitch, loudness, adduction, and register glides are elicited to determine the range, speed, accuracy, and stability of phonation within the VRP.

When laryngological pathology is present, it is standard practice in many clinics to ask for a measure of frequency and intensity or a VRP. Often, little thought is given as to why this has been requested but it is generally considered that vocal impairment reduces the frequency/intensity range in some instances such as Reinke's edema. In other cases, such as mutational falsetto, the problem may change the habitual level of production. It is also considered to be a good means of tracking changes in organic conditions because, as the lesion is corrected, the acoustic area profiled expands. The simplest way to collect this information is using a microphone computer system with software specifically designed to play stimulus notes and record responses. Clinicians who do not have this dedicated equipment can use a piano keyboard for the stimulus and a portable sound level meter to record the intensity level of each response and hand plot the VRP. Thus, recording of the VRP need not be expensive or complicated.

Nevertheless, there are many problems associated with clinical collection and interpretation of intensity and frequency data. The first problem is time. The complete VRP, done in a standardized manner suggested by the European Phoniatrics Society (Schutte & Seichner, 1983), takes 45 minutes to complete. This is not always clinically practical because of the necessity of obtaining case history and other test information. Guidelines are needed to help direct clinicians when to select this test over others when time is a consideration. Moreover, it is necessary to clearly establish the value of this time-consuming measure if it is to be used routinely. A second problem is that many factors critical to interpretation have not been well defined. Critical values for normal male and female speakers at different age levels have not been established. In addition, factors such as singing training, test instructions, and other such variables likely to affect the test outcome have not been established. Ques-

Table 6–2. Test utterances recommended by the National Center for Voice & Speech acoustics standards meeting participants in 1995 for clinical recording and analysis of acoustic signals.

NONSPEECH

Voice Range Profile defines test frequencies and intensitites (low = 10% of F range, medium = 450% of F range, high = 80% of F range; soft = 10% of intensity range, medium = 50% of intensity range; loud = 80% of intensity range)

Sustained [a], [i], [u] Vowels
1. low, soft, 2s
2. low, loud, 2s
3. high, soft, 2s
4. high, loud, 2s
5. medium high, medium loud, 2s
6. comfortable pitch and loudness, 2s
7. comfortable pitch and loudness, maximum duration

Sustained [s] Consonant
comfortable pitch and loudness, maximum duration

Sustained [z] Consonant
comfortable pitch and loudness, maximum duration

Pitch Glides
1. low-high-low, one octave, 0.25 Hz
2. low-high-low, one octave, 1.0 Hz
3. low-high-low, one octave, maximum rate

Loudness Glides
1. soft-loud-soft, 0.25 Hz
2. soft-loud-soft, 1.0 Hz
3. soft-loud-soft, maximum rate

Adductory Glides [a] and [ha]
1. onset-pressed-offset, 0.1 Hz
2. onset-pressed-offset, 2.0 Hz
3. onset-pressed-offset maximum rate

Register Glides
1. modal-pulse-modal, 0.1 Hz
2. modal-falsetto-modal, 0.1 Hz
3. modal-falsetto-modal, maximum rate, as in yodeling

SPEECH

Counting from 1 to 100, comfortable pitch and loudness
All voiced sentence, "Where are you going?" soft, medium, loud
Sentence with frequent voice onset and offset "The blue spot is on the key again," soft, medium, loud
Oral reading of "Rainbow Passage"
Descriptive speech, "Cookie Theft" picture
Parent-child speech, "Goldilocks and The Three Little Bears"
Dramatic speech involving deep emotions (fear, anger, sadness, happiness, disgust)
Singing part of "Happy Birthday to you," modal and falsetto register

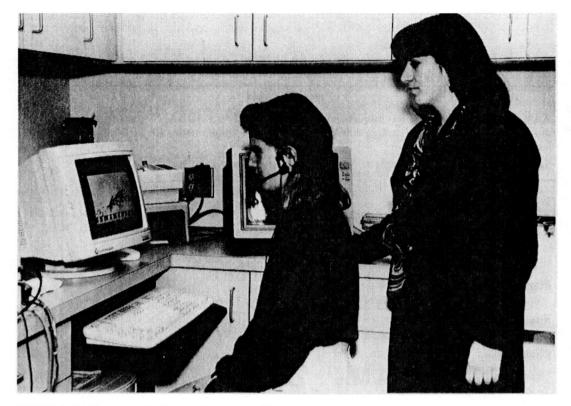

FIGURE 6–9. Photograph of a vocal range profile being recorded while the patient *(left)* and the clinician *(right)* monitor the frequency and intensity range displayed on the computer screen.

tions have been raised concerning maximum performance levels and what they reflect, or even if they can be achieved with heroic clinical efforts. Finally, test-retest variations can be considerable but also have not been well established.

Perturbation

Traditionally, two types of perturbation measures have been used to assess voice: jitter and shimmer. *Jitter* refers to cycle-to-cycle variations in time or period, and *shimmer* refers to cycle-to-cycle variations in amplitude. Perturbations are thought to reflect factors such as asymmetries in mass, neural control, tension, and biomechanical characteristics of the vocal fold. Measures of jitter and shimmer are determined for habitual speaking

levels using commercially available computer programs (see Figure 6–10). Perturbation values obtained with different software generally are not comparable because different algorithms are used for the calculations.

The inexpensive nature of obtaining and analyzing vocal perturbations has made them widely popular measures that are routinely used in many clinics. It is assumed that most clinicians have obtained normative data with their equipment prior to using it in the clinic because of the problems in making comparisons with data reported in the literature.

Perturbation measures have recently come under fire. Guidelines concerning equipment characteristics, test conditions, sampling rate, and other testing variables are sorely needed in this area of vocal function assessment. After several

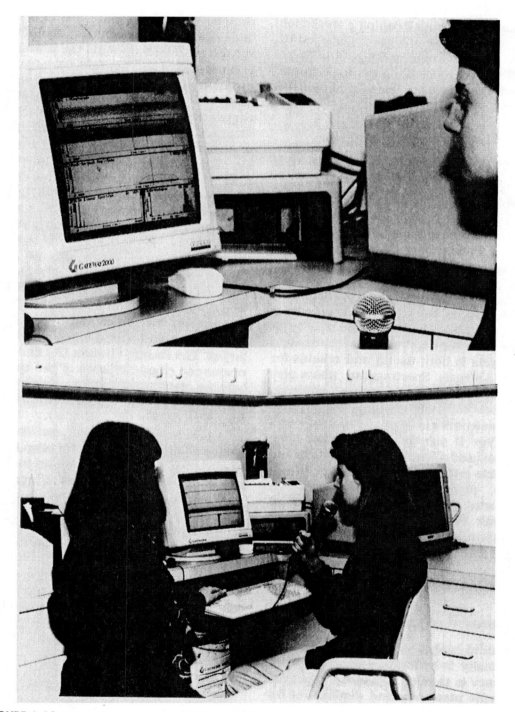

FIGURE 6–10. One of many commercially available computer programs designed to make perturbations measures.

days of debate and years of correspondence, scientists attending a workshop on acoustic voice analysis, sponsored by the National Center for Voice and Speech (NCVS), concluded that prior to perturbation analysis, voice signals should be classified into three types:

Type I signals are nearly periodic;

Type II signals contain intermittency, strong subharmonics, or modulations;

Type III signals are chaotic or random.

Voices can be classified using a spectrogram, a phase portrait, or a cyclic parameter contour.

According to the recommendations offered by the workshop participants, classification into voice type is necessary to determine which methods of assessment are most appropriate. Perturbation analysis is both useful and reliable for Type I signals. Spectrograms, phase portraits, or next-cycle parameter contours are best for understanding the physical characteristics of vocal vibration in Type I or Type II signals. Perturbation measures, used alone, were thought to be unreliable and ill-advised. For Type III signals, perceptual ratings (Gerratt & Kreiman, 1995; Rabinov, Kreiman, & Gerratt, 1995) of roughness or phase portraits to provide visual confirmation of high dimensionality (Herzel, Berry, Titze, & Saleh, 1994) are indicated. An example appears in Figure 6–11.

Spectral Analysis

Spectral analysis is to voice quality what intensity is to loudness and what frequency is to pitch. Spectrum analyzers provide measures and displays of frequency, intensity, and time. The complex acoustic waveform is converted into an easy visualization of relationships among the amplitude, frequency, and time of individual acoustic components. This plot of energy in each of the frequencies in a complex tone allows clinicians to determine changes in the configuration of the vocal tract, and determine the presence of noise, formants, formant transitions, duration of speech segments, and voice onset time. Studies have shown positive correlations between perceptual judgments of voice qualities and spectral analysis. Characteristics important in identifying quality deviations include the presence of noise and the loss of harmonic components (Yanagihara, 1967), increased formant fill and noise, and overall levels of spectral noise (Fritzell & Fant, 1986; Hirano, 1981). Changes in tongue positioning patterns can also be discerned from spectrograms and provide information about phonosurgery patients who no longer rely on maladaptive patterns to produce voice and hyperfunctional patients who need to reposture the larynx. The second formant (F_2) denotes resonance characteristics of the cavity between the tongue and lips. F_2 rises as the tongue moves forward and falls as the tongue recedes in the oral cavity.

Considerable information can also be gained about specific vocal function from spectrographic analysis as shown in Figure 6–12, which compares a normal speaker with a case of vocal nodules and a case with unilateral vocal fold paralysis on a broad and narrow filter bandwidth where both qualitative and quantitative differences are evident.

Using the broad band filter, vertical striations representing each glottal pulse are evident. From these acoustic vocal tract excitations, clinicians can quantitatively obtain measures of fundamental frequency and perturbations, format structure, nasalance, and noise. Qualitative judgments of the presence or absence of perturbation and voice or frequency breaks are also possible from wideband spectrograms. Formants are clearly evident and help clinicians gain an appreciation for coordination of the vocal tract structures. Presence

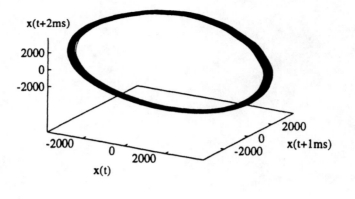

(a)

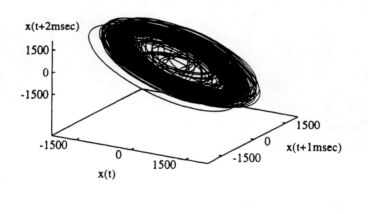

(b)

FIGURE 6-11. An illustration from the acoustic standards report (Titze, 1995) of a phase portrait for a normal speaker and speaker with vocal fold paralysis.

of noise in higher harmonics or formant fill and nasalization can also be discerned and described from the visual image. In contrast, the narrow band does not show formants, but it does provide information concerning the harmonic structure, the presence of vocal tremors, and information about pitch contours.

Voice onset time (VOT) can also be obtained from a spectrographic analysis. *VOT*

is defined as the length of time between the production of a vowel and the onset of the following consonant. VOT may be abnormally long in patients with poor arytenoid adduction or neurogenic disease.

Despite the fact that sound spectrography has been around for over 60 years and its potential clinical relevance for describing vocal function, it has never become well accepted as a routine part of

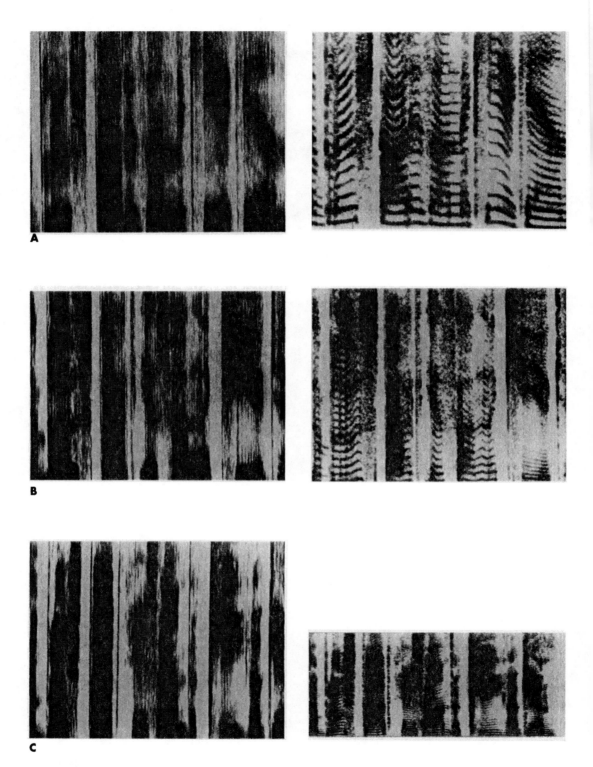

FIGURE 6–12. A series of narrow *(left)* and wide band *(right)* spectrograms of a normal speaker (A), a speaker with nodules (B), and a speaker with unilateral vocal fold paralysis (C) demonstrating qualitative and quantitative differences between speakers.

standard clinical assessment. Whether this is related to the time needed for analysis, expense of equipment, or other measures appearing to have more explanatory value is unclear. For additional information on measurements, analysis, and clinical applications, the reader is urged to see Kent and Read (1992) and Baken (1987).

Velopharyngeal Influence

The influence of the velopharynx on voice production, and vice versa, is yet another consideration in voice assessment. Poor velopharyngeal valving can lead to compensatory movements at the level of the larynx and vocal hyperfunction. Typically, when velopharyngeal function problems are suspected, velopharyngeal port func-

tion is assessed as part of the voice evaluation. Figure 6–13 shows typical examples of assessment of nasal resonance and kinematics of the velopharyngeal port.

Assessing velopharyngeal port function parallels assessment of laryngeal function in the types of procedures used, the need for rigorous test protocols, and the body of literature describing procedures and outcomes, and it is deserving of a chapter devoted solely to the topic. For this reason, the reader is referred to other sources for details of VP assessment which is only mentioned here. Moon (1995) provides a comprehensive review and analysis of procedures used to evaluate velopharyngeal function, stressing the importance of listeners' judgments of the presence of hypernasality. He also discusses the pros

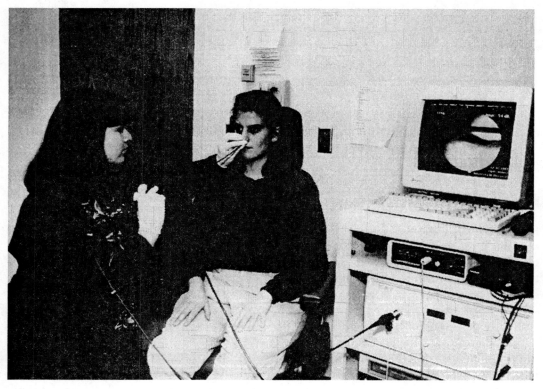

A

FIGURE 6–13. Typical examples of assessment of nasal resonance and kinematics of the velopharyngeal port. In **A.** Nasalendoscopy is used to visualize the velopharyngeal port from above. *(continued)*

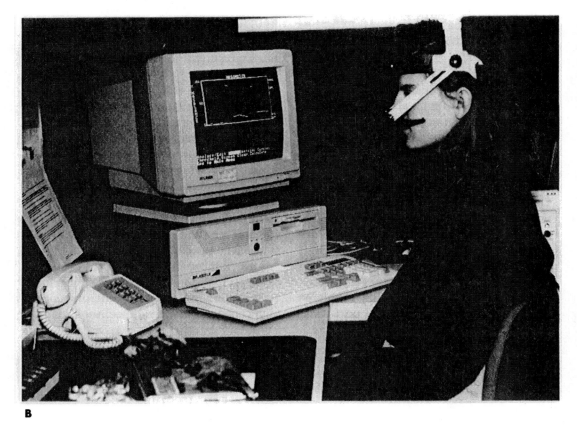

B

FIGURE 6–13. *(continued)* **B.** A measure of nasal resonance is determined from the Kay Nasomater.

and cons of using kinematic, acoustic, and aerodynamic measurements to quantify listeners' judgments.

Psychological Considerations

Psychological considerations in the assessment of voice disorders have long been recognized. Yet, with few exceptions, they have also largely been neglected in standard test batteries. Far too often we see descriptions of voice problems artificially divided into either functional or organic disorders. Muscle tension dysphonia, considered to be a problem of living in today's stressful world, and other problems with no obvious organic disorder are assumed to be functional. Problems such as paralysis are considered to

be organic. Ignoring the impact of the psyche as either a primary or secondary cause of the presenting dysphonia is naive. Loss of communication in today's society is a significant impairment for anyone, but is even worse for professional voice users who are dependent on their voices for income. Clinicians need to consider how psychological processes affect assessment and information receptivity. This is particularly true when the implication of the information given to the patient at the end of a diagnostic interview suggests that surgery is indicated.

The common psychological reaction to stress is to deny or minimize problems, an obvious defense mechanism. A classic example is that the average laryngeal cancer patient presents to the clinic 16 months following the onset of the symptoms. In this case of denial, the patient perceives that he has a voice problem developing. This causes him anxiety so he rejects his perception, or, in other words, he goes into denial. Anxiety is a universal reaction to illness. Fortunately, knowledge helps reduce anxiety. Knowing this, we must educate patients about what we plan to do in testing, about test outcomes, clarify what can and cannot be treated, and how the patient can take control. For voice problems, one of the major causes of anxiety is loss of function. Loss of voice is a threat to a person's social and professional well-being.

One of the factors that affects how one responds psychologically to voice problems, and even to the questions we ask when taking a case history, as well as to the information we give in making a diagnosis, is the patient's basic personality (Blumenfield & Thompson, 1985). Kahana and Bibring (1964) describe seven personality types in terms of their reactions to illness:

1. The overdemanding, dependent personality who fears helplessness but has a great need for personal care and demands endless attention;
2. The orderly, controlled, compulsive personality who becomes more psychologically rigid and overcontrolling in the face of an illness;
3. The dramatic, captivating, histrionic or hysterical personality who becomes overly dramatic about his or her illness and is emotionally labile;
4. The long-suffering, self-sacrificing masochistic personality who precipitates or perpetuates illness to receive love and attention;
5. The suspicious, querulous, paranoid personality who blames others for both the illness and failure to improve;
6. The narcissistic personality who becomes vain, arrogant, and superior to his or her health care providers and disdainful of their attempts to help;
7. The shy, aloof, schizoid personality who becomes increasingly withdrawn.

These types are generalizations, and the divisions are not pure; however, most clinicians are familiar with patients who fit these classic descriptions, or some combination or mixture of similar reactions. They are important to recognize because each responds to the news of an illness, treament, and health care providers in different manners.

Phonosurgery is designed to improve organic voice disorders and is considered by some to be a cosmetic procedure. Whether or not one considers it a cosmetic procedure, it is considered to be elective surgery. Elective surgeries are more psychologically stressful and generally are scheduled some time in the future, giving the patient more time to worry. Also, patients undergoing these procedures must sign informed consent. By law, consents must present the worst-case scenarios. Patients learn that, while their voice is likely to get better, it may also get worse. Naturally, this adds to the patient's threat of body integrity, fears of mutilation, and dependence on others for communication. In many institutions, it is the speech-language pathologist who does most of the explaining about the procedure. Not only does the speech-language pathologist need to consider patients' psychological reactions to elective surgery, but he or she must also recognize the patients who are at risk for adverse psychological reactions. Extra precautions may be necessary to make sure that the patient does not have unrealistic expectations. For others, extra documentation of what was told to the patient may be indicated. These adverse reactions and patient risks also hold for patients who develop voice problems secondary to upper respiratory infections and abuse. If they deny the problem and continue to abuse their voices, and if they appear to welcome the extra attention they get from having a laryngitis, a chronic problem can develop. What began as a mild irritation of the larynx can conclude as a case of vocal fold nodules.

ASSESSMENT LINKS TO TREATMENT

As previously stated, successful treatment of persons suffering from vocal dysphonias depends on the clinician's ability to assess the type and degree of vocal impairment and monitor the person's subsequent progress through treatment. Using a treatment response form (Figure 6–9) helps both the clinician and the patient because each can easily see where change is taking place and when parameters are approaching normal. This helps to motivate the patient and helps clinicians determine if treatment is moving in the right direction. Response forms are also helpful in measuring the responsiveness to treatment probes. This is accomplished by making measures while applying facilitating techniques such as digital manipulation of the larynx and while eliciting different pitch and loudness levels. From this testing the clinician is able to determine whether tension needs to be reduced, glottal closure improved, the airway enhanced, or symmetry of vibration improved. Clinicians can then use the data obtained to educate the patient as to what changes are likely to occur with treatment (Figure 6–3). Thus, armed with these charted measures and tables, clinicians can better counsel patients as to what they can expect to change with treatment, whether it is medical, surgical, or behavioral.

SUMMARY

In summary, the responsibility of all testing rests with the voice care team: the otolarygologist provides medical clearance and diagnosis and the speech-language pathologist provides a description of the vocal function as it relates to probable causal factors obtained from the case history. Clinicians need to ask themselves what limitations the tests have and what questions to ask about vocal function. The rapidly changing knowledge base and developing technology require that clinicians be ever vigilant to new applications and opportunities for applications of tests and measures. Comprehensive voice assessment is tailored to the individual needs of the patient who may need minimal monitoring or a detailed description of vocal function during various vocal gymnastics performed in the clinic and work setting. Critical to all vocal function assessment is an ongoing assessment of the medical/health history, general physical status, psychological well-being, and auditory perceptual judgment of the voice. No single measure adequately describes vocal function, but testing must be done to provide unique information in a manner that is as cost-effective as feasible. And, as always, the clinician must be mindful of Gottfried's (1983) law that you cannot test a test and a person at the same time. "Diagnosis rests in the final analysis, on the abilities of a single super-instrument: a competent professional" (Baken, 1987).

To reiterate, in recent years new technologies have been combined with clinical acumen to develop assessment protocols that provide more information relating vocal structure to function than was previously possible. Results of assessment of voice can be used to suggest treatment programs, make prognostic statements, and evaluate the efficacy of existing therapy. Nevertheless, in the last quarter of a century, voice assessment has not progressed as far as clinicians had hoped. Assessment standards are nonexistent, and many questions remain to be answered. Most importantly, systematic study to determine which combination of techniques is most useful for detecting disorders, documenting changes resulting from treatment, and identifying persons at risk for developing voice disorders has not been completed.

In 1993, the National Institute on Deafness and Other Communication Disorders published a National Strategic Research Plan. The research questions posed in that document still need to be addressed, and are as relevant today as when initially posed. Moreover, although some of these questions evolved from recent applications of new technologies, many others, first posed in G. P. Moore's book, *Organic Voice Disorders*, have been recognized for decades as important questions to address, but have not been answered because of lack of financial resources. For clinical purposes, it is essential that valid, reliable, and standardized methods for objective voice assessment be established, and that these methods have normative studies for the general population, including its cultural diversity, and for professional speakers and singers referenced to age and gender variables from the entire range of human vocal responses. More specifically, the National Strategic Research Plan suggests NIH should devote resources to address the following research aims:

1. Study the nature of respiratory, laryngeal, and upper aerodigestive tract actions and interactions in voice production and determine the principles that govern adaptive and maladaptive behaviors in response to laryngeal disorders or diseases.

2. Gather data on voice production that encompass various domains, including neural, muscular, structural, aeromechanical, acoustical, and perceptual domains.

3. Conduct research to delineate further the effects of bolus characteristics, respiratory parameters, and voluntary control on timing and extent of laryngeal elevation and closure, and pharyngeal contraction during swallowing.

4. Conduct studies on the mechanisms involved in the control of vocal pitch, loudness, quality, and register, including mechanisms associated with singing.

5. Delineate the acoustic to perceptual transformation in voice quality disorders, with special attention to those aspects of the voice signal that give rise to the perception of disorder and its quantities.

6. Study the timing mechanisms of laryngeal behavior in coordination with respiratory and articulatory activity.

7. Conduct studies on the exceptional (trained) singer to specify the limits of the human voice and its optimal efficiency.

8. Determine the effects of lifestyle choices (diet, smoking, drug use, exercise, and alcohol consumption) on the function of the larynx and upper aerodigestive tract.

9. Conduct studies of neural control of the larynx for voice production, respiration, and swallowing in humans and animals, including the elucidation of reflex mechanisms for each.

10. Specify the nature of voice production as it relates to the developing structure of the entire respiratory system, upper aerodigestive tract, and larynx in particular.

11. Obtain data on laryngeal and upper aerodigestive function of normal octogenarians, nonagenarians, and centenarians for voice production and swallowing.
12. Obtain information on the effects of drugs (alone or in combination with other therapy) on the voice.
13. Study the role of psychogenic factors in the pathogenesis of voice disorders and response to treatment, and develop criteria for distinguishing psychogenic from organic voice disorders.
14. Study the effects of aging on voice production to establish the true nature of age-related voice (not pathologic) changes and develop treatment to forestall or prevent such changes.
15. Study the effects of respiratory disorders on the voice.
16. Conduct studies on large populations of normal and disordered speakers to clarify the relations between quantitative measures and perceptual vocal characteristics to determine how to use quantitative measures in making treatment decisions.
17. Determine the usefulness of aeromechanical measurements in the differential diagnosis and assessment of treatments for vocal disorders and evaluate the contribution of the respiratory system to aerodynamic measures.
18. Develop meaningful parameters to quantitatively evaluate laryngeal visual images.
19. Study the impact on laryngeal electromyography of variations in electrode configuration, interaction of electrode configuration, interactions of electrodes with muscles, techniques used to verify electrode placement, and testing protocols.
20. Develop techniques for nonvoluntary activation of laryngeal nerves as a means of verifying the integrity of laryngeal nerves in uncooperative or anesthetized patients.
21. Develop and determine the usefulness of techniques for intraoperative

monitoring and assessment of vocal function in improving surgical results and preventing complications.

We applaud the aims and hope that NIH and workers in the field of voice will combine intellectual and financial resources to answer these questions within the next decade to further improve assessment and treatment of vocally challenged individuals.

REFERENCES AND RECOMMENDED READINGS

A Report of the Task Force on the National Strategic Research Plan.(1993, April). National Institute on Deafness and Other Communication Disorders. MD: National Institutes of Health Bethesda, Maryland.

Allen, K.E.(l982). *Aerodynamics, The science of air in motion.* (2nd ed.). New York: McGraw-Hill.

Aronson, A. E. (l990a). *Clinical voice disorders,* (3rd Ed.). New York: Thieme-Stratton.

Aronson, A. E. (1996b) "Voice signs of neurologic disease throughout the lifespan." Unpublished handout distributed at the Pacific Voice Conference, San Francisco, CA.

Baken, R. J. (1987). *Clinical measurement of speech and voice.* Boston: College-Hill Press.

Baken, R. J. (l992). Electroglottography. *Journal of Voice,* 6, 95–98.

Billings, J. A., Stoeckle, J. D. (l989). *The clinical encounter: A guide to the medical interview and case presentation.* Chicago: Year Book Medical Publishers.

Bless, D. M. (l991). Measurement of vocal function. *Otolaryngologic Clinics of North America,* 24,1023–1033.

Bless, D. M. (1988). Voice assessment. In R. D. Kent, & D. E. Yoder.(Eds.), *Decision making in speech-language pathology.* Philadelphia: B.C. Decker.

Bless, D. M., & Baken R. J. (1992). Introduction: Assessment of voice. *Journal of Voice* 6, 95–98.

Blumenfield, M, & Thompson, T. L. (1985). The psychological reactions to physical illness. In R. C. Simons, (Ed.), *Understanding* human behavior in health and illness (3rd ed.) Baltimore: Williams & Wilkins.

Boone, D. R. (1983). The voice and voice therapy (3rd ed.). Englewood Cliffs, NJ: Prentice-Hall.

Brown, W. S., Morris, R. J., Hicks, D. M., & Howell, E. (1993). Phonation profiles of female professional singers and nonsingers. Journal of Voice, 7, 219–226

Colton, R. H., & Casper, J. K. (1990). Understanding voice problems: A physiological perspective for diagnosis and treatment. Baltimore: Williams & Wilkins.

Coulehan, J. L., & Block, M. R. (1992). The medical interview: A primer for students of the art (2nd ed.). Philadelphia: F.A. Davis.

Cousins, N. (1979). Anatomy of an illness as perceived by the patient. New York: W. W. Norton.

Dubovsky, S. L. (1985). The psychophysiology of health, illness, and stress. In R. C. Simons, (Ed.), Understanding human behavior in health and illness (3rd ed.). Baltimore: Williams & Wilkins.

Eckel, F., & Boone, D. (1981). The s/z ratio as an indicator of laryngeal pathology. Journal of Speech and Hearing Disorders, 46, 147–149.

Fritzell, B., & Fant, G. (Eds.). (1986). Voice acoustics and dysphonia. Journal of Phonetics, 14.

Gerratt, B. R., & Kreiman, J. (1995). The utility of acoustic measures of voice quality. In D. Wong, (Ed.), Workshop on acoustic voice analysis. Iowa City: National Center for Voice and Speech.

Gottfried, E. L., & Wagar, E. A. (1983). Laboratory testing: A practical guide. EM, 29, 9.

Gray, S. D., Hammond, E., & Hanson, D. F. (1995). Benign pathologic responses of the larynx. Annals of Otology Rhinology Laryngology, 104, 13–18

Gray S. D., Hammond, T. H., Zhou, R., & Hammond, E. (in press). An analysis of cellular location and concentration in vocal fold lamina propria. Laryngoscope.

Gray, S. D., Titze, I., & Lusk R. P. (1987). Electron microscopy of hyperphonated vocal cords. Journal of Voice, 1, 109–15.

Herzel, H., Berry, D. A., Titze, I. R., & Saleh, M. (1994). Analysis of vocal disorders with methods from nonlinear dynamics. Journal of Speech and Hearing Research, 37, 1008–1019.

Hicks, D., (1990 September). Functional voice assessment: What to measure and why. Assessment of Speech and Voice Production:

Research and Clinical Applications. Proceedings of a Conference September 27–28, 1990 Bethesda, Maryland. National Institute on Deafness and Other Communication Disorders National Institutes of Health Bethesda, Maryland NIH Publication #92-3236.

Hirano, M. (1981). Clinical examination of voice. New York: Thieme.

Hirano, M. (1989). Objective evaluation of the human voice: Clinical aspects. Folia Phoniatrica. 41, 89–144.

Hirano, M., & Bless, D. M. (1993). Videostroboscopic examination of the larynx. San Diego: Singular Publishing Group.

Kahana, R. J., & Bibring, G. L. (1964). Personality types in medical management. In N.E. Zimberg (Ed.), Psychiatry and medical practice in a general hospital. New York: International Universities Press.

Karnell, M. P., & Finnigan, E. M. (1994). Tools for voice measurement. Current Opinion in Otolaryngology and Head and Neck Surgery, 2, 240–246.

Karnell, M. P., Scherer, R. S., & Fischer, L. B. (1991). Comparison of acoustic voice perturbation measures among three independent voice laboratories. Journal of Speech and Hearing Research, 34, 781–790.

Kent, R., & Read, C. (1992) The acoustic analysis of speech. San Diego: Singular Publishing Group.

Koschkee, D. (1991, April 12–13). Planning and monitoring therapy. Presented at the American Speech-Language Hearing Association Scientific Advances in the Treatment of Voice Disorders Workshop, Madison, WI.

Koschkee, D. L. (1993). Treatment of voice disorders. Presented at ASHA Workshop on Instrumental Assessment and Treatment of Voice, Madison, WI.

Koschkee, D. L., & Rammage, L. (in press). Voice therapy in the medical setting. San Diego: Singular Publishing Group.

Koschkee, D., & Swift, E. (1991, April 12–13). Use of instrumentation: Planning and monitoring therapy. Presented at the American Speech-Language Hearing Association Scientific Advances in the Treatment of Voice Disorders Workshop, Madison, WI.

Koschkee, D. L., & Swift, E. (1993). Treatment of voice disorders. Presented at ASHA Workshop on Instrumental Assessment and Treatment of Voice, Madison, WI.

Koufman, J. A. & Blalock, P. D. (1988). Vocal fatigue and dysphonia in the professional voice user: Bogart-Bacall syndrome. *Laryngoscope, 98,* 493–498.

Kreiman, J., Gerratt. B. R., Kempster, G. B., Erman, A., Berke, G. S. (1993). Perceptual evaluation of voice quality: Review, tutorial, and a Framework for Future Research, *Journal of Speech and Hear Research, 36,* 21–40.

Löfqvist, A., Carlborg, B., & Kitzing, P. (1982). Initial validation of an indirect measure of subglottal pressure during vowels. *Journal of the Acoustical Society of America, 72,* 633–635.

Moon, J. B. (1995). Evaluation of velopharyngeal function. In R. Sprintzen (Ed.), *Cleft palate* (p. 251–304).

Moore, G. P. (1971). *Organic voice disorders.* Englewood Cliffs, NJ: Prentice-Hall.

Morris, R. J., Brown, W. S., Hicks, D. M., & Howell, E. (1995). Phonation profiles of male trained singers and nonsingers. *Journal of Voice, 9,* 142–148.

Peppard, R. C., & Bless, D. M. (1991). The use of topical anesthetic in videostroboscopic examination of the larynx. *Journal of Voice, 5,* 57–63.

Poburka, B., & Bless, D. M. (1995). Computer aided instruction for videostroboscopic training. *Asha, 36,* 107.

Rabinov, C. R., Kreiman, J., & Gerratt, B. R. (1995). Comparing reliability of a perceptual and acoustic measures of voice. In D. Wong, (Ed.), *Workshop on acoustic voice analysis.* Iowa City: National Center for Voice and Speech.

Ramos, A. C. (1996). *Endocrine changes and voice in pre and perimenapausal women.* Unpublished doctoral dissertation, University of Wisconsin-Madison. 1996.

Rothenberg, M. (1973). A new inverse-filtering technique for deriving the glottal air flow waveform during voicing. *Journal of the Acoustical Society America, 53,* 1632–1645.

Sataloff, R. T. (1991). *Professional voice: The science and art of clinical care.* New York: Raven Press.

Sataloff, R. T., Spiegel, J. R., Carroll, L. M., Schiebel, B. R., Darby, K. S., & Rulnick, R. (1988). Strobovideolaryngoscopy in professional voice users: Results and clinical value. *Journal of Voice, 1,* 359–364, 1988.

Saxon, K. G., & Schneider, C. M. (1995). *Vocal exercise physiology.* San Diego: Singular Publishing Group.

Scherer, R. C. (1990, September). Aerodynamic assessment in voice production in assessment of speech and voice production: Research and clinical applications. *Proceedings of a Conference.* NIH Publication No. 92-3236.

Scherer, R. C. (1991). Physiology of phonation: A review of basic mechanics. In C. N. Ford, & D. M. Bless (1991). *Phonosurgery assessment and surgical management of voice disorders.* New York: Raven Press.

Scherer, R. (1988). Preliminary evaluation of selected acoustic and glottographic measures for clinical phonatory function analysis. *Journal of Voice, 2,* 230–244.

Scherer, R. C., Titze, I., Raphael, B. N.,Wood, R. P., Ramig, L. A., & Blager, R. F.(1991). Vocal fatigue in a trained and an untrained voice user. In T. Baer, C. Sasaki, & K. S. Harris, (Eds), *Laryngeal function in phonation and respiration.* Boston: Little, Brown.

Schutte, H. K. (1992). Integrated aerodynamic measurements. *Journal of Voice, 6,* 127–134.

Schutte, H. K. *The efficiency of voice production.* Groningen.

Schutte, H. K., & Seichner, W. (1983). Recommendations by the Union of the European Phoniatricians (UEP): Standardized voice area measurement/phonetograph. *Folia Phoniatrica, 35* 286–288.

Shipp, T. (1973). Intraoral air pressure and lip occlusion in midvocalic stop consonant production. *Journal of Phonetics, 1,* 167–170.

Smitheran J. R., Hixon, T. J. (1981). A clinical method for estimating laryngeal airway resistance during vowel production. *Journal of Speech and Hearing Disorders, 46,* 138–146.

Stemple, J. C. (1993). Voice research: So what? A clearer view of voice production, 25 years of progress; the speaking voice, *Journal of Voice, 7,* 293–301.

Stemple, J. C. (1993). *Voice therapy clinical studies.* St. Louis: Mosby Year Book.

Stemple, J. C., Stanley, J., & Lee, L. (1995). Objective measures of voice production in normal subjects following prolonged voice use. *Journal of Voice, 9,* 127–133.

Titze, I. (1991, April). *Acoustics: Inverse filter.* Presented at the American Speech-Language Hearing Association Scientific Advances in the Treatment of Voice Workshop, Madison, WI

Titze, I. (1993). Current topics in voice production mechanisms. *Acta Otolaryngologica (Stockh), 113,* 421–427.

Titze, I. (1986). Mean intraglottal pressure in vocal fold oscillation. *Journal of Phonetics,* 14, 359–364.

Titze, I. (1989). On the relation between subglottal pressure and fundamental frequency in phonation. *Journal of the Acoustical Society of America, 85,* 901–906.

Titze, I. (1994). *Principles of voice production.* Englewood Cliffs, NJ: Prentice-Hall.

Titze, I. (1988). The physics of small-amplitude oscillation of the vocal fold. *Journal of the Acoustical Society of America, 83,* 1536–1552.

Titze, I. (1996). *Workshop on acoustic voice analysis summary statement.* Iowa City: National Center for Voice and Speech.

Titze, I., & Talkin, D. T. A theoretical study of the effects of various laryngeal configurations on the acoustics of phonation. *Journal of the Acoustical Society of America, 66,* 60–74.

Verdolini-Marston, K., Titze, I., & Druker, D. (1990). Changes in phonation threshold pressure with induced conditions of hydration. *Journal of Voice, 4,* 142–151.

Von Leden, H. (1991). History of phonosurgery. In C. N. Ford, & D. M. Bless, (Eds), *Phonosurgery assessment and surgical management of voice disorders.* New York: Raven Press.

Woo, P., Colton, R., Casper, J., & Brewer, D. (1991). Diagnostic value of stroboscopic examination in hoarse patients. *Journal of Voice, 5,* 231–238.

Yanagihara, N. (1967). Significance of harmonic changes and noise components in hoarseness. *Journal of Speech and Hearing Research, 10,* 166–181.

LIST OF APPENDIXES

On the following pages are example case history forms developed by Koschkee (in press) summarizing factors thought to be important for interpretation of causal factors and their interactions with voice production.

Appendix 6–A

Typical Adult Voice History Form

History of the Voice Problem

Symptoms
- What is the chief complaint?
- What changes in voice have been noticed (e.g., hoarseness, breathiness, vocal fatigue, loss of vocal range)?
- Are there associated sensations or symptoms (e.g., pain in the throat when using voice, tickling or choking sensation, breathing problems, swallowing difficulties, heartburn, weight loss, coughing)?

Onset
- When did the symptoms first begin?
- Was the onset sudden or gradual in nature?
- What did the parent think was causing the problem?

Duration
- Is the problem acute (days or weeks) or chronic (months or years)?

Variability
- Is the problem constant or does it wax and wane?
- If it varies, what factors seem to aggravate or relieve the symptoms (e.g., weather, amount of speaking, coughing, episodes, time of day)?

Progression of Symptoms
- Since the time of onset, have the symptoms worsened, improved, or remained the same?
- What development prompted evaluation?

Previous evaluations, treatments, results
- Have there been previous evaluations or treatments (e.g.,
- surgery, voice therapy, radiation therapy, acupuncture, homeopathy?
- What were the effects of treatment?

Past Medical History

Major illnesses
- Have there been previous physical or mental illnesses?
- What was the length of each illness, extent of incapacity, types and effects of treatments?

Surgeries
- What surgeries have been performed?
- Was intubation or tracheotomy required?
- Were there complications (e.g., recurrent laryngeal nerve section, airway obstruction, hemangioma)?

Accidents or injuries
- Have there been traumatic injuries to the head or neck?
- Blunt or penetrating traumas (e.g., sport injuries, strangulation, automobile accidents)?
- Foreign body aspiration (e.g., choking on foods or small objects)?
- Ingestion of caustic agents (e.g., acids, alkalines)?
- Inhalation injuries or burns?

(continued)

Appendix 6–A. *(continued)*

Past Medical History *(continued)*

Accidents or injuries (continued)
- Iatrogenic injuries (from irradiation, prolonged intubation, or tracheotomy)?

Allergies
- Are there allergies to foods? drugs? environment?

Review of Symptoms
- Are other symptoms present that might be associated with the voice disorder?
- Are there problems in general health, ear, nose and throat, breasts, musculoskeletal, respiratory, cardiovascular, genitourinary, or neurologic systems?
- Is there an identifiable symptom complex or pattern?

Current Health Practices

Medications
- Are any drugs being used on a regular or intermittent basis? prescription drugs? non-prescription drugs (e.g. aspirin, laxatives, vitamins, cold tablets, over-the-counter sleeping pills or nerve pills?)

Recreational drugs
- Is there past or present use of street drugs such as marijuana (pot), speed (amphetamines) Dexedrine, Ritalin), LSD (acid), PCP (angel dust), cocaine, heroin, mushrooms, etc.?

Tobacco
- What type and amount of tobacco is used?
- How long has the patient been smoking or chewing tobacco?
- Is there exposure to second-hand smoke?

Alcohol
- How much and what types of alcoholic beverages does the patient drink?
- Are there beneficial effects on the voice from drinking?

Caffeine
- Is there use of caffeine-containing drinks (e.g., coffee, tea, soft drinks, hot chocolate)? foods (e.g., chocolate bars, cocoa), or medications (e.g., Excedrin™, Anacin™, Vanquish™, Triaminicin™, Coricidin™, Sinarest™, No-Doz™, diet pills)?

Dietary patterns
- Is a special or restricted diet used?
- Would the present diet promote gastroesophageal reflux (e.g., spicy foods, high fat foods, caffeine)?
- Is there evidence of an eating disorder such as anorexia nervosa or bulimia?

Voice usage
- In what ways is the voice typically used (e.g., cheering at a child's hockey game, professional or public speaking, talking over noise in a factory, singing, yodeling, crying)?

Stress management
- In what ways is stress managed (e.g., exercise, medication, counseling, meditation, support groups, primal scream therapy?

Family/Work History

Hereditary conditions
- What inheritance patterns are present in the family history?

(continued)

Appendix 6–A. *(continued)*

Family/Work History (continued)

Hereditary conditions (continued)	• Are there similar problems in parents, siblings, offspring?
Family dynamics/Learning	• Do environmental influences seem to account for the voice problem (e.g., is the patient from a large family that "always talked too loudly")?
	• What current family interaction patterns exist (e.g., shouting matches, verbal competitions at the dinner table)?
Major life changes	• What events have happened in the past 12 months that might increase stress?
Emotional reactions to illness	• Is there a family history of "throat cancer"?
	• Is over-reaction to the current voice problem based upon past family experiences.

Psychological Considerations

Psychological history	• What is the patient's mental health history?
	• Does it include depression, mania, suicide attempts, alcohol abuse, an eating disorder, schizophrenia, "nervous breakdowns", sexual abuse, or other psychological problems?
	• What past or present treatments have been used (e.g., psychotherapy, pharmacotherapy, electroconvulsive therapy, in-patient hospitalization)?
Current stress levels	• Have recent problems or circumstances elevated stress levels at home or work (e.g., financial problems, divorce, an illness or death in the family, a change in jobs, moving to a new city)?
Voice disability index	• What impact is the voice problem having on daily living activities?

Appendix 6–B

Family History (From Adult Voice History). Please indicate if any family members have had any of the following illnesses. If so, who?

	Yes	No	Unsure	Who (e.g., mother, brother, aunt, etc.)
Heart disease				
High blood pressure				
Stroke				
Cancer				
Alcoholism				
Drug abuse				
Thyroid disorder				
Seizures (epilepsy)				
Migraines				
Allergies				
Asthma				
Ulcers				
Depression				
Neurologic disease				
Psychiatric problems				
Other (please list)				

Appendix 6–C

Review of Systems (From Adult Voice Case History)

HAVE YOU BEEN TROUBLED OR ARE YOU TROUBLED NOW BY ANY OF THE FOLLOWING?

GENERAL: <u>Yes</u>   <u>No</u>

Excessive fatigue

Unexplainable weight change

Excessive thirst

Intolerance for hot weather

Unexplainable perspiration

Persistent pain in any part
of the body

Lumps or swelling

Exercise related health or
breathing problems

SKIN AND HAIR:

Recurrent skin rash

Recurrent sores

Patches of hair falling out

Swollen glands

Excessive coarseness of hair

Persistent or recurrent
itching

Excessive drying of skin

EYE, EAR, NOSE, & THROAT:

Facial pain

Blurred or double vision

Loss of vision

Loss of hearing

Ringing in ears

Ear pain

Trouble with nose or sinuses

Teeth or gum problems

Voice changes

Swallowing problems

HEART:

Abnormal chest x-ray

Chest pain

Discomfort in chest on exertion

Palpitation of the heart

Heart murmur

Other heart trouble

Leg cramps while walking

Ankle swelling

High blood pressure

RESPIRATORY: <u>Yes</u>   <u>No</u>

Sleep apnea

Cough

Sputum (phlegm) production

Pneumonia or pleurisy

Shortness of breath with activity

Wheezing or asthma

Pulmonary emboli (blood clot
to the lung)

Exposure to toxic dusts, chemicals

SKELETON AND JOINTS:

Swollen or painful joints

Neck pains

Gout

Frequent back stiffness

Back trouble

Severe leg cramps

Difficulty walking

INTESTINAL SYSTEM:

Change in eating habits

Frequent indigestion

Heartburn

Frequent belching

Recurrent abdominal pain

Frequent nausea or vomiting

Bitter or acid taste in mouth

NERVOUS SYSTEM:

Frequent or severe headaches

Attacks of staggering or
loss of balance

Unexplained dizziness

Loss of consciousness

Head injury

Weakness or heaviness of
limbs

Persistent or recurrent
numbness or
tingling of hands
or feet

	Yes	No
Episodes of difficulty talking	—	—
Increasing irritability and mood swings	—	—
Prolonged periods of feeling depressed or blue	—	—
Difficulty in concentrating	—	—
Difficulty in memorizing	—	—
Difficulty in sleeping	—	—
Uncontrollable tension	—	—
Twitching or tremors	—	—
Personal problems that cause you great concern	—	—
Suicidal thoughts	—	—

	Yes	No
GENITOURINARY:		
Gonorrhea or syphilis	—	—
Herpes	—	—
(Women only)		
Possibly pregnant	—	—
Change in menstrual pattern	—	—
IMMUNE SYSTEM:		
Unexplainable bruising	—	—
Lymph nodes swelling or pain	—	—
HIV positive	—	—
Other immunologic problems	—	—

Adapted by Koschkee (1994) from the Allergy Clinic Intake Form, UW Hospital and Clinics, Madison, Wisconsin.

Appendix 6–D

The pediatric voice history: contributions to the voice problem

History	Factors
Voice history	• Past and present symptoms • Onset and duration • Clinical course and variability • Previous evaluations and/or treatments
Medical history	• Major illnesses • Surgeries • Accidents and/or injuries • Allergies • Drug/medication use • Relevant medical problems
Voice usage	• Excessive loudness • Voice strain/tension • Abusive habits • Affective voice usage
Family history	• Familial diseases, illnesses, conditions • Family dynamics, learning, environment
Developmental information	• Hearing history • Gross and fine motor development • Associated speech/language delays or disorders • Cognitive development
Child's personal profile	• Personality • Social interaction patterns • Personal habits, behaviors, stresses

CHAPTER 7

PRINCIPLES OF TREATMENT

DOUGLAS M. HICKS, Ph.D.
DIANE M. BLESS, Ph.D.

Management of voice disorders has changed dramatically over the years, with behavioral, medical, and surgical care being the consensus options. Knowledge of vocal fold tissue properties and vibratory mechanics, along with improved surgical techniques and tools, has led to more physiologically based treatment programs. This change in clinical orientation has resulted in clinicians from different professional orientations working together to determine the most effective treatment based on (a) what the patient is capable of doing with his or her existing laryngeal mechanism; (b) knowledge of what can be changed with behavioral exercises; (c) knowledge of what is possible to surgically change; (d) recognition of the complex nature of voice production, and (e) incorporation of modern technology to increase therapeutic efficiency or improve outcome. Emphasis on laryngeal physiology has created more effective and prescriptive treatments for patients.

Laryngeal physiology is the critical bridge that reconciles a patient's symptoms and the underlying pathology (Moore, 1971). Clinical experience tells us that the same vocal symptoms can be caused by a variety of different pathologies; and, conversely, the same pathology can produce various dysphonias. It is only when the nature and extent of laryngeal dysfunction are accurately identified that treatment efficiency is enhanced. This requires the careful evaluation of vocal physiology as described in Chapter 6. Furthermore, this physiological orientation is the most useful basis to discuss principles of treatment.

At its simplest level, normal voice performance results from periodic, in-phase vibration of the true vocal folds with complete medial compression of at least the membranous portion of the folds. Violation of vibratory periodicity, phase, or compression tends to alter the loudness or quality of the voice. Changes in the effective vibrating mass or shape of the vibratory margin of the vocal folds create pitch alteration. Although not approaching a perfect relationship, predictable patterns of impact exist between violations of physiology and resultant voice symptoms. For example, glottal gapping usually creates sufficient excess air turbulence to produce a breathy type dysphonia. Aperiodicity of vocal fold vibration is typically associated with vocal roughness. The combination of glottal gapping and vibratory aperiodicity typically creates hoarseness. Increasing fold mass can result in lowering of perceived pitch. The subjective attribute of disorder severity appears related to the magnitude of physiologic disruption and the speaker's ability to compensate. These scientific tenets have emerged from the laboratory where both objective analysis and synthesis of voice are employed to investigate both normal and disordered voice production (Childers, Alsaka, Hicks, & Moore, 1986; Childers, Hicks, Moore, & Alsaka, 1986; Childers, Hicks, Moore, Eskenazi, & Lalwani, 1990; Moore, Hicks, & Childers, 1986).

Treatment confidence can be built on physiologic relationships by altering structure and function of the larynx to create certain vocal changes. Traditional voice therapy attempts to manipulate laryngeal function through behavioral adjustments and compensation, while medical and surgical management directly address tissue status and its vibratory characteristics.

The remainder of the chapter will be organized around the three logical treatment options: behavioral voice therapy, medicine, and surgery. Focusing on organic disorders alone limits both treatment principles and specific techniques that might otherwise be addressed if all types of voice disorders were covered. Furthermore, all management for organic dysphonias is guided by the general goal of compensation versus restoration. Return of normal voice is not always possible with organic disorders. Instead, clinicians are better served to recapture the best possible voice performance allowed by the organic condition. Finally, the ultimate goal is to create desirable change regardless of the method used to achieve it. Hopefully, treatment will accomplish at least functional adequacy for the patient.

It is not the intent of this chapter to provide a "how to" guide book nor to create a new set of therapy techniques. That would be redundant in light of previously published textbooks (Aronson, 1990; Boone & McFarlane, 1994; Colton & Casper, 1990; Morrison & Rammage, 1994; Stemple, Glaze, & Gerdeman, 1995). More useful would be an attempt to clarify and justify the appropriate use of behavioral options available to the clinician as they apply to organic voice disorders. For each technique presented, the organic voice disorder(s) for which the treatment is applicable, a rationale for its use, and a description of the treatment are presented.

BEHAVIORAL THERAPY

Patient Education

Patient education is the foundation for treatment for all organic voice disorders, because it provides the necessary knowledge base for the patient to respond to treatment with motivation and commitment. Regardless of the technique, ultimate therapy effectiveness is built on patient cooperation, which is achieved through patient education. The patient becomes an informed consumer of the options for treating his or her problem and thus is more likely to become an active, rather than passive, participant in the remediation of the voice problem. Reduction of fear of the unknown, as well as elimination of misconceptions, are critical goals to achieve. Effective education is accomplished through the following steps:

1. Thorough review of the laryngeal structure and function utilizing diagrams, drawings, or playback of videoendoscopy/stroboscopy films;
2. Explanation of the mechanical basis of voice symptoms, enabling the patient to reconcile the laryngeal findings and the voice performance;
3. Explanation of the role(s) various contributing factors play in perpetuating and/or exacerbating vocal difficulties

(i.e., past surgical history, general health, lifestyle choices, diet, medicines, emotions/stress, allergies, gastroesophageal reflux);

4. Clarification of prescriptive conclusions, recommendations, and prognosis, as well as probable therapeutic outcomes;
5. Clarification and justification of patient-specific therapy goals, including an estimate of the therapy time frame.

Voice Monitoring

Like patient education, voice monitoring is applicable to all organic voice disorders, and it, too, can help facilitate an efficient response to therapy techniques. In fact, the ability to accurately monitor one's own voice performance is a skill that is relevant to the behavioral management of all dysphonias. Without that skill, both therapy efficiency and effectiveness are compromised. Unfortunately, focus on this clinical area is frequently overlooked due to the misperception of it as an archaic therapy component. Voice monitoring is often equated with the traditional goal of ear training (Fisher, 1966). In reality, this skill is an essential prerequisite for optimal behavioral change rather than a true therapy technique. Voice monitoring does not require listening to sounds/noises, contrasting high and low tones, or even listening to the voices of others. It requires training the speaker to be able to hear when he or she has hit the relevant voice target. This can be accomplished by direct training or as a by-product of working directly on changing a specific vocal characteristic such as pitch or loudness.

The goal is to help the patient develop a trained ear atuned to the problem area(s) of the voice, as well as to identify changes in vocal performance created by different therapy techniques. The rationale is quite simple: How can one expect the patient to successfully modify vocal behavior until he or she is capable of accurately and consistently identifying when and in what way the actual vocal performance differs from the desired vocal performance? It is precisely at those times that implementation of therapy techniques can be most effective. If a speaker is able to achieve this identification, no further work on voice monitoring is indicated. However, for speakers who are unable to tell when facilitating techniques yield vocal improvement, voice monitoring may be required.

It must be emphasized that focus on this skill is short-term, just sufficient to verify the patient's success. Steps to accomplish adequate voice monitoring skills include:

1. Educate the patient on the relevant voice performance parameters that comprise the dysphonia (e.g., problems of laryngeal quality, pitch, loudness, and nasal resonance);
2. Require the patient to demonstrate ability to differentiate among the parameters, as well as to recognize problem instances;
3. Utilize structured compare/contrast activities based ideally on immediate feedback and live voice samples. Recorded samples are less desirable because the recorded voice does not provide a faithful production of how the patient hears his or her own voice;
4. Move from gross distinction initially to more subtle contrast in order to refine the patient's ability to monitor his or her own voice.

Once accomplished, voice monitoring is a skill that rarely needs subsequent attention in therapy.

Improved Breath Support for Speech

Like the prior two techniques, improved breath support is applicable to all organic voice disorders by creating sufficient power to initiate and maintain efficient phonation. Too often, focus on breath support has been associated with detailed instruction on abdominal versus chest breathing to the exclusion of training respiratory coordination. Review of common breathing "exercises" confirms that dichotomy, as well as the professional preoccupation with teaching breathing. Breaking the act of breathing into its component parts is artificial, cumbersome, and potentially disruptive to therapy success. Aside from the rare patient with significant pulmonary and/or abdominal problems, the vast majority of voice patients demonstrating poor breath support for speech are really reflecting poor coordination between respiration and phonation.

Voice patients generally do not exhibit abnormal lung volumes, and respiratory dynamics typically fall within normal limits. Moreover, Hixon and his colleagues (Hixon, Goldman, & Mead, 1973; Hixon, Mead, & Goldman, 1976; Hixon, Watson, Harris, & Perlman, 1988; Hoit & Hixon, 1986) have clearly demonstrated there are many ways to move the air volumes around to achieve the same levels of voice production. Some speakers are more naturally rib cage breathers, while others achieve the same speaking objective primarily with abdominal movement. The treatment challenge is to determine when breath support focus is necessary to increase efficiency or to help compensate for laryngeal inadequacies. In reality, the primary culprit is simply poor breath "pausing" strategies for speech. In other words, the patient functions with inadequate or inefficient breath recharging behavior that is insufficient to initiate and sustain phonation. Because human speech is considered a low pressure phenomenon, even patient populations with bonafide respiration problems can learn functionally adequate compensatory strategies to support speech.

Normal lung volumes and adequate respiratory flexibility to produce normal voice do not negate the benefits from working on abdominal control. This may actually be part of the strategy for teaching improved voice control. One long-standing technique, the accent method (Smith & Thyme, 1976), focuses initially on abdominal movement but eventually capitalizes on rhythm to teach coordination of the entire vocal apparatus. Treatment begins with work on physiological abdominal movements to facilitate free airflow during phonation and to change the locus of phonatory attention. Later, sound is superimposed as gentle pulses allowing transition from abdomen to whole body movement to teach coordination of structures and avoid developing counterproductive tension. Research by Kotby and colleagues (Kotby, El-Sady, Basiouny, Abou-Rass, & Hegazi, 1991) and Smith and Thyme (1976) has demonstrated that this technique reduces vocal complaints, reduces the size of nodules, and improves vocal quality and intensity of high harmonics in the vocal output at frequencies below 1000 Hz.

The keys to successful therapy require accurate identification of the particular breath support inefficiency. In general, difficulties relate to one or a combination of the following: inadequate inhalation compounded by hyperfunctional or pressed compensation, premature exhalation prior to phonation, and talking too long on one breath. These problems are common and simply reflect inefficient timing habits. Therefore, rather than teaching patients how to breathe, therapy for breath support focuses on properly executed breath control and pausing strategies.

Success in developing these strategies is accomplished through:

1. *Development of Good Sustained Phonation Ability:* Despite literature emphasis that 20 seconds of sustained phonation ability is "normal," virtually no

normal discourse demands more than 10–12 seconds of sustained ability. Therefore, a more clinically useful target is the lower duration.

Focus should not be placed primarily on the mechanics of breathing but rather on the efficient conversion of airflow into voice through vocal fold vibration. An exception might be the purposeful elimination of clavicular breathing habits for patients relying on that maladaptive behavior as the primary breath support strategy for speech. For organic conditions that involve significant glottal gapping (medial edge mass lesions, fold immobility, webbing), sustained phonation ability of even 2 seconds may be impossible. The use of true fold medial compression or pressed techniques, as well as supplementation by electronic amplification devices, might allow sufficient compensation to obtain that temporal goal. Amplification devices relieve the patient somewhat of maintaining functional loudness through extraordinary expenditure of aerodynamic forces.

2. *Development of Proper Breath Pausing Habits:* Initially, use of marked reading passages that require a recharging breath at appointed times during oral reading will begin to retrain predictable breath support habits. Liberal use of visual feedback through videotape playback of the patient's efforts should reinforce effective skills. Experimenting with various pausing schemes should help the patient develop comfort with the versatility of skills and gain confidence in his or her ability to maintain breathing control.

Once reasonable success is accomplished in the structure of oral reading passages, the focus of therapy should change to spontaneous conversation. Maximum effectiveness at this stage will occur only through the review of taped video and/or audio samples of the patient's productions. Examples of poor support should be repeated until effective breath support

is achieved. Ultimately, therapy should shape predictable, consistent pausing skills.

3. *Building Up the Patient's Awareness of Improper Breathing Cues (Kinesthetic and Auditory):* Such cues include audible gasping, increased speaking rate, decreased speaking pitch, evidence of vocal fry or pressed voice, loudness trailing off, sense of running out of breath, and changes in thoracic cavity configuration. The more accurately and consistently patients can recognize breath support difficulty, the more effective they will be at implementing helpful modifications.

Elimination of Vocal Abuse(s)

Vocal abuse can be a factor in a variety of voice disorders, including those due to irritative factors, nodules/polyps, intracordal lesions, and contact ulcers. The elimination of abuses is essential to reversing their negative causal or contributory impact on laryngeal structures, which, in turn, facilitates spontaneous recovery and response to treatment.

It is important to understand that vocal abuse is comprised of two components: misuse and overuse. Typically an abusive patient will have evidence of both components, although frequently one is predominant. Of the two components, overuse is often misunderstood and overlooked. It is imperative, however, to identify and treat significant overuse.

Misuse is intuitively what patients and clinicians think of when referring to "abuse." It involves pushing the larynx beyond it physiologic limits and is commonly illustrated by severe coughing, throat clearing, yelling, or screaming. Overuse, in contrast, involves a wearing down or fatiguing process. It can be conceived of as using the larynx within appropriate physiologic boundaries, but for extensive, uninterrupted periods of time. Constant telephone conversations, long lectures or public address, and chronic mild coughing are illustrative. Again, it must be emphasized that, even though overuse behavior is harder to recognize and appreciate, it is still detrimental.

All individuals have a threshold of abuse, which, once violated, leads to various pathologic tissue changes. Variable tolerance to abuse both within and across patients emphasizes that an individual's abuse threshold is not static and may reflect a genetic predisposition. In fact, abuse tolerance frequently changes as a function of many factors including age, physical health, emotional health, hormonal factors, vocal training, occupation, and lifestyle choices. One should never lose proper perspective, however, and forget that the larynx is inherently a robust organ which readily handles a heavy demand and even a certain amount of abuse without permanent damage. The typical mild dysphonia experienced by many spectators after enjoying a sporting event quickly resolves back to normal within hours for most speakers, thereby confirming laryngeal heartiness. Unfortunately, an already structurally compromised larynx may display reduced tolerance for vocal abuse. This creates the all-too-common pattern of worsening voice with minimal use/abuse. This vicious physiologic cycle takes relatively little phonation to perpetuate the particular organic condition. The typical abuse-related changes of the larynx, like edema, erythema, and various mass lesions, do not have sufficient recovery time, even with a night's sleep, to avoid the exacerbating effect of continual, even modest, voice demand.

Management of this therapy focus can be accomplished by the following:

1. Help the patient generate a comprehensive voice use profile corresponding to a detailed daily schedule over 1 week.

2. Independently, patient and clinician generate a list of the 5–10 worst "abuse" activities.
3. Generate a mutually agreeable list and ranking of the worst five abuses.
4. Negotiate (not dictate) strategy options designed to change abusive behavior via elimination, reduction, or modification to a nonabusive form.
5. Implement and monitor compliance with these strategies.
6. Adjust or include additional strategies until perceived vocal targets are obtained.

Once the improvement process begins, encourage continued compliance and patience. The ultimate goal is to require as few permanent lifestyle changes as necessary to achieve and maintain the desired vocal change. Additionally, therapy focus for this area will establish a patient's awareness of abuse factors for the future and help habituate new proper vocal hygiene behavior. The ultimate proof of success is desired vocal performance, although structural improvement usually parallels the voice improvement.

Direct Vocal/Laryngeal Manipulation

As a therapeutic technique, direct vocal/laryngeal manipulation is appropriate for patients who exhibit irritative factors, nodules/polyps, intracordal lesions, contact ulcers, immobility, spasmodic dysphonia, or neurological dysphonias. The principle that underlies this technique is that it changes specific voice parameters (pitch, loudness, and laryngeal quality) in specific directions to create the desired improvement in vocal performance. Treatment in this area is accomplished via a number of exercises designed to manipulate laryngeal physiology to effect a specific vocal outcome. The most recognized group of such exercises has been described by Boone and McFarlane (1994) as "facilitating techniques." They should be applied creatively and prescriptively as tools for change and must be viewed strictly as a means to an end. Although the exercises/tasks are fairly simple and straightforward to administer, accomplishing successful change is not always easy. After all, organic lesions impose certain physiologic restrictions which dictate the extent of ultimate compensation and resultant voice change.

Reduction of Vocal Fold Medial Compression

Several of the organic lesions (i.e., edema, inflammation, nodules, polyps, lesions of the lamina propria, and contact ulcers) owe their genesis or maintenance to tissue trauma associated with excessive medial compression of the true folds. Therapeutic benefit will occur only by counteracting this destructive physiology with reduced medial compression. The decreased adductory forces limit vocal fold impact forces, which is believed to both prevent and reverse traumatic injury to the larynx.

The strict version of that principle involves complete voice rest, replacing verbal communication with gestures and writing. This is an extreme measure to be reserved for a select few conditions such as acute laryngitis, the immediate post-phonosurgery phase, extreme laryngeal trauma, and hemorrhagic lesions.

A less severe application of this treatment principle involves soft phonation with an easy onset attack and breathy quality that is not adequate beyond an arm's distance from listeners. This is achieved through incompletely adducted true vocal folds with a tiny, consistent glottal gap or barely touching folds, but not with a whisper. The reduced vibratory collision allows functional verbal communication while promoting tissue recovery. Associated vocal changes will include re-

duced loudness, increased breathy quality, and reduced sustained phonation. Generally, these techniques are viewed as short-term strategies to be used until tissue recovery has occurred.

Common facilitating exercises include the yawn-sigh technique, use of aspirate onset (/h/-initiated words), soft phonation, and purposeful breathy phonation as used in confidential voice therapy, resonant voice therapy, and flow mode therapy, all described in a recent National Center for Voice and Speech (NCVS) booklet (1994). Whispering should be avoided as an alternative "voice" strategy due to its physiology. Several studies have confirmed the physiologic basis of whispering to involve tight medial compression of the anterior true folds except for a small posterior glottal chink that creates "noise" on which to talk (Hicks & Sweat, 1984; Monoson & Zemlin, 1984; Solomon, McCall, Trosset, & Gray, 1989). It is a nonphonatory voice mode and is believed to inhibit tissue recovery.

The reduced compression technique also has potential application to adductor spasmodic dysphonia. Rather than reduction of trauma or promotion of healing, reducing true fold adduction can stabilize the phonatory disruption underlying this disorder. Unfortunately, empirical observations suggest functional improvement in no more than 50% of cases treated by a behavioral approach.

Clinicians now realize that, in cases of excessive adductory forces, without concomitant treatment of factors like gastroesophageal reflux, even the best-applied therapy may fail. Koufman (1991) has stated that gastroesophageal reflux is implicated as a causal or maintaining factor for many organic lesions. Koufman argues that reflux irritates the laryngeal tissue which then promotes the appropriate conditions for organic lesions to occur. He further claims that aggressive, concomitant behavioral and medical management must be instituted if the voice problems are to be remediated.

A final application of the reduced vocal fold compression techniques is embodied in resonant voice therapy, described in a 1994 publication of the National Center for Voice and Speech. The focus is on increasing oral vibratory sensations with a corresponding decrease in vocal fold adduction forces. Clinicians use combinations of nasals and consonants with different inflection patterns to lower the velum and get better phonatory balance. Empirically, the results are a strong vocal output with low vocal fold closing impact.

Laryngeal Reposturing

Many patients with iatrogenic scarring, nodules, or paralysis develop musculoskeletal tension in attempts to compensate for the underlying pathology. One form of musculoskeletal tension is chronic posturing of the larynx in an elevated position. Aronson (1990) and Roy and Leeper (1993) suggest this elevated position leads to cramping and stiffness of the hyoid-laryngeal musculature, which contributes to the cause and maintenance of the dysphonias. Aronson claims that indirect tension reduction techniques often fail, whereas manual repositioning of the larynx to a lower position by kneading the circumlaryngeal area is successful in reducing the tension. Roy and Leeper have confirmed these assertions with clinical studies of speakers with nodules, stiffness, and unilateral vocal fold paralysis.

Increased Vocal Fold Medial Compression

The physiologic opposite of reduced fold adduction involves increased medial compression. Its therapeutic utility is reserved for true fold immobility problems, whether by paralysis or joint fixation. The ultimate benefit is dictated by factors such as unilateral versus bilateral immobility, position of the immobile fold(s), extent of compensation by the mobile fold(s), size of glottal gapping, and vocal fold morphology and tonus.

An overriding consideration of this technique is the understanding that immobile vocal folds (even paralyzed ones) will vibrate if approximated closely enough to be engaged by aerodynamic forces. Furthermore, immobile folds are not traumatized or fragile. There is no need for protective strategies; and, in fact, more harm than good comes from vocal reservedness. The patient must be instructed and encouraged to use his or her voice without reservation. Maximum compensation benefit will come only with the unreserved use of the voice. Patients will more likely heed these recommendations if they can visualize the mechanical basis of their problem via video monitoring and subsequent playback of the endoscopic examination. Counseling patients to use their voices, regardless of how they sound, will help curtail the natural tendency to protect the "broken" larynx through self-imposed "holdback" strategies.

The increased medial compression principle is commonly achieved by a group of isometric exercises that involve pushing, pulling, and pressing with the arms. The result is an increase in thoracic and cervical tension that generalizes to the larynx and promotes closer approximation of the true vocal folds. Ultimate success with the technique occurs when the patient can induce the laryngeal behavior on demand without upper body isometrics. These exercises capitalize on the primary valving function of the larynx to build intrathoracic pressure for such activities as weight bearing, waste elimination, and child bearing. As one might logically expect, caution must be exercised in using these techniques to avoid overcompensation harm to the larynx. This is particularly true for patients with concomitant, uncontrolled gastroesophageal reflux where irritated tissues are less tolerant of increased impact and pressure forces.

Typical vocal gains include increased conversational and maximum loudness, improved stability of phonation, reduced aphonia and breathy phonation, reduced vocal fatigue, improved sustained phonation, and reduced vocal effort. Vocal benefits can be supplemented with other techniques such as digital, laryngeal pressure to the immobile side (improves medial position of the vocal fold), rotation of the head opposite to the immobile side (stretches the affected vocal fold to improve position and tonus), use of portable amplification devices (improves functional loudness without laryngeal strain), and use of an animated, enthusiastic voice style (naturally promotes optimal coordination of breath support and vocal fold vibration).

Another application of this technique is with abductor spasmodic dysphonia and certain neurological dysphonias, like those associated with Parkinsonism. As was true for adductor spasmodic dysphonia, empirical observation suggests no more than 50% of patients with abductor spasmodic dysphonia attempting a behavioral approach alone derive functional benefit. Recently, documented improvement for the weak, soft, and breathy voice characteristic of a patient with Parkinson's disease has occurred with the Lee Silverman Voice Treatment (LSVT) method (Ramig, Countryman, Thompson, & Horii, 1995). Although consciously increased loudness is the therapy focus, physiologically this involves increased medial compression forces during phonation.

Voice Care "Prescription"

Voice care "prescriptions" are applicable for all organic lesions requiring phonosurgery. Several of the organic disorders are not likely to respond to traditional behavior modification alone. Those that require phonosurgery, where the vocal fold cover is violated, need a period of carefully controlled voice use postsurgery. This approach to therapy provides a carefully graded voice rest/conservation schedule to allow laryngeal recovery after surgery. See a suggested model in Table 7–1.

The entire process takes a minimum of 6 weeks and frequently takes 8 to 12 weeks. Initially, many voice specialists prescribe complete voice rest for the first week to 10 days following surgery; others require no more than 24 hours followed by modified voice rest. The difference in practice centers around the patient's ability to comply with "complete" vocal rest and whether or not the muscle atrophy that may co-occur with tissue healing, under a complete rest protocol, is a good clinical tradeoff. Determining whether

Table 7–1. Voice care "prescription" following phonosurgery.

Weeks Post-Op	Voice Use
7–10 days	Complete voice rest
2nd and 3rd weeks	Unrestricted quiet talking but only in subdued conversational settings
4th week	Normal conversational voice in controlled/recreational settings, avoiding any overt misuse or overuse
5th week	Normal voice use in social settings with some competing background noise
6th week	Unrestricted voice use in social settings with the exception of overt use

absolute long-term postoperative voice rest is advantageous is difficult because data on the topic are nearly nonexistent. Koufman and Blalock (1989) reported that appropriate vocal therapy was the only variable that resulted in significantly reduced postoperative dysphonia. Patients on absolute voice rest had less postoperative dysphonia than those on vocal conservation but the difference was not statistically significant. As suggested by Zeitels (1995), one of the major advantages of voice rest may be as a means of preventing individuals from returning prematurely to a vocally demanding workplace.

In the total voice rest program, the initial complete voice rest is followed by unrestricted quiet talking in quiet conversational settings for weeks 2 and 3. During week 4, the patient is allowed to use a normal conversational voice in controlled/recreational settings, avoiding any overt misuse or overuse. In week 5, normal voice use in social settings with some competing background noise is permitted. Finally, during week 6, the patient is allowed unrestricted voice use in social settings, with the exception of overt misuse. In any stage of vocal re-entry, the patient needs to be sensitive to vocal or sensory indications of voice failure. If perceived, the patient should revert back to the prior week's restriction. No whispering or yelling is allowed at any time during recovery.

An alternative method of accomplishing a graded return of voice after surgery is to dictate the total amount of quiet voice use allowed each day. Again, this phase would follow 7–10 days of complete voice rest and it would begin with five minutes of quiet talking for 2 days. Every 2 days, there would be a doubling of the daily allowance so that the following progression would occur: 5 minutes, 10 minutes, 20 minutes, 40 minutes, 1.5 hours, 3 hours, 6 hours, and 12 hours. Once the 12-hours-per-day level has been reached, the patient expands his or her voice use into social settings, but avoids overt abuse.

In reality, all of these voice rest options are simple variations on a common theme, differing only in the voice use schedule. All begin with no voice and, over time, gradually increase vocal demands until optimal functioning has returned.

Occasionally, voice rest is supplemented with vocal exercises involving tongue or lip trills which keep the vocal muscles active and tissues loose, while maintaining proper aerodynamic coordination. This technique may be particularly important following phonosurgery when the patient may have edema and attempts to use higher aerodynamic driving pressures to set the folds into vibration. The technique appears to offer a kind of respiratory conditioning without creating secondary hyperfunctional behavior.

Lifestyle Changes

Lifestyle changes are frequently implemented to counteract the tissue irritation process and promote spontaneous recovery. For individuals with contact ulcers, or an irritated larynx, this is a necessary therapy approach. Although much of the treatment related to lifestyle issues ultimately requires medical management, therapeutic intervention in the form of counseling is important. Patients frequently will not understand the unavoidable connection between these factors and their voice problems. They need to be educated about the inflammatory tissue changes that occur and disrupt vocal physiology.

The external and internal true vocal fold irritation created by hot smoke and chemical absorption promotes a double liability from cigarette smoking. Even the danger of exposure to passive smoke is not routinely understood. The impact of alcohol on systemic tissue is another common irritant. Unfortunately, these two lifestyle choices are frequently together in social settings, magnifying their negative effects. Patients should be thoroughly counseled regarding the need for complete smoking cessation as well as reduction of alcohol consumption to a modest level. Patients need to know there is a dangerous synergistic effect with these two substances which have been implicated as causal factors in laryngeal carcinoma.

Uncontrolled gastroesophageal reflux (GER) has become a recent "hot" topic in medical otolaryngology. Although sophisticated diagnostic evaluation and aggressive prescriptive medications are available, a conservative antireflux regimen is frequently all that is necessary to promote tissue recovery. It is imperative that counseling on GER explains the close physical proximity of the larynx to the upper esophageal opening. Furthermore, patients need to be apprised that damaging GER frequently occurs without overt symptoms of heartburn or indigestion, as the caustic stomach juices regurgitate during sleep. As a result, the basic antireflux instructions given to the patient should include the following:

1. Avoid large meals.
2. Avoid late night eating. Attempt to restrict eating beyond normal dinner hours.
3. Avoid lying down immediately after meals. Attempt to maintain an upright posture for at least 2 hours following meals.
4. Avoid alcohol and tobacco products.
5. Eliminate any documented troublesome foods.
6. Avoid aspirin and ibuprofen. Use acetaminophen instead.
7. Lose weight if you are overweight.
8. Avoid the following foods: fatty or fried foods, citrus juices, tomato products, caffeinated coffee, tea, and soda, chocolate, and carbonated beverages. These foods are particularly irritating in the presence of decreased lower esophageal sphincter pressure.
9. Elevate the head of the bed at least 6 inches. Elevation can be accomplished through the use of a pillow wedge or by placing blocks of wood under the headboard. "Pillow stacks" should not be used to accomplish elevation.
10. Use medications as indicated by your physician on a preventive basis after each meal and before bedtime.

The therapeutic goal of these suggestions is to eliminate the symptoms rather than provide after-the-fact relief. Benefits to tissues and the voice usually require a minimum of several weeks before they are realized.

Uncontrolled allergies, particularly airborne irritants, frequently are associated with tissue edema and erythema, either directly or secondary to postnasal drip. "Living with them" may represent admirable courage on the patient's part but does nothing to promote tissue stability. Irritated true vocal folds commonly create vocal problems with pitch (usually too low) and laryngeal quality (breathy, rough, or hoarse). Even the self-prescribed use of off-the-shelf medications can be counterproductive if they severely disrupt the lubricating function of normal secretions. Medical evaluation and prescriptive treatment is the proper recommendation to neutralize this irritative factor. Ultimately, treatment will involve a combination of medical management and substance avoidance.

MEDICAL TREATMENT

The second major treatment option for organic voice disorders, medical management, is the responsibility of the physician. The goal of this option is to address laryngeal tissue status and influence improved vocal performance. More detailed discussions of these topics are provided in individual chapters specific to particular organic conditions. However, presentation of the theoretical principles of medical management is appropriate in this chapter.

Pharmacology

"Drugs" (whether prescription, illegal, off-the-shelf, or common food stuffs) can have both beneficial and detrimental effects on the voice. Awareness of this fact will assist the physician/clinician in either adding or removing a substance from the treatment plan. For example, reduction of caffeine in the diet is appropriate due to its drying affect on the mucous membranes. Because it is a common diuretic substance found in coffee, tea, colas, and chocolate, simple diet recommendations can counteract excessive dryness of tissues and thick secretions. Conversely, increased hydration through water intake, along with increased humidification, is thought to be beneficial to laryngeal tissue lubrication.

Drugs have multiple effects, sometimes impacting on body functions other than those intended. For example, administration of androgens in female patients may have a permanent virilizing effect on the voice. Once changed, the masculine effects cannot be reversed.

Patient sensitivity to drugs is highly variable and requires careful monitoring of effects to avoid allergic reactions or undesirable side effects. Standard dosages are a helpful starting point but prescriptive adjustments are important to attain the best result with the least liability.

Effective medical management of organic voice disorders is accomplished by eliminating or reducing the negative effects of certain drugs. Knowledge of voice and drug interaction is crucial to that end. F. G. Martin (1983, 1984, 1988, 1992) provides detailed information to assist clinicians in avoiding such problems. He divided the voice-related effects of drugs into seven categories: coordination and proprioception, airflow, fluid balance, secretions of the upper respiratory tract, structural changes of the vocal folds, and hearing.

Surprisingly, many of the drugs used for helping voice patients also have a potentially damaging impact. For example, bronchodilators (to improve breath support) and decongestants (to decrease edema) can create tremor and nervousness that can disrupt phonatory stability. Local anesthetic sprays or lozenges to relieve sore throats can reduce pain sensitivity and lead to overall stressing of the voice. Antihistamines can relieve bothersome cold or allergy symptoms but at the cost of excessive drying of mucous membranes.

Typically, pharmacologic management of organic voice disorders encompasses a finite number of options. Generally, there are nine categories of drugs which can be used in the treatment of organic voice disorders.

Antibiotics

Antibiotics are designed to counteract infection and the resulting edema and erythema associated with tissue irritation. Tissue change can occur from direct infection or secondary to postnasal drip and coughing. Antibiotics can be useful in treating irritative factors due to infection, particularly of the upper airway.

Cough Suppressant

Cough suppressants are designed to reduce or eliminate vocal fold trauma associated with severe coughing. Coughing can be associated with several organic disorders including irritative factors, nodules/polyps, lesions of the lamina propria, and contact ulcers.

Mucolytic Agents

Designed to liquify the natural secretions of the upper airway and promote better lubrication, mucolytic agents are relevant to irritative factors, nodules/polyps, lesions of the lamina propria, and contact ulcers.

Antireflux Medications

Antireflux medications are designed to eliminate the regurgitation of caustic stomach juices that irritate laryngeal tissue. They are relevant to irritative factors and contact ulcers.

Decongestants

Decongestants were developed to reduce edema of the upper airway. They are relevant to irritative factors.

Anti-inflammatory Agents

Anti-inflammatory agents are designed to reduce edema and erythema of the upper airway. Aqueous sprays are desirable over aerosols due to the potentially irritating effect of the pressurized delivery substance associated with aerosols. These corticosteroids can also be administered by injection or via a tapering pill dosage and are relevant to irritative factors and contact ulcers.

Antitremor Chemicals

These drugs were designed to reduce neuromuscular tremors and to promote vocal fold vibratory stability. They are relevant to spasmodic dysphonia and other neurological conditions associated with vocal tremor.

Botulinum Toxin

Botulinum toxin (BOTOX®) is designed to interrupt neural signals at motor end plates to reduce neuromuscular contractions of intrinsic laryngeal muscles and to promote phonatory stability. In other words, the toxin produces a paresis of muscles in which it is injected. Botulinum toxin is used to treat both adductor and abductor spasmodic dysphonia.

Myo-neural Junction Facilitators

These drugs were designed to re-establish efficient chemical transmission across the myo-neural junction. They are relevant to neurological disorders such as myasthenia gravis.

SURGERY

The third treatment option for organic voice disorders, surgical intervention, is the responsibility of the head and neck surgeon. The group of relevant procedures is classified as phonosurgery, whose goal is to restore and improve vocal performance. Again, more detailed discussion will be supplied in individual chapters dedicated to specific disorders. In this chapter, an overview of these procedures and their rationale is presented.

The hallmark of phonosurgery is surgical precision, mucosal preservation, and maintenance of the vocal ligament integrity (Ossoff & Courey, 1993). The various types of procedures can be divided into six different categories: tissue excision, tissue injection, tissue vaporization, framework procedures, neuromuscular adjustment, and conservation.

Tissue Excision

Tissue excision is the removal of pathologic tissue and is accomplished through either microdissection tools or the laser. Violation of as little of the surrounding tissue is important, as is maintenance of the layered morphology of the vocal folds. Loss of the body/cover profile through surgical trauma, tissue removal, and/or scarring will destroy the essential mucosal wave dynamics underlying normal voice production.

Surgical removal of nodules is rare and should be reserved for advanced, fibrotic lesions that do not respond favorably to voice therapy. Polyps, in contrast, frequently will not respond to therapy and require surgical removal. This is particularly true for hemorrhagic lesions and intracordal cysts. Contact ulcers do not respond well due to the reduced vascularity of the region which does not promote healing. Furthermore, the basis of contact ulcers may be hyperfunctional phonatory strategies and esophageal reflux which are amenable to behavior modification and medical management.

Tissue Injections

This group of procedures utilizes a variety of injectable materials to change the shape or position of the vocal fold. Gelfoam⁸ provides temporary benefits, as it is readily absorbed by the body. It provides the patient and physician a "test ride" of possible benefits to be derived by using more permanent materials. Teflon⁸ is such an option and has a long history of use with acceptable outcomes except for the potential of either migration or an inflammatory reaction. There is no predictive test to determine the patient's susceptibility for occurrences of either complication. Two other substances providing injection benefits are collagen and autologous fat. Injection techniques have relevance for repair of defects due to tissue loss, scarring, sulcus vocalis, reduction of medial edge bowing, or repositioning the immobile vocal fold closer to midline.

Tissue Vaporization

Accomplished through the use of the laser, organic defects like vocal fold varices and papilloma can be successfully addressed through a procedure known as tissue vaporization. When a tissue sample is not required for biopsy, even mass lesions can be vaporized by the laser.

Framework Procedures

Several different procedures are included in this group, the intent of which is to change the position, shape, or tonicity of the vocal fold. The most common application involves medialization of an immobile vocal fold via an externally inserted implant (Hoffman, 1996; Isshiki, 1977; Koufman, 1986; Tucker, 1990). The implant may be constructed of various materials such as silastic, hydroxyapatite, and Gore-Tex®. Some of the implants are preformed; others must be custom carved at the time of surgery. The ability to adjust the size, shape, and position of the implant, along with the patient's ability to produce voice during the procedure, provides potentially excellent results.

With recent and continuing advances in surgical treatments for laryngeal paralyses, the potential benefits of voice therapy may seem to pale, but data collected by Leonard (1995) suggests otherwise. Twenty-two patients with unilateral paralysis who had not undergone medialization or augmentation were observed twice within 15 months post-onset of paralysis. During the second evaluation, patients who had undergone three to nine sessions of voice therapy were compared with those who had received none. Various objective acoustic and aerodynamic measures were all better in the therapy group, suggesting that voice therapy can improve voice even in the presence of vocal fold paralysis.

To counteract vocal fold flaccidity or the presumed abductory spasms underlying AB spasmodic dysphonia, two types of framework procedures have emerged. Isshiki (1977) described a cricothyroid approximation procedure while Tucker (1985) championed an anterior commissure advancement procedure. In both cases, the vocal folds are stretched, increasing tension that elevates pitch, improves fold approximation, and improves phonatory stability.

To reduce vocal fold tension or counteract adductor spasms (i.e., AD spasmodic dysphonia), an anterior commissure retrusion procedure has been described (Isshiki, 1977; Tucker, 1989). Vocally, the benefits typically involved lower pitch and improved phonatory stability.

Neuromuscular Adjustment

Two distinctly different types of phonosurgery fall under this category: reinnervation for vocal fold paralysis and nerve lysis for AD spasmodic dysphonia. The former type describes the use of a nerve-muscle pedicle inserted into various intrinsic laryngeal muscles (Tucker, 1978, 1993) or actual nerve anastomosis (Crumley, 1985) to restore muscle tone and function. Objective vocal fold performance data are lacking.

Since 1976, lysis of the recurrent laryngeal nerve has been utilized for the treatment of AD spasmodic dysphonia (Dedo, 1976). Despite generally good vocal benefits immediately postsurgery, long-term benefits have been disappointing due to the return of phonatory disruptions (Aronson & DeSanto, 1981, 1983). As confidence in the use of BOTOX® to treat AD spasmodic dysphonia has grown, use of surgical intervention of all types (framework and nerve lysis) has dwindled.

Conservation

Along with growing confidence in the therapeutic management of laryngeal malignancies via radiation and chemotherapy, phonosurgery has fostered more conservative surgical procedures. The use of total laryngectomy as a primary treatment for laryngeal cancer has dropped. The various partial laryngectomy procedures, in addition to cordal and isolated

lesion techniques, have emerged. Their number and variety are beyond the scope of this chapter, but they are beginning to change the vocal rehabilitation process from the traditional postlaryngectomy protocols (see Chapter 13). Retention of part of the laryngeal complex creates challenging dysphonia and dysphagia symptoms not previously seen. Compensatory voice and swallowing techniques, augmentative communication devices, and subsequent phonosurgery are all now part of the treatment mentality for patients with laryngeal cancer.

TREATMENT EFFICACY

Recent focus on health care reform has directed attention to the effectiveness of all treatment, including that for voice disorders. The efficacy of our clinical services, whether behavioral, medical, or surgical, is not well-documented with controlled, systematic investigation. Few studies have used random assignment of treatment groups, control groups, sufficient patient numbers for robustness, and systematic, well-defined intervention methods. This leads primarily to anecdotal, subjective assessment of success, providing neither confidence in results nor generalized ability to larger patient populations.

The basis for this fault is not simple naiveté or lack of motivation. Addressing treatment efficacy through outcome measure is fraught with problems including the following:

1. difficulty isolating phonatory behaviors because of the complex nature of voice production and an individual's ability to compensate, cope, and respond to changes
2. difficulty defining appropriate measures to monitor those behaviors
3. difficulty coordinating the different expectations of the various professional

disciplines involved (surgical, medical, allied health, pedagogical) who each approach treatment and success differently

4. variance in patient expectations
5. limitations imposed by the current technology
6. insurance coverage/service reimbursement issues
7. limitations in the number of patients with a particular disorder seen at any single institution
8. lack of funding to conduct large scale efficacy studies
9. lack of funding to investigate epidemiology of voice disorders.

Ultimately, successful outcomes must be judged contingent on the goals of treatment which can vary greatly. As discussed earlier, the only options for managing voice disorders include behavioral, medical, surgical, or a combination of the three. Furthermore, the basic goal for treating some organic voice disorders is compensatory, achieving the best voice consistent with the laryngeal status. This may, but does not necessarily, include functional restoration to normal. There is also general agreement that future outcome studies will address functional adequacy of voice by requiring measure of success to combine both objective and subjective criteria (Hicks, 1994).

Although the dilemma over treatment efficacy poses a real challenge for future research activity, a complete scholarly void does not exist. Review of the available information regarding voice therapy benefits will be illustrative. Although voice therapy is frequently an integral part of medical and surgical treatment, similar review of medical and surgical benefits is beyond the scope of this chapter. Suffice it to state that similar data exist and are fraught with the same problems that have resulted in limited publications that are sporadic historically and, for the most part, are not scientifically

rigorous. Traditionally, the medical literature on treatment benefits for voice has lacked objective criteria. Recently, technological advances that readily objectify voice and frequent collaboration with voice scientists/clinicians have changed that tradition. Systematic, scientific inquiry is now becoming the standard for validating clinical practice (Hicks, 1993).

No complete review of the voice therapy efficacy literature was available prior to 1993 and the American Speech-Language-Hearing Association's (ASHA) Task Force on Treatment Efficacy in Speech-Language Pathology. At the request of ASHA, Dr. Lorraine Ramig (1994) undertook the task of systematically reviewing the scientific literature from 1921 to the present to identify published information pertaining to treatment efficacy of laryngeal-based voice disorders. She discovered a larger core of relevant literature than one might expect; there were 129 publications, including 55 data-based, peer-reviewed articles; 53 treatment reviews or professional issues articles; and 21 books reporting voice treatment efficacy.

Across all these publications, therapy efficacy was reported in three forms: experimental studies, program evaluation, or case studies. Only the first type, because of design controls, allows the attribution of therapy success to the actual treatment provided. Neither program evaluations nor case studies allows such direct clinical interpretation. Instead, they only support experimental findings by documenting clinical trends and individual experience.

As a group, the identified efficacy publications document therapy benefits attributed to reduction of vocal abuse and hyperfunctioning, compensation for organic laryngeal conditions, and compensation for psychological dysphonias. The largest number of studies related to abuse and hyperfunctioning, addressing primarily vocal nodules, polyps and contact ulcers. Compensation for organic conditions was limited to Parkinson's disease and vocal fold paralysis. Discussion of the psychological dysphonias, without concomitant lesions, is not directly relevant to our focus on organic voice disorders.

Although the current efficacy literature represents both a helpful and hopeful beginning in documenting voice therapy benefits, there is no room for complacency. Documenting the effectiveness of treatment is a current health care mandate which will require future scientific investigation. Without such investigation, the continued viability of specific rehabilitation specialties may be in jeopardy.

QUESTIONS REGARDING CLINICAL ISSUES AND RESEARCH PERSPECTIVES

As is generally true for the pursuit of knowledge, the more one learns, the more questions and uncertainties arise. This is no less true for the human voice and its disorders than for any other part of the body. The list of possible relevant research questions and clinical issues is virtually endless. A comprehensive review of the possibilities is not feasible here but listing a few options might help stimulate and guide future research endeavors.

Efficacy/Outcome Studies

There is a need for controlled, systematic investigation of treatment effectiveness related to all organic and functional dysphonias. The research should include comparison between different treatment options (behavioral vs. surgical) for the same pathology (e.g., intracordal cyst).

The Role of Gastroesophageal Reflux (GER) in Dysphonia

It is essential to determine if the gastroesophageal reflux has a causal, contributory or maintenance impact on dysphonia, and then to clarify if chronic, uncontrolled GER is a predisposing factor to cancer of the larynx and pharynx. It must also be determined if a conservative diet and over-the-counter antacid medications are sufficient to control GER or whether aggressive medical management is necessary to derive sufficient benefit.

Neuromuscular Basis of Spasmodic Dysphonia

Research is needed to establish both quantitative and qualitative evidence of the muscular contractions or imbalance underlying spasmodic dysphonia. It is also necessary to develop alternative strains of Botulinum toxin that produce less prominent side effects and longer acting benefits, or alternate strains of neurotoxins that only require a single injection.

Sulcus Vocalis

The clinical significance of sulcus vocalis with regard to dysphonia needs to be clarified, and effective treatment for the condition needs to be established.

Diplophonia

Questions regarding the physiological basis of diplophonia need to be answered, and effective treatment strategies need to be developed.

Aerosol Propellants of Inhaled Medicines

The effects of aerosol propellants on a variety of disorders, and on the environment, has been the subject of much discussion and debate. With regard to organic voice disorders, research is needed to determine the deleterious effects of these agents on voice production.

Diet Factors

Although we often recommend diet management to patients with dysphonia, we need to research and document the presumed counterproductive effects of common food stuffs such as dairy products, spicy foods, and foods and drinks containing caffeine.

Musculoskeletal Tension

The most efficacious method of reducing a common cause of dysphonia, musculoskeletal tension, needs to be established. Research comparing therapy options such as digital manipulation, imagery, differential tension/relaxation exercises, massage, biofeedback, hypnosis, and muscle relaxers needs to be conducted.

Paradoxical Vocal Cord Motion (PVCM)

Questions exist about the physiological basis of paradoxical vocal cord motion and why it responds well to treatment. By finding and explaining the reasons PVCM typically responds to treatment, the question of how the treatment effectiveness can be generalized to other voice disorders can be explored.

Vagal Dysfunction

Establishing how the vagus nerve is involved in asthma, gastroesophageal reflux, paradoxical vocal cord motion, and hoarseness can possibly provide clarification on how this vagal dysfunction can be treated with a combination of behavioral and medical management.

Molecular Biology

The role of cellular disease mechanisms in laryngeal pathologies such as laryngeal webs and papilloma needs to be explored and documented.

SUMMARY

Typically, the treatment hierarchy in voice begins with the most basic behavioral target at the last complex production level followed by rapid progression to conversational speech and generalization to daily routine use. When patients struggle at higher levels, clinicians go back one step to assure mastery before progressing to increasingly difficult levels.

Treatment techniques are rarely used in isolation. The complexity of voice disorders demands clinicians consider the physiology, psychology, and general well-being of each patient in order to develop a prescriptive treatment program as described in this chapter. This usually means that vocal hygiene concepts are incorporated into the treatment program and that, simultaneously with direct symptom management, the patient may be seen for counseling or treatment of physical health problems.

In developing treatment programs for organic voice disorders, clinicians need to be mindful of the unique abilities and characteristics each patient brings to the clinic. Some are unable to comply with requests for initiating vocal hygiene programs; others make major lifestyle changes. Some find following directions difficult and must move slowly through treatment hierarchies; others jump from isolated sound to conversational speech or singing. Some learn better by visual methods, others by auditory channels. Some are anxious because they must miss work or classes to attend therapy; others are eager. Some are fearful of surgical alternatives while others seek them out. Some have had extensive voice training before entering treatment and hope to attain a better than normal voice; others are satisfied with functional improvement, regardless of the quality. These distinctions are not trivial, and successful treatment requires clinicians to incorporate individual differences into treatment plans. As stated at the beginning of this chapter, each pathology and its presenting dysphonia may be expressed in several different ways. Furthermore, superimposed on the degree and severity of the dysphonia are the personal characteristics of the patient that must be addressed in treatment.

One major change impacting on the behavioral treatment of voice disorders over the last decade is availability of equipment and computer technology. This has afforded most clinicians the opportunity to provide biofeedback for their patients who are experiencing dysphonia. This visual feedback of vocal parameters may be direct visualization of the vocal folds or graphic representation of aerodynamic and acoustic signals. These monitoring techniques generally are most beneficial at the beginning of treatment to facilitate auditory and proprioceptive feedback; patients frequently have not learned to use feedback available to them. Visual feedback helps circumvent old vocal patterns and develop new phonatory habits. Whether the clinician uses yawn-sigh, confidential voice, or some other technique, reliance on visual feedback allows the patient to concentrate more on how voice production feels and sounds when hitting a behavioral target. This tends to improve the accuracy and efficiency of learning the new behaviors.

Technology has also provided clinicians a means of tracking progress, and determining clinical outcomes for specific organic disorders. By entering data for each treatment session, clinicians can chart progress and make comparisons of their treatment results with those reported in the literature. Objective monitoring techniques also provide clinicians a means of comparing efficacy among different techniques. In this age of accountability, efficacy data, both for individual clinicians and across specific organic disorders, becomes extremely important in justifying length of treatment programs and in obtaining reimbursement.

Finally, the evolution of a multidisciplinary collaboration model has revolutionized the care of voice disorders. Combining the benefits of medicine, allied health, and vocal pedagogy in an integrated fashion has provided patients with careful, comprehensive, and sophisticated voice disorder management. Advances in technology, reliance on a physiological perspective, improvements in phonosurgical techniques, and progress in behavioral management efficacy have all contributed to the treatment benefits enjoyed by patients with voice disorders.

In keeping with the interdisciplinary framework recommended by G. Paul Moore (1971) for the diagnosis and treatment of voice disorders, the treatment approach outlined in this chapter reflects the need for consultation among a variety of team members. Primarily, this team should consist of the otolaryngologist, the speech-language pathologist, the patient, and other individuals affected by the patient's voice disorder. Together, they must decide whether the voice therapy approach, the medical approach, or the surgical approach is the best method to resolve the patient's voice disorder. Indeed, within each major treatment group, the options are many, and the team as a whole should decide which approach may be warranted for each individual patient.

REFERENCES

Aronson, A. E. (1990). *Clinical voice disorders: An interdisciplinary approach* (3rd ed.). New York: Thieme.

Aronson, A. E., & De Santo, L. W. (1981). Adductor spasmodic dysphonia: 1½ years after recurrent laryngeal nerve resection. *Annals of Otolology, Rhinology, and Laryngology, 90*, 1–6.

Aronson, A. E., & De Santo, L. W. (1983). Adductor spasmodic dysphonia: Three years after recurrent laryngeal nerve resection. *Laryngoscope, 93,* 1–8.

Boone, D. R., & McFarlane, S. C. (1994). *The voice and voice therapy* (5th ed.). Englewood Cliffs, NJ: Prentice-Hall.

Childers, D. G., Alsaka, Y. A., Hicks, D. M., & Moore, G. P. (1986). Vocal fold vibrations in dysphonia: Model versus measurement. *Journal of Phonetics, 14,* 429–434.

Childers, D. G., Hicks, D. M., Moore, G. P., & Alsaka, Y. A. (1986). A model for vocal fold vibratory motion, contact area, and the electroglottogram. *Journal of the Acoustical Society of America, 80,* 1309–1320.

Childers, D. G., Hicks, D. M., Moore, G. P., Eskenazi, L., & Lalwani, A. L. (1990). Electroglottography and vocal physiology. *Journal of Speech and Hearing Research, 33,* 245–254.

Colton, R. H., & Casper, J. K. (1990). *Understanding voice problems: A psychological perspective for diagnosis and treatment.* Baltimore: Williams & Wilkins.

Crumley, R. (1985). Update of laryngeal reinnervation concepts and options. In B. J. Bailey & H. F. Biller (Eds.), *Surgery of the larynx* (pp. 135–147). Philadelphia: W. B. Saunders.

Dedo, H. H. (1976). Recurrent nerve section for spastic dysphonia. *Annals of Otology, Rhinology, and Laryngology, 85,* 451–459.

Fisher, H. B. (1966). *Improving voice and articulation.* Boston: Houghton-Mifflin.

Hicks, D. M. (1993). Assessment and documentation of voice disorders. *Operative Techniques in Otolaryngology—Head and Neck Surgery, 4,* 196–198.

Hicks, D. M. (1994, November). *Using outcome measures for assessing treatment effectiveness.* Short course presented at the Annual Convention of the American Speech-Language-Hearing Association, New Orleans, LA.

Hicks, D. M., & Sweat, L. L. (1984). Whisper: Help or hindrance to the professional voice. In V. Lawrence (Ed.), *Transcripts of the Twelfth Symposium: Care of the Professional Voice* (pp. 56–60). New York: The Voice Foundation.

Hixon, T. J., Goldman, M. D., & Mead, J. (1973). Kinematics of the chest wall during speech production: Volume displacements of the rib cage, abdomen, and lung. *Journal of Speech and Hearing Research, 16,* 78–115.

Hixon, T. J., Mead, J. & Goldman, M. D. (1976). Dynamics of the chest wall during speech production: Function of the thorax, rib cage, diaphragm, and abdomen. *Journal of Speech and Hearing Research, 19,* 297–356.

Hixon, T. J., Watson, P. J., Harris, F. P., & Perlman, N. B. (1988). Relative volume changes of the rib cage and abdomen during prephonatory chest wall posturing. *Journal of Voice, 2,* 13–19.

Hoffman, H. T. (1996, January). *Thyroplasty: Gore–Tex technique.* Paper presented at the Clinical Laryngology Update meeting of the National Center for Voice and Speech, Iowa City, IA.

Hoit, J. D., & Hixon, T. J. (1986). Body type and speech breathing. *Journal of Speech and Hearing Research, 29,* 313–324.

Isshiki, N. (1977). *Functional surgery of the larynx: With special reference to percutaneous approach.* Tokyo: Maeda Press.

Kotby, M. N., El–Sady, S. R., Basiouny, S. E., Abou-Rass, Y. A., & Hegazi, M. A. (1991). Efficacy of the accent methods of voice therapy. *Journal of Voice, 5,* 316–320.

Koufman, J. (1986). Laryngoplasty for vocal cord medialization: An alternative to Teflon[®]. *Laryngoscope, 96,* 726–731.

Koufman, J. A. (1991). The otolaryngologic manifestations of gastroesophageal reflux disease (GERD): A clinical investigation of 225 patients using ambulatory 24-hour pH acid and pepsin in the development of laryngeal injury. *Laryngoscope, 101*(Suppl. 53), 1–78.

Koufman, J. A., & Blalock, P. D. (1989). Is voice rest never indicated. *Journal of Voice, 3,* 87–91.

Leonard, R. (1995, December). *Challenges for the voice clinician—1995.* Paper presented at the Annual Convention of the American Speech-Language-Hearing Association, Orlando, FL.

Martin, F. G. (1983). Drugs and the voice. In V. Lawrence (Ed.), *Transcripts of the Twelfth Symposium: Care of the professional voice* (pp. 124–132). New York: The Voice Foundation.

Martin, F. G. (1984). The influence of drugs on voice. In V. Lawrence (Ed.), *Transcripts of* the *Thirteenth Symposium: Care of the Professional Voice* (pp. 191–201). New York: The Voice Foundation.

Martin, F. G. (1988). Tutorials: Drugs and vocal function. *Journal of Voice, 2,* 338–344.

Martin, F. G. (1992, November). *Drugs and voice.* Paper presented at the Annual Convention of the American Speech-Language-Hearing Association, San Antonio, TX.

Monoson, P., & Zemlin, W. R. (1984). Quantitative study of whisper. *Folia Phoniatrica, 36,* 53–65.

Moore, G. P. (1971). *Organic voice disorders.* Englewood Cliffs, NJ: Prentice-Hall.

Moore, G. P., Hicks, D. M., & Childers, D. G. (1986). Some physiologic correlates of phonatory quality. In V. Lawrence (Ed.), *Transcripts of the Fourteenth Symposium: Care of the Professional Voice* (pp. 222–230). New York: The Voice Foundation.

Morrison, M., & Rammage, L. (1994). *The management of voice disorders.* San Diego: Singular Publishing Group.

National Center for Voice and Speech. (1994). *A vocologist's guide: Voice therapy and training.* Iowa City, IA: NCVS.

Ossoff, R. H., & Courey, M. S. (1993, October). *Microlaryngeal surgery in the professional voice patient.* Instruction course presented at the Annual Meeting of the AAO-HNS, Minneapolis, MN.

Ramig, L. O. (1994). Treatment efficacy of laryngeal-based voice disorders. Unpublished manuscript.

Ramig, L. O., Countryman, S., Thompson, L. L., Horii, Y. (1995). Comparison of two forms of intensive speech treatment for Parkinson disease. *Journal of Speech and Hearing Research, 38,* 1232–1251.

Roy, N., & Leeper, H. A. (1993). Effects of the manual laryngeal musculo-skeletal tension reduction technique as a treatment for functional voice disorders: Perceptual and acoustic measures. *Journal of Voice, 7,* 242–249.

Smith, S., & Thyme, K. (1976). Statistic research on changes in speech due to pedagogic treatment (the accent method). *Folia Phoniatrica, 28,* 98–103.

Solomon, N. P., McCall, G. N., Trossett, M. W., & Gray, W. C. (1989). Laryngeal configuration and constriction during two types of whispering. *Journal of Speech and Hearing Research, 32,* 161–174.

Stemple, J. C., Glaze, L., & Gerdeman, B. (1995). *Clinical voice pathology: Theory and management* (2nd ed.). San Diego: Singular Publishing Group.

Tucker, H. M. (1978). Human laryngeal reinnervation: Long-term experience with the nerve-muscle pedicle technique. *Laryngoscope, 88,* 598–604.

Tucker, H. M. (1985). Anterior commissure laryngoplasty for adjustment of vocal fold tension. *Annals of Otology, Rhinology, and Laryngology, 94,* 547–549.

Tucker, H. M. (1989). Laryngeal framework surgery in the management of spasmodic dysphonia: A preliminary report. *Annals of Otology, Rhinology, and Laryngology, 98,* 52–54.

Tucker, H. M. (1990). Combined laryngeal framework medialization and reinnervation for unilateral vocal fold paralysis. *Annals of Otology, Rhinology, and Laryngology, 99,* 778–781.

Tucker, H. M. (1993). *The larynx* (2nd ed.). New York: Thieme Medical Publishers.

Zeitels, S. M. (1995). Premalignant epithelium and microinvasive cancer of the vocal fold: The evolution of phonomicrosurgical management. *Laryngoscope, 105*(3, Pt 2), 1–51.

CHAPTER 8

THE IRRITATED LARYNX: EDEMA AND INFLAMMATION

PEAK WOO, M.D.

INTRODUCTION AND DEFINITIONS

Acute Laryngitis

Acute inflammation of the upper airways is one of the most common causes of organic voice disorders. The effects of the common cold and other viruses result in temporary but troublesome dysphonia. Such afflictions are usually only a transient annoyance unless one is a voice professional or singer. Repeated episodes of vocal disability interfere with livelihood. The desire to meet financial needs and maintain a professional reputation with regard to voice usage may bring the patient to a health care professional. If the problem fails to resolve over weeks to months, a chronic problem may be present, and this, in turn, may progress to disabling and permanent dysphonia. When a condition results in effortful and/or painful communication, it brings even the most recalcitrant patient to seek care.

The term *laryngitis* is a clinical descriptive term that covers the entire spectrum of disorders of the larynx that involve the pathophysiologic process of inflammation.

Laryngitis loosely encompasses the spectrum of disorders from acute inflammatory edema to scar formation, scar being the sequelae of tissue inflammation and repair. Because inflammatory response is a physiologic process, laryngitis is often classified as acute, subacute, chronic, or recurrent. This helps to describe the clinical course and prognosis of these disorders. Table 8–1 lists the various acute and chronic inflammatory disorders that are commonly found in a laryngologist's practice.

Common to all forms of laryngitis is the basic pathophysiologic process of inflammation and repair. With acute inflammation and repair, fluid and hemodynamic changes occur in vocal folds, altering their mass and vibratory characteristics, thereby producing dysphonia. Pharmacologic treatment and speech therapy can be used to blunt the severity of the response. Speech therapy may be used to decrease the inciting injury from vocal fold trauma due to voice abuse. Corticosteroids may be used to reduce the severity of the body's response to injury. Inflammation, when it is persistent, may progress to chronic inflammation resulting in permanent tissue changes and permanent dysphonia.

Table 8-1. Laryngitis and its variants: acute and chronic inflammatory disorders of the larynx.

Acute Disorders

    Common laryngitis (viral)

    Bacterial laryngitis

    Allergic laryngitis

    Traumatic laryngitis of voice abuse

    Mucosal hemorrhage with laryngitis

    Other: radiation laryngitis, smoke inhalation

Chronic Disorders

    Infectious laryngitis

        Bacterial

        Tuberculosis, leprosy

        Fungal (Candida, blastomycosis, histoplasmosis, coccidioidomycosis)

    Infiltrative disorders with systemic disease

        Amyloidosis

        Bullous pemphigus

        Bechets disease

        Rheumatoid arthritis

        Wegener

        Sjögrens syndrome

        Sarcoidosis

    Irritative laryngitis without epithelial hyperplasia

        Nonspecific laryngitis

        Reinke's edema with polypoid degeneration

        Microangioma and varix

        Hemorrhage and scarring after exudative laryngitis

    Irritative laryngitis with epithelial hyperplasia

        Hyperplastic laryngitis

        Sulcus vocalis

        Laryngitis sicca

        Pachydermia laryngitis

        Reflux laryngitis

        Contact granuloma

    Atrophic laryngitis associated with aging

Endocrine and Metabolic Changes

    Menstrual cycle changes

    Virilization drugs

    Hypothyroidism

    Senile and postmenopausal changes

An understanding of inflammation, repair, and local homeostasis is important to managing organic voice disorders. The organic voice disorders that will be addressed in this chapter deal with the pathologic process of inflammation. Inflammation is a reaction of vascularized living tissues to local injury. Like all living tissue, vocal folds are dependent on blood supply and bathed in a fluid environment. Besides inflammation, fluid homeostasis changes associated with endocrine and aging changes can affect the voice. Similarly, hemodynamic changes due to hemorrhage and thrombosis may affect laryngeal tissue.

Because phonation depends on oscillation of delicate vocal folds, even small alterations in local tissue homeostasis can result in changes in perceived vocal quality. It is the voice care professional's duty to be aware of the varieties of causative factors that may bring the patient to consultation. To be successful, a search of causative factors requires a healthy investigative spirit.

Chronic Laryngitis

Chronic laryngitis refers to inflammatory conditions of the larynx distinguished by chronic inflammatory cellular infiltration. Histopathologically, there is little to distinguish the various clinical forms. Thus, reflux laryngitis and pachydermia of long-term smoking look similar histologically (Bain, Harrington, Thomas, & Schafer, 1983; Wilson, White, von Haache, & Maran et al., 1989). Both are characterized by acute and chronic inflammatory cellular infiltrate with or without epithelial hyperplasia. Chronic laryngitis refers to a broad category of disorders that result in a chronic inflammatory response. Patterns of the chronic tissue response can take one or several forms. These include (a) infiltrative disorders such as amyloidosis (Charrow, Pass, Ruken, 1971; Hughes,

Paonessa, Conway, 1984); (b) chronic granulomatous diseases affecting the larynx such as sarcoidosis, tuberculosis, and fungal laryngitis; (c) chronic nonspecific inflammation (e.g., contact ulcer, bacterial laryngitis, laryngitis sicca) (Brodnitz, 1961); and (d) proliferative processes involving the epithelial layer (e.g., varix, hyperplastic laryngitis, keratosis, sulcus vocalis) (McGavran, Bauer, & Ogura, 1960).

Factors contributing to chronic laryngitis may include (a) environmental exposures to dust, chemicals, or toxins; (b) immune and autoimmune disorders; and (c) chronic infection or inflammation in organs contiguous with the larynx (e.g., chronic reflux laryngitis, chronic sinobronchial infections).

PATHOGENESIS

Laryngitis is inflammation and reaction of the vascularized tissue of the larynx to injury. The tissue response sets into motion a complex sequence of events which involves tissue defense and cellular repair. The inflammatory response is a highly organized series of steps to destroy, wall off, and repair the damage. In the process of repairing injury, an often undesirable functional side effect for the larynx is scar formation. Common laryngeal disorders such as laryngeal edema, acute and chronic laryngitis, and vocal fold scarring are results of attempts to alleviate inflammation. These processes cause dysphonia. Although it is common to think of bacteria or viral diseases as causes for acute laryngitis, many forms of injury to the larynx exist. These include thermal injury, radiation injury, chemical injury, and trauma from vocal misuse and abuse. The larynx, by virtue of its anatomy, sits at a critical point in the aerodigestive tract. Therefore, acute and chronic inflammation of these sites may also affect the larynx by local contamination. Examples of these problems include: (a) sino-bronchial infection causing laryngitis (bacterial and viral); (b) reflux laryngitis (chemical and acid); (c) traumatic laryngitis (voice abuse); and (d) inhalation laryngitis (thermal). Figure 8–1 is a schematic diagram of the pathophysiology of acute and chronic inflammatory changes of the larynx.

It is useful to classify inflammatory disorders of the larynx into acute and chronic inflammatory patterns. Such a classification schema is useful for prognosis and treatment purposes. The differential diag-

noses for patients presenting with acute versus chronic laryngitis are as varied as are the extent of workup and treatment.

Acute Laryngitis

Acute laryngitis applies to an inflammatory disorder of the larynx, usually of short duration lasting hours to days, which affects the otherwise healthy patient. During the early phase, the normal laryngeal mucosa experiences vascular dilation, increased blood flow, and vascu-

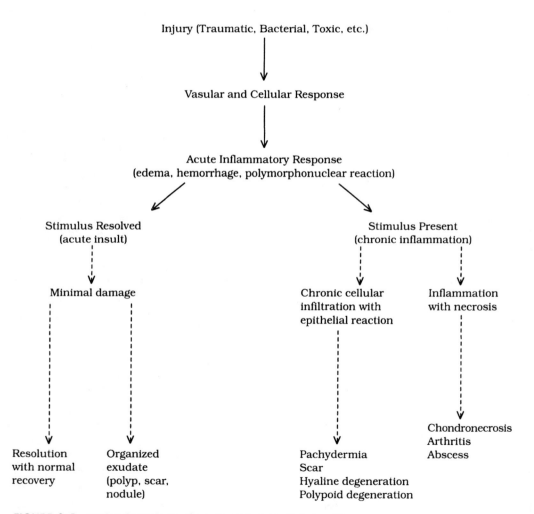

FIGURE 8-1. Pathophysiology of acute and chronic laryngitis.

lar stasis. The vascularized tissue of the vocal folds undergoes increased vascular permeability with exudate of protein-rich fluid into the extravascular space. The increased vascular permeability results in laryngeal edema. Permeability changes in the tissue are then followed by infiltration of white blood cells into extravascular space. This corresponds to the classic observations of erythema (rubor), pain (dolor), and heat (color).

Acute inflammation of the larynx is a common disorder encountered by laryngologists. Laryngeal edema after intubation, shouting at rock concerts, and severe coughing are often accompanied by transient voice changes. The extent of the injury to tissue is quite variable. Acute inflammation may result in one of the four possible outcomes: (a) complete resolution, indicating restoration of the site of injury to normal; (b) healing by scar formation; (c) abscess formation and necrosis; and (d) progression to chronic inflammation.

Ideally, a patient will have limited injury and little tissue destruction, and the tissues will heal with little or no evidence of permanent damage. However, as indicated in the previous paragraph, healing is frequently marked by the formation of scar tissue. When mucosal injury is extensive, or if an exudative process results, the healing process often involves fibrosis and scarring with collagen deposition. In the delicate vocal folds, especially in the superficial layer of the lamina propria, dense collagen fibers are noticeably absent. When unwanted collagen is deposited due to the inflammatory response, it may interfere with the normal vibration of the vocal folds during phonation. One example is the nonvibratory segments seen in singers after multiple vocal fold hemorrhages (Baker, 1962).

Abscess formation and necrosis further complicate the recovery process. In normal tissue, white blood cells and macrophages scavenge the site of tissue injury. From this exudate formation, abscess and necrosis of tissue may result. With antibiotics, abscess and necrosis are increasingly rare in the larynx. Except for life-threatening infections such as epiglottitis and radiation-induced chondronecrosis, acute infections progressing to abscess and necrosis are now unusual.

There are also instances in which the inciting stimulus persists, and the inflammatory response becomes protracted and goes from recurrent acute inflammation to a chronic inflammatory response. Chronic inflammation may be due to ongoing stimulation which promotes laryngeal tissue reaction and repair or a repair process that persists after the initial causative agent has been removed. An irritating stimulus such as smoke or alcohol may be an agitant resulting in pachydermia laryngica, or it may be due to acid reflux resulting in chronic reflux laryngitis (Ward & Berci, 1982). The irritation may be due to an autoimmune response resulting in rheumatoid arthritis, or it may be due to a host of bacterial and fungal agents that promote a chronic inflammatory response. (Haar, Chandhry, Kaplan, & Milley, 1980). Tuberculosis, fungal, and other agents producing granulomatous laryngitis are examples of bacterial and fungal agents which produce chronic laryngitis (Levenson, Ingerman, Grimes, & Robett, 1984).

Acute Viral Laryngitis

Acute viral laryngitis is usually a consequence of viral inflammation of the upper respiratory tract. The common rhinovirus and influenza virus are common pathogens. Multiple other viral agents have been implicated as causes of viral laryngitis.

The incidence of acute laryngitis is difficult to estimate because most patients with acute laryngitis do not present for evaluation. Being a disease that is usually of limited duration, the average person undertakes a period of expectant treatment while they "wait out" a cold or laryngitis. The same can be said for the acute laryngitis that follows overusing the voice at a sporting event or rock concert. Traumatically induced edema of the larynx lasts up to 2 or 3 days and gradually returns to normal with complete or modified voice rest. Two exceptions to this scenario are (a) patients with bacterial suppurative laryngitis that results in fever and supraglottitis and (b) patients with special voice needs. This is because patients with supraglottitis progress to airway compromise and voice professionals seek out care for treatment due to professional and vocational needs.

When a patient presents for evaluation of acute voice loss and acute viral laryngitis is suspected, the chronological history and identification of the inciting agent is most important in the appropriate diagnosis and treatment. Because acute laryngitis is a nonspecific inflammatory response, a careful history should help the clinician to differentiate among the various possibilities. These possibilities include voice abuse, nonspecific laryngitis, and bacterial or viral laryngitis.

Complaints of vocal dysfunction in laryngitis are centered on complaints of limitation of vocal range and/or phonatory function and pain or discomfort associated with voice production. Cough and a painful irritated larynx are symptomatology which more commonly bring the patient to evaluation.

Professional voice patients who are well-trained usually think of a medical or organic condition as the cause for their vocal complaints (Baker, 1962; Rubin, 1967; von Leden, 1960). Although vocal fold hemorrhage, nodules, and acute inflammation do occur, the finding of hyperfunction or functional voice abuse leading to an organic laryngeal problem is very common. Therefore, it is important for the voice health professional to carefully differentiate traumatic laryngitis and functional voice disorders from laryngitis due to viral illnesses.

Acute viral laryngitis is usually associated with other respiratory symptoms such as coryza, rhinorrhea, and cough. A sore throat may herald the presence of pharyngitis prior to laryngitis. Fever, pain when swallowing, and generalized throat irritation often accompany voice changes. Interestingly, voice changes are often later in onset and voice quality is frequently worse during the resolution stages of the acute upper respiratory infection. Occasionally the tracheo-bronchial tree is spared and the patient may present with only pain and sore throat to be followed by a husky poor voice quality. A low grade fever is common, but a high fever with dysphagia should lead the clinician to suspect bacterial laryngitis or supraglottitis. If the infectious etiology is viral, the vocal symptoms rapidly clear in 4–6 days. During the resolution stage of acute laryngitis, the patients often complain of increased phlegm. Throat clearing and irritative symptoms lasting up to 2 weeks are not uncommon after acute laryngitis.

Bacterial infections such as *Beta Streptococcus*, *Hemophilus Influenza* and *Pneumococcus* may complicate the course of viral laryngitis and prolong the course of illness. Figure 8–2 shows an example of hyperemia of the vocal folds with areas of suppuration below the vocal folds. Note that the vocal folds are darkened and thickened. These infections are often associated with rigor, fever, and chills. Tenacious thick phlegm with cough often prevents a good night of sleep and brings the patient to the physician's office after several days of home treatment. Such a history is easily differentiated from laryngitis due to other causes.

Vocal Fold Tear and Hemorrhage

Mucosal tear and submucosal hemorrhage are two feared complications of acute la-

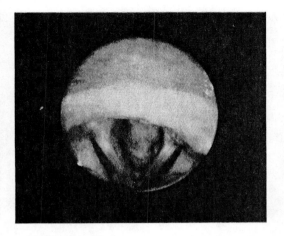

FIGURE 8-2. Acute suppurative laryngitis.

ryngeal inflammation and may result in permanently altered voice.

Mucosal tear results from microtrauma when patients aggressively phonate or cough. The consequence of such a tear is often healing by secondary intention and vocal fold scarring. Unlike soft vocal fold nodules which are reversible, microtears may result in a residual scar and a nonvibratory segment. Such an adynamic segment of the vocal folds results in some further decrement in voice elasticity and may be permanent.

Noninfective or Nonspecific Laryngitis

Acute inflammations of the larynx not attributable to viral or bacterial etiologies have been termed noninfective laryngitis. These include: allergic laryngitis; traumatic laryngitis of vocal abuse; and thermal, chemical, and caustic irritation of the larynx. Although the presentation and clinical course of this spectrum of disorders is variable, the pathogenesis and treatment of information and tissue response is sufficiently similar to be included together.

Chronic Laryngitis

Chronic inflammation of the larynx appears to cause changes at two major sites. These changes occur in the epithelial and subepithelial layers of vocal folds. Benign mucosal disorders may result in changes in normal epithelial proliferation and maturation. These epithelial proliferative disorders include hyperkeratosis, dyskeratosis, parakeratosis, acanthosis, and cellular atypia. Figure 8–3 is an example of benign keratosis in a chronic heavy smoker. Figure 8–4 is an example of chronic laryngitis with false vocal fold hypertrophy.

Chronic inflammation in the subepithelium has an important role in the development of Reinke's edema and polypoid degeneration (Kambic, Rodsel, Zargi, & Acko, 1981). Other submucosal proliferative disorders which may represent a response to trauma and inflammation are microangiomas of the vocal folds. Figure 8–5 is an example of posterior pachydermia laryngica and Reinke's edema with polypoid degeneration in a heavy smoker.

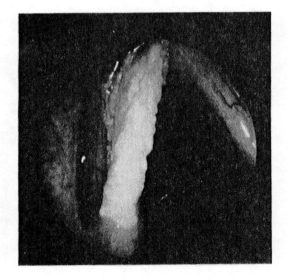

FIGURE 8-3. Benign epithelial hyperplasia in a heavy smoker.

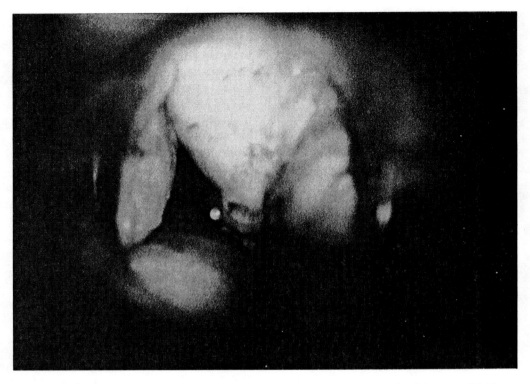

FIGURE 8–4. Chronic laryngitis with localized amyloidosis involving the false vocal folds.

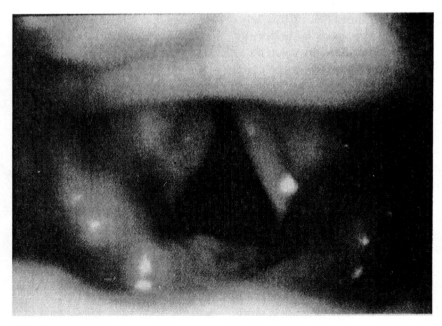

FIGURE 8–5. Pachydermia laryngica and polypoid degeneration in a chronic heavy smoker.

Besides local tissue response to chronic irritation, systemic chronic inflammatory disorders may cause chronic laryngitis. Rheumatoid arthritis, systemic lupus erythematosus, and mucosal ulcerative disorders such as pemphigus and Bechets may affect the laryngeal mucous membrane and joints. (Charrow et al., 1971). Airway and voice compromise occasionally complicate these systemic inflammatory disorders. To diagnose these disorders, a high level of suspicion followed by biopsy, culture, and special histopathologic studies may be necessary.

Chronic Nonspecific Laryngitis

This form of laryngitis is a disease of adults in their 40s to 60s. This age group is more commonly afflicted due to their higher incidence of smoking and environmental exposure to fumes and work-related irritants.

Chronic nonspecific laryngitis is found in heavy smokers and drinkers (McGavran et al., 1960). These patients rarely complain of dysphonia despite their severe symptoms. Occupational factors may play a role in pathogenesis of chronic nonspecific laryngitis. A work-related entity should be considered in patients who work in foundries, beauty shops, paper mills, printing shops, and other sites where chemical, thermal, and fine foreign particulates may be inhaled.

Medication side effects often contribute to chronic nonspecific laryngitis. Patients on psychotropic drugs with anticholinergic side effects have a dry throat with a hoarse, rough sound. Allergic and bacterial rhinosinusitis with laryngeal involvement may progress to chronic nonspecific laryngitis if antigen exposure is prolonged.

Chronic Hyperplastic Laryngitis

Chronic hyperplastic laryngitis is a condition often seen in males and females with chronic laryngitis. These patients have vocal fold epithelial changes associated with chronic inflammation. These changes can vary from mild epithelial hyperplasia to severe dysplasia. Clinically, chronic hyperplastic laryngitis often cannot be differentiated from chronic laryngitis or early carcinoma. The incidence of this disorder is high in patients with risks for epithelial neoplasia and chronic laryngitis. Patients typically have a long history of smoking or drinking. They are often abusive of their voices and typically spend time in dry or dusty environments. Unlike patients with nonspecific chronic laryngitis, these patients have obvious epithelial changes of the vocal folds which mimic a laryngeal mass.

ONSET AND COURSE OF THE DISORDER

Acute Laryngitis

Acute laryngitis is usually preceded by symptoms of chills and malaise. The throat typically is dry and irritated. Due to interstitial edema, the fundamental frequency of the voice often drops, and sustained phonation may become unreliable. If left untreated, the laryngeal inflammation may progress and result in severe dysphonia.

During acute laryngitis, vocal folds have a pink color with an appearance of fine velvet. The fine capillaries on the surface of the vocal folds are dilated as a result of increased blood flow. As the infection progresses, the suppurative stages of inflammation result in copious secretions which cause frequent expectoration and cough. The patient often has excessive secretion and expectoration, and coughing and throat clearing become increasingly painful. As the amount of secretions and the accompanying pain increase, sleep becomes impossible.

The suppurative stage is usually limited to 48–72 hours. This is followed by gradual resolution. During the resolution stage, the secretions become less viscous, though still copious. Voice function returns but retains a veiled quality. Throat irritation is less although a scratchy irritated throat often is present for many weeks after the acute inflammation has subsided. Full restitution of vocal function usually occurs in 7 to 10 days.

Vocal Fold Tear and Hemorrhage

Vocal fold hemorrhage due to vascular leakage may result in normal healing without damage. Extensive macrophage and fibroblast stimulation followed by healing may change the layered viscoelastic properties of the vocal folds and reduce vocal fold pliability.

Noninfective or Nonspecific Laryngitis

Mild traumatic laryngitis is often present after exhaustive voice use (Zhao, Cai, & Wang, 1991). Figure 8–6 is an example of nodular diathesis with mucous stranding seen frequently in patients with traumatic laryngitis and phonasthenia. The teacher who spends his or her day lecturing and speaking often has mild transient mucosal edema with voice loss. Nonspecific irritants such as second-hand smoke, hair spray, dry temperatures, and sudden temperature changes also may result in mild laryngeal edema with irritation. Medications that have drying effects on the mucosa include diuretics, antihypertensives, antihistamines, and psychotropic drugs with anticholinergic side effects.

Nonspecific laryngitis is suspected when voice loss and laryngeal irritation are present without the usual symptoms of upper respiratory infection. The clinical course of nonspecific laryngitis is variable and may range from brief to prolonged. The causative agent of nonspecific laryngitis is usually identified as a laryngeal irritant. Appropriate identification of the inciting agent and avoidance is the best course of treatment. In the patient with habitual loud speaking voice and traumatic laryngitis, vocal re-education by a speech-language pathologist is the best approach. Patients with dry throats due to medication side effects are best treated by aggressive vocal hygiene, hydration, and changes in medication regimen.

Chronic Nonspecific Laryngitis

The history of chronic laryngitis is one of the recurrent episodes of dysphonia with progressive inability to return to normal voice. The severity of vocal difficulties may fluctuate, but voice quality does not return to normal. The voice gradually deteriorates over weeks to many months. In the majority, pain and dysphonia are not prominent features. The patient may exhibit chronic throat clearing but rarely will complain of pain or discomfort. When the patient coughs, thick tenacious fluid is not present. The thick mucous is a sign of infection or inflammation. In some patients, this is accompanied by a sensation of a "lump in the throat." The voice in these patients is often poor and ventricular phonation is a common finding (Figure 8–7).

A bacterial etiology for chronic laryngitis should be suspected if there is transient improvement while on antibiotics followed by recurrent relapses when the course of antibiotics is concluded.

Chronic Hyperplastic Laryngitis

Histologically, there are variable degrees of epithelial hyperplasia with atypia. Production of keratin may be prominent along with acanthosis and parakeratosis. Involvement of the subepithelial layer by acute and chronic inflammatory infiltrates is common. There are variable amounts of

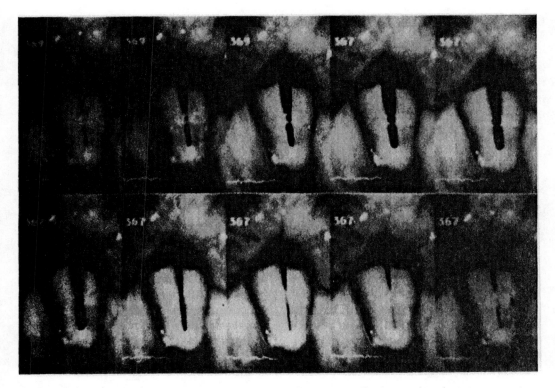

FIGURE 8–6. Nodular diathesis in a teacher with nonspecific laryngitis due to excessive demands on her voice.

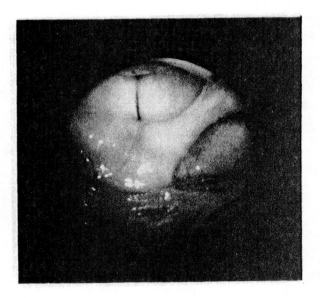

FIGURE 8–7. Ventricular phonation as a compensatory mechanism for stiff nonvibrating folds.

fibroblasts and collagen in the stroma. The malignant potential of benign keratosis of the larynx is low. However, intermediate degrees of cellular atypia and its malignant transformation potential have not been thoroughly studied. The uncertain prognosis for these lesions leads most physicians to recommend their complete removal, thereby popularizing the concept of vocal fold stripping.

It is generally agreed that chronic inflammation and irritation represent one important factor in production of chronic hyperplastic laryngitis. Epithelial hyperplasia is one form of tissue reaction to chronic irritation and inflammation. Clinical terms that have been used to describe this condition in the larynx include laryngitis sicca, chronic hyperplastic laryngitis, pachydermia of the larynx, leukoplakia, benign keratosis, and others. Histological examination of tissue often fails to differentiate between the aforementioned clinical forms. Chronic hyperplastic laryngitis may be thought of as a variant of chronic inflammation disorder that has progressed to vocal fold epithelial changes.

MEDICAL CONSIDERATIONS

Acute Viral Laryngitis

The history should include a careful review of symptoms of the gastrointestinal tract, pulmonary system, nasal-sinus passages, and neurological disorders. Table 8–2 is a partial list of common symptoms which may have relationships to, and may cause, laryngeal inflammation.

The medical history should also include a review of prescription medications. Medications taken by the patient may promote mucosal drying and mucositis (e.g., diuret-

Table 8–2. Organ symptoms associated with laryngeal inflammation.

Organ System	Symptom
Gastrointestinal tract	Regurgitation
	Dyspepsia
	Nocturnal cough
	Chronic throat clearing
	Lump in throat sensation
Pulmonary	Wheezing
	Shortness of breath
	Cough
	Sputum production
Sinus	Postnasal drip or discharge
	Chronic honking or sniffing
	Thick tenacious secretions
	Facial pain and pressure
Endocrine	Changes in sex drive
	Excessive heat or cold
	Change of voice with menses or during menopause

ics, antihypertensives, psychotropic drugs). Over-the-counter medications also may cause local drying and mucosal injury (e.g., antihistamines and aspirin). Table 8–3 is a list of medications that have the potential to create xerostomia.

Table 8–3. Medications associated with xerostomia (dry mouth).

Classification	Generic Name	Product Name
Anticholinergics	Atropine	Enlon-Plus
	Scopolamine Propanthetine	Transderm Scope®
		Pro-Banthine
Antihypertensives	Guanethidine	Ismelin
	Clonidine	Catapres
Antihistamines	Diphenhydramine	Benadryl
	Chlorpheniramine	Chlor-Trimeton
Antipsychotics	Chlorpromazine	Thorazine
	Promazine	Sparine
	Thioridazine	Mellaril
Anorectics	Amphetamines	
	Diethylpropion	Tenuate and Tenuate Dospan
Narcotics	Meperidine	Demerol
	Morphine	
Anticonvulsants	Carbamazepine	Tegretol
	Lithium Carbonate	Lethane®
Antiparkinsonian	Benztropine	Cogentin
	Trihexyphenidyl	Artane
Antineoplastics	Busulfan	Myleran
	Procarbazine HCl	
Antispasmodics	Dicyclomine hydrocloride	Bentyl
	Hyoscyamine sulfate	Levsin and Levsinex
		Paxil
Sympathomimetics	Ephedrine	Primatene, Quadrinal, Quelidrine, Tedral
Antidepressants	Tricyclic	Doxepin, Amitriptyline,
	MAO Inhibitors	Isocarboxazid, Phenelzine
Antianxiety agents	Meprobamate	Miltown
	Benzodiazepines	Valium, Librium, Serax, Antivan
	Hydroexzine	Atarax
Muscle Relaxants	Orphenadrine	Norflex
	Cyclobenzaprine	Flexeril
Diuretics	Hydrochlorothiazide	HydroDiuril
Antiemetics	Metoclopramide	Reglan

Work history should include inquiries as to smoking and exposure to second-hand smoke; exposure to fumes, dyes, and petrochemical distillates, photochemical acids and bases; and rapid changes in cold and warm environments. Nonspecific allergies to environmental irritants are a common source of throat irritation which can progress to disabling dysphonia.

If appropriate, a voice history and log of difficulties associated with specific vocal activities should be started. Besides the duration of voice use, the environment where voice difficulties occur should also be noted. Also, for patients who are singers, differentiation between vocal qualities of the speaking voice versus the singing voice should be noted. Patients with extraordinary voice needs should have a thorough search of factors that may contribute to laryngeal irritation. This may take the form of a questionnaire or be accomplished through the use of direct questioning. Table 8–2 is a list of common complaints which may be elicited in patients with acute and chronic laryngeal inflammation. The interaction between organic illness and hyperfunctional voice disorder in voice professionals often warrants a multidisciplinary approach to diagnosis and treatment, involving the speech-language pathologist, voice coach, and physician. Such an approach is often helpful in reducing the duration of diagnosis and treatment for the more difficult cases.

Chronic Nonspecific Laryngitis

Chronic bacterial laryngitis is suggested by findings of diffuse inflammation with suppuration. The larynx is swollen and dry. Pachydermia of the interarytenoid area is often present. Tissue response to infection of the false vocal folds, arytenoid, and interarytenoid areas may be so intense that a mass lesion is suspected. Patients may be advised to have a microla-ryngeal examination to rule out neoplasia. Erythema of the aerodigestive tract is rarely limited to the larynx. Pharyngeal inflammation is often obvious. Thick mucus collects in the posterior pharynx. The posterior pharyngeal wall appears thickened and has an uneven pebble stone appearance due to areas of lymphoid hypertrophy.

The otolaryngologist will look for infections of the tonsil, nasopharynx, and sinus areas as primary sites of infection. The lung and tracheo-bronchial tree should also be considered as potential sites of infection. Sputum samples should be sent for cultures of bacteria, fungus, and tuberculosis. When inhaled steroids have been used for prolonged periods, or if the patient is immune compromised due to HIV infection, candida laryngitis should be suspected. Flexible laryngoscopy often shows a mixture of organic disease and hyperfunctional voice disorder. This is summarized in Table 8–4.

The bacteriology of chronic infectious laryngitis is different than acute laryngitis. The most common pathogenic organism isolated in chronic laryngitis is *Staphylococcus aureus*. Appropriate antibiotic treatment should include coverage for common gram-positive and -negative pathogens. If tuberculosis or fungal laryngitis is suspected, treatment should be guided by endoscopic biopsy and culture results.

Surgical intervention may be necessary to establish the diagnosis. Endoscopy, biopsy, and culture may be necessary for management of chronic laryngitis. Histoplasmosis, tuberculosis, and sarcoidosis are causes of granulomatous laryngitis that should be diagnosed by tissue biopsy and culture. Autoimmune disorders such as amyloidosis, Wegner's granulomatosis, lupus erythematosus, and rheumatoid arthritis with laryngeal involvement should be suspected in patients with laryngeal findings consistent with chronic laryngitis but refractory to antibiotic and medical treatment. Early

Table 8–4. Flexible laryngoscopy findings in chronic laryngitis.

1. Hypophonia or whisper aphonia
2. Ventricular dysphonia with hypertrophy
3. Short antero-posterior diameter with short vocal folds
4. Excess mucous stranding with pebble stone appearance of posterior pharynx
5. Hypopharyngeal squeezing with laryngeal elevation

diagnosis and treatment may help prevent complications that can cause permanent damage to the larynx.

Chronic Hyperplastic Laryngitis

Early epithelial changes may be subtle. Examination of the larynx by a magnified telescope offers the best view. The vocal fold epithelium achieves a frosted glass appearance with edema and surface stippling. This change may be patchy or localized and may occur over several sites of the endolarynx. When viewed by mirror examination, early vocal fold thickening may be difficult to distinguish from retained thick mucus. Conversely, thickened mucus which is retained on one site of the vocal folds is easily misinterpreted to be a white keratotic lesion. In these patients, stroboscopic examination is most useful. In a small percentage of patients, cessation of smoking, aggressive mucosal hygiene, and treatment of gastroesophageal reflux may reverse the hyperkeratotic changes. However, in the majority, overt changes of the vocal folds are treated by endoscopic biopsy and removal.

Histologically, nonkeratinizing epithelium of the vocal fold has been transformed to thickened, nonpliable keratinized squamous epithelium. There is often prominent vascularity, epithelial hyperplasia, and variable degrees of inflammatory infiltrate. Cellular atypia is usually present and varies from mild to severe.

The differentiation of benign versus malignant vocal fold lesions cannot be definitively made by clinical methods alone. In some patients with risk factors for neoplasia, a biopsy and operative treatment is the logical course of action. Preoperative counseling should always include discussion of the possibility of cancer. Furthermore, the necessity of histologic examination of tissue may supersede other voice considerations. It is important to recognize that, in the majority of white patches on the vocal fold, the potential for malignancy is low. Appropriate treatment should balance factors such as the lesion's potential for malignancy with the voice needs of the patient.

THE VOICE EVALUATION

Voice Characteristics

Acute Viral Laryngitis

Unreliability of the voice is a common complaint and may prompt the patient to seek the assistance of either a speech-language pathologist or physician. There is often a husky, brassy voice characteristic which is often recognizable to the lay person as "laryngitis." The patient also may complain about voice breaks, particularly when attempting pitch changes. Speaking is accomplished only with great effort, resulting in short bursts much like a croak. Speaking may become progressively more painful, and the patient may cease to speak. Despite voice cessation, the throat remains red and irritated which causes the patient to frequently clear the throat. Of course, this results in further abuse of the larynx, and could exacerbate the problem.

Examination of the vocal folds during laryngitis shows some typical findings. During the early hyperemia stage, the vocal folds may look quite normal except for a pink rose color. However, attempts at phonation often result in vocal folds that fail to oscillate. During the suppurative stage of inflammation, copious thick secretions are present throughout the larynx and at the vocal fold contact area (see Figure 8–1). Thickened strands of mucus between vocal folds are often seen. If coughing is severe, the arytenoid and interarytenoid area may be erythematous and swollen. During the height of inflammation, singers and other voice users are most susceptible to vocal fold hemorrhage. Vocal fold hemorrhages are usually a result of mechanical trauma to the dilated vascular bed of the vocal folds. This can result in a submucosal hemorrhage. Such mechanical trauma may be due to excessive voice use or to harsh throat clearing.

If the patient is a singer, differentiation of vocal quality during speaking versus singing is useful. Singers with mild laryngeal edema may have a normal speaking voice but demonstrate an impaired singing voice. The high vocal range in singers is especially affected with mild laryngitis. Difficulty with control of the passage and a loss of their brilliant tone in the mid range are the other common complaints.

Noninfective or Nonspecific Laryngitis

Vocal characteristics of nonspecific laryngitis are indistinguishable from acute laryngitis. Voice loss in nonspecific laryn-gitis follows a more variable clinical course than acute laryngitis. Vocal symptoms often have an indolent, subacute form which neither progresses to aphonia nor resolves to total restitution of the voice.

Chronic Hyperplastic Laryngitis

The prominent voice symptom is a hoarse rough voice quality that fails to improve. There may be some fluctuation, but voice quality never becomes normal. Even when the patient reverses some of the abusive habits (e.g., stops smoking), the voice does not return to normal. This prompts most patients to seek the care of an otolaryngologist.

Endoscopy

Acute Viral Laryngitis

Stroboscopic examination shows vocal fold oscillation to be affected. Although not diagnostic for acute inflammatory laryngitis, stroboscopic examination helps to stage the course of the disease as well as to offer some prognostic signs as to return of vibratory function. Figure 8–8 is a series of stroboscopic photos which show the extensive thick mucous strands across thickened vocal folds during acute laryngeal inflammation. Table 8–5 summarizes some typical stroboscopic features associated with the various stages of laryngitis and its sequelae.

Vocal Fold Tear and Hemorrhage

Submucosal fibrosis results in a nonvibratory segment. Stroboscopically, the vocal fold hemorrhage causes localized stiffness of the affected fold, resulting in unilateral reduction in amplitude and mucosal wave. Because of the asymmetric tension, vocal fold vibration may be associated with phase shift as one vocal fold opens and closes before the other.

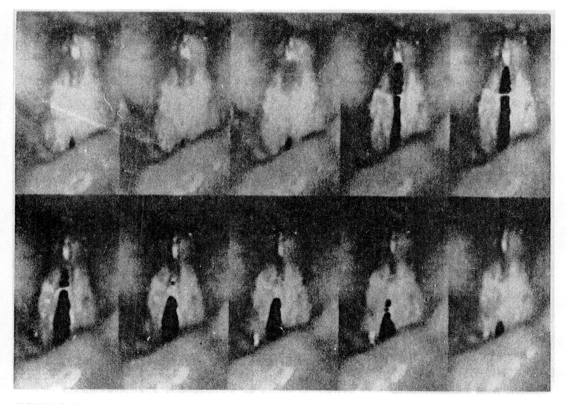

FIGURE 8–8. Stroboscopy example of acute laryngitis.

Phase shifts result in a to-and-fro vibratory pattern of the vocal folds which looks like a snake dancer.

Noninfective or Nonspecific Laryngitis

Endoscopic examination can differentiate between acute laryngitis and nonspecific laryngitis. Allergic laryngitis has laryngeal findings that resemble the normal larynx. There is little erythema or increased mucus production. The only hint of abnormality is the pale bluish color of the vocal fold edge with a hint of vocal fold edema. Erythema located over the posterior interarytenoid area may be present in patients with acid reflux laryngitis or habitual chronic throat clearing.

Stroboscopic examination also helps differentiate between acute and chronic laryngeal irritation. With prolonged irritation, the superior surface of the vocal fold loses its glistening smooth appearance. The smooth glossy surface is replaced by a stippled surface which can be easily detected by stroboscopy. It looks like salt or pepper has been sprinkled on the surface. Figure 8–2 shows an example of "salt and pepper" larynx in a patient with chronic laryngeal inflammation. Another stroboendoscopic feature that helps to identify early nonspecific laryngitis is persistent mucus stranding. This is usually accompanied by decreased mucosal vibratory amplitudes and decreased mucosal waves.

Chronic Nonspecific Laryngitis

The ability of stroboscopy to look at mucosal vibration is one of the most sensitive measures of mucosal function during health and disease.

Table 8-5. Stroboscopic finding in patients with acute laryngitis and vocal fold hemorrhage.

Acute Laryngitis—Early

Glottic configuration: midcord contact (posterior chink, bowing)

Symmetric reduction in mucosal wave

Symmetric reduction in amplitude

Prolonged (breathy) open phase during oscillation

Delay in mucosal wave propagation during vocal fold opening; aperiodicity

Acute Laryngitis—Suppurative

Copious vocal fold secretions

Edema with "hot dog" appearance of vocal folds

Rocking motion of vocal fold cover

Loss of mucosal wave

Incomplete closure

Aperiodicity

Acute Laryngitis—Resolution

Mucus stranding across vocal folds

Long open phase

Phase shifts may be present

Sluggish mucosal wave propagation

Vocal Fold Hemorrhage

Loss of amplitude on side of hemorrhage

Reduced mucosal amplitude

Characteristic dark color: dark red/green/yellow (color dependent on duration of hemorrhage)

Aperiodicity

In patients with mild inflammation, the mucosal vibratory amplitude remains good despite excessive secretion and color change. Propogation of the mucosal wave may be erratic and jerky, imparting a sensation that there is increased inertia to movement. In patients with more severe mucosal inflammation, the mucosal amplitude of vocal fold vibration becomes progressively diminished. The mucosal wave often is absent. When there is severe stiffness of the vocal folds, vibration of the vocal folds ceases. In severe laryngitis, the vocal folds fail to vibrate during phonation, showing absence of vibratory amplitude and mucosal wave.

In addition, stroboscopic examination is useful for differentiation of mucosal stiffness due to epithelial hyperplasia or Reinke's edema. In patients with epithelial thickening, mucosal wave propagation is disturbed but the folds continue to oscillate. The thickened epithelial layer will exhibit a rocking motion on an otherwise normal Reinke's layer. Much as a boat will ride the crest of a wave in a storm, the vocal fold will still oscillate in a to-and-fro manner. When there has been extensive epithelial and subepithelial inflammation, the rocking motion subsides and the vocal folds become stiff and immobile (see Table 8–6).

Table 8–6. Effects on vocal folds seen by stroboscopy.

Inflammation State	Physiologic Effect	Stroboscopic Finding
Laryngitis		
Acute phase	Decreased mass	Decreased F_0
	Decreased tension	Reduced amplitude
	Edema	Reduced mucosal waves
	Asymmetric swelling	Sluggish mucosal propagation
		Asymmetric vocal fold vibration with phase shift
		Brief closure
		Mucous stranding
Chronic phase	Decreased mass	Decreased F_0
Reinke's edema	Asymmetric mass loading	Aperiodic voice source
		Reduced amplitude
		Segmental loss of mucosal wave
		Rocking motion
		Incomplete or irregular closure
Scar/Nodule	Increased stiffness	Asymmetry of motion
	Increased mass	Incomplete or irregular closure
		Brief contact
		Reduced amplitude on one side
		Segmental loss of mucosal wave
Epithelial	Increased stiffness	Decreased F_0
	Increased mass	Mucosal wave
		Amplitude change
		Loudness to maintain onset of voice
		Asymmetric motion
		Boat on a wave appearance

Chronic Hyperplastic Laryngitis

On endoscopy, a nonspecific unilateral or bilateral thickening of the vocal fold is seen. The color is usually white and irregular but may be pink to reddish in color. Demarcation between the normal vocal folds and the mucosal lesion may be well defined.

Acoustic Analysis

Although acoustic measures have been used in assessment of other laryngeal pathologies (e.g., nodules and polyps), data on acute laryngitis have been largely anecdotal. Voice spectrogram studies usually show an increase in interharmonic noise and a loss of energy in the higher frequencies. The use of signal-to-noise ratio, jitter, shimmer, and other measures help to document the acoustic product but does not help in diagnosis. A larger database correlating other physiologic measures to acoustic analysis may be fruitful in future investigations.

Aerodynamics

Aerodynamic measures using a constant temperature hot wire anemometer (CTHWA) have been done in some laboratories. The CTHWA method measures flow variations at the lips and gives some indication of the efficiency of laryngeal air flow conversion. Studies of pathologic voices in patients with polyps, nodules, and paralysis show a decrease in the fluctuant flow component relative to the mean flow equipment (AC to DC ratio). Although the mean flow value is not significantly altered, the AC/DC ratio in laryngitis is significantly reduced, indicating a lowered glottal efficiency. Visual inspection of the airflow signal in individual cases confirms these findings.

Electroglottography (EGG)

Another technique that has been used to investigate vocal fold vibratory function is electroglottography (EGG). Because of its noninvasive nature, EGG has recently become more popular as a diagnostic tool. The procedure gives the investigator some indication of change in glottal contact during phonation. The shape of the EGG may be interpreted as to the duration of vocal fold contact, the rapidity of vocal fold opening and closing, and the smoothness of vocal fold opening and closing. During acute laryngitis, there is an increase in the open phase and slower rates of vocal fold opening and closing.

Because of the variable amplification used to obtain the EGG waveform, EGG cannot be used to compare treatment groups. It may be useful as a biofeedback method to track an individual's vocal fold function during treatment. EGG findings appear to correlate to stroboscopic findings.

SOCIAL IMPLICATIONS

The emotional and psychosocial adjustments made to acute inflammation are variable. For singers, this often depends on the importance of voice restoration within a limited time frame. Distress is often attributable to either voice qualities that conflict with his or her schedule or the fear of irreversible voice damage due to laryngeal tumor or hemorrhage. Heightened fear of vocal fold injury may prompt a demand for a quick "cure" and bring on urgent consultations from singers before a major performance. This psychological aspect of voice should be recognized and understood. It should not be trivialized or overtreated by the voice care professional.

TREATMENT: OPTIONS AND OUTCOMES

General Management

Acute Viral Laryngitis

The majority of patients with acute viral laryngitis have a self-limited course. Voice rest and supportive measures are all that is necessary. To soothe the irritated dry throat, steam inhalation in moderate amounts may be useful. This is done by commercially available units or home remedies such as inhaling through a hot wet towel.

To decrease thick secretions and reduce irritation, many popular remedies other than medications exist (Punt, 1979). Herbal tea, lemon flavoring, and honey are favorites among many singers. Strong irritative antiseptic mouth wash should be avoided. Warm salt water gargles used frequently can help to mechanically remove thick viscous secretions and reduce pharyngeal irritation. Hydration remains one of the best, if not the best, remedies for acute laryngitis.

Vocal Fold Tear and Hemorrhage

Mucosal tears and submucosal hemorrhages are absolute indications for voice rest. It is critical that further injury to the delicate vocal folds be avoided. Voice rest, along with medical treatment to reduce cough and throat irritation, is used to allow uneventful healing and avoid further mucosal damage. Needless to say, for professional voice users such as singers and teachers, it may be necessary to cancel performances and lectures until healing has completed.

Noninfective or Nonspecific Laryngitis

The primary treatment of nonspecific laryngitis lies in identification of the inciting agent and establishing a plan to decrease or eliminate exposure. Voice rest, hydration, and mucolytics are useful adjuncts in the treatment of nonspecific laryngitis. Inhaled steroid spray or systemic steroid use may be indicated to bring about rapid symptomatic improvement.

Patients with throat pain and irritation often develop harmful voicing gestures. Chronic hypophonia with bowed, incompletely closed vocal folds is often seen in patients with contact granuloma. Ventricular phonation is often a compensatory gesture for immobile or nonpliable true vocal folds. In patients with these harmful voicing gestures, behavioral speech therapy used in conjunction with the appropriate medical supportive measures can result in better long-term function.

Chronic Nonspecific Laryngitis

Besides medical and surgical treatment, supportive measures for patients with chronic laryngitis should include aggressive management of mucosal hygiene. Local rheologic factors contributing to mucosal stiffness and dryness should be reversed. A vocal hygiene program begins by identifying the local irritants to the larynx and planning for reduced exposure. The simple use of a filtered mask and saline nasal douching often works and may greatly reduce local irritation. Allergy or irritation caused by noxious fumes and organic solvents is more complicated. In the management of these patients, limitation of exposure and change of work environment may be necessary. Second-hand smoke in the home and work place is increasingly being implicated as a nonspecific laryngeal irritant and should be addressed as part of the environmental assessment.

Besides optimization of environmental factors, hydration plays an important role in improving local mucosal hygiene. Hydration should include a minimum of 48 ounces of fluid intake per day. Limitation of caffeinated beverage intake is advisable. The use of a mucolytic to produce thin clear mucus is often helpful.

Chronic Hyperplastic Laryngitis

The treatment of hyperplastic laryngitis incorporates surgical and medical modalities. Biopsy proven benign keratosis is best treated by microlaryngoscopy and careful removal of the affected epithelium. Using modern microlaryngeal surgical techniques, it is often possible to find a plane between the abnormal epithelium and the normal subepithelial layer. The importance of selected epithelial removal while leaving the jelly-like Reinke's layer intact should be emphasized. Figure 8–9 is a schematic representation of careful epithelial cover resection. Unlike vocal fold stripping, careful epithelial removal leaves intact the vocal ligament and the superficial layer of the lamina propria.

The surgical technique for resection of epithelial lesions has been described well by Kleinsasser and others (Kleinsasser, 1990). The preferred technique used by the author is to make an incision, grasp the lesion with microcup forceps, and gently tease the epithelial layer away with a sharp pick. When the abnormal

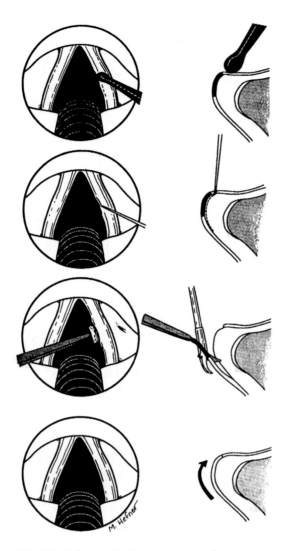

FIGURE 8–9. Epithelial resection by micro-laryngoscopy should leave the lamina propria and vocal ligament intact.

epithelium has been dissected free, the microscissors are used to remove the epithelium for histologic examination. The residual epithelial mucosal tags are then trimmed with the microscissors or CO_2 laser used on microspot mode. This creates a linear vocal fold edge and allows smooth epithelial resurfacing.

Careful removal of epithelial lesions offers the best chance for functional voice return. Figure 8–10 is an example of epithelial resection without dissection or removal of structures deep to the basement membrane.

Despite such a careful surgical approach, some residual vocal disabilities can be anticipated after extensive epithelial cover resection. Some vibratory amplitude decrement can be observed despite excellent healing and reepithelization. The voice quality usually improves but may remain decreased in loudness and dynamic range. These results should be anticipated and discussed with the patient prior to surgical treatment. The presence of mucosal vibratory changes in these patients should not be construed as a poor surgical result.

The patient with recurrent benign mucosal lesions after previous micro-laryngoscopic removal represents an especially challenging problem. These patients may have already had multiple previous microlaryngoscopic excisions for benign vocal fold lesions. Despite this, epithelial lesions may continue to develop. If laryngeal irritants have been adequately removed and mucosal hygiene has been maximized, the decision whether to perform repeat laryngeal excision must be individualized. Although complete removal of the offending lesion offers the best chance for cure, involvement of the anterior commissure and subglottic areas may make complete resection difficult without the risk of web and scar formation. In some patients with benign keratosis, it is reasonable to follow the lesion by selected biopsy rather than repeated vocal fold cover resection. This approach demands careful follow-up and frequent visits by a compliant patient.

Pharmacological Management

Acute Laryngitis

Pharmacologic treatment of acute laryngitis is occasionally necessary. Such ther-

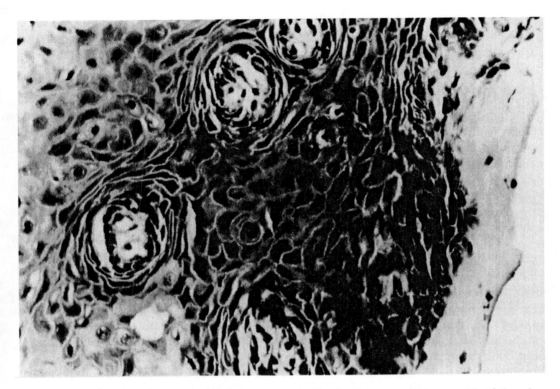

FIGURE 8–10. Epithelial resection without injury to the lamina propria is possible if the plane deep to the basement membrane is used as the plane of dissection.

apy is tailored to the individual needs of the patient. In patients with simple viral laryngitis, no pharmacologic intervention is necessary for a limited illness. In patients with significant symptoms, several drugs may be used.

To decrease the heavy cough and throat clearing which may interfere with sleep and spirit, a cough suppressant and mucolytic used in combination are useful. Organidin and codeine used in combination help to hydrate the airway and reduce the cough reflex. If there is an associated hypersecretory state such as viral rhinitis, a decongestant may also be used as a supplement. Antihistamines, however, should be used with caution due to their drying effect.

Mouthwash and sprays have been used by noted laryngologists over the centuries to reduce inflammation and edema. Afrin or epinephrine are occasionally sprayed on the vocal folds to achieve mucosal vasoconstriction and provide transient relief from dysphonia. Regular applications risk the development of systemic adrenergic effect that may manifest in the voice as vocal tremor.

Atropine and its derivatives and systemic corticosteroids are occasionally used to blunt the physiologic effects of inflammation. Atropine decreases the secretion; corticosteroids blunt the inflammatory response. Drugs like these should always be strictly monitored by the treating physician.

Acute Viral Laryngitis

Antibiotics have been used with increasing frequency for treatment of acute viral and bacterial laryngitis. When laryngitis is associated with bacterial tonsillitis, sinusitis, or bronchitis, antibiotic therapy is justified. For laryngitis associated with high fever, suppuration, and toxemia, bacterial etiologies must be considered. There is an increasing incidence of drug resistance to traditional antibiotics such as ampicillin and penicillin. *Branhamella Catarrhalis, strep pneumococcus, H influenza,* and *Staphylococcus* are common pathogens which have shown increasing drug resistance to antibiotics. Cultures and close follow-up after antibiotic treatment are necessary in cases suspected of antibiotic resistance.

Patients on antibiotic therapy should have their medications reviewed periodically. Side effects of long-term antibiotic therapy include candida laryngitis and nonspecific laryngitis. These pathogens could contribute to chronic laryngeal inflammation.

Noninfective or Nonspecific Laryngitis

Nonspecific laryngitis is often difficult to manage. The specific inciting agent may be difficult to identify. In its subacute form, frequent exacerbations of voice may occur at the most injudicious times. Drugs such as corticosteroids may be useful to temporize the symptoms. Definitive treatment depends on a successful search for the inciting agent. Because of their intermittent complaints and paucity of physical findings, these patients may be labeled as having functional or psychogenic dysphonia. In such cases, an interdisciplinary evaluation with an otolaryngologist and a speech-language pathologist can be most helpful.

Chronic Hyperplastic Laryngitis

In the postoperative period (following resection of epithelial tissue), careful avoidance of trauma, irritants, and edema is necessary to decrease scarring and fibrosis. Corticosteroids and antibiotics are given in the postoperative period to reduce vocal fold inflammation and edema. Voice rest for 1 week is advisable. Antireflux and antitussive regimens to reduce cough and throat clearing are routinely employed to further reduce laryngeal trauma. In all patients undergoing microlaryngeal surgery, conrol of the mucosal environment to permit satisfactory healing is as important as the technical skills employed during microlaryngeal surgery.

Speech Pathology

Acute Viral Laryngitis

Psychological counseling and speech therapy do not have a role in acute laryngitis except in patients with special voice demands (Khz, Biebl, & Rauchegger, 1988). If a singer must perform with a minor ailment, it is wise to first document the pathology. Female singers who phonate with laryngitis often exhibit large posterior chinks with excessive mucus retention (see Figure 8–11). The efficiency of this system for airflow conversion during singing is poor. A few emergency training sessions with a voice coach or speech-language pathologist with training and experience in such treatments may be useful. The purpose of these sessions is not to teach the patient proper voice use but rather to provide these voice professionals with techniques designed to (a) avoid vocal injury, (b) produce the least effortful yet acceptable sound, and (c) address the special psychosocial needs of the patient.

Chronic Nonspecific Laryngitis

Speech pathologists are often called on to assist with care of patients with nonspecific laryngitis (Bloch, Gould, & Hirano,

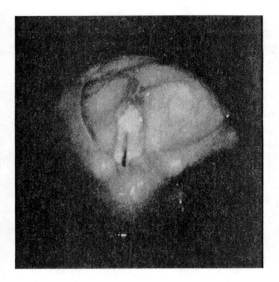

FIGURE 8–11. Singer with mild laryngitis. Note the large posterior chink and anterior mucous retention.

1981; Brodnitz, 1961). Although hyperfunctional voice disorders are rarely a cause of chronic laryngitis, continued chronic laryngitis often promotes hyperfunctional voice disorder. Compensatory mechanics during voicing often become necessary for the patient to talk.

The role of the speech-language pathologist in the rehabilitation of patients with chronic nonspecific laryngitis is to reeducate the patient as to appropriate voice production. Table 8–7 summarizes the speech-language pathologist's role in the management of chronic laryngitis. When the medical aspects of a chronic organic voice disorder have been reversed, reversal of habitual hyperfunction by the speech-language pathologist can return the patient to better function. Aerodynamic, acoustic, and vocal function measures help to document the progress with therapy but have little to offer in terms of diagnosis. Patients with chronic laryngitis typically have shortened phonation time, increased effort, and limited dynamic loudness and pitch range. Serial

recordings and measures of phonatory function help to document improvements in function as the patient undergoes therapy. They also are useful as tools for feedback on a patient's progress.

Prognosis

Prognosis for return of voice in acute laryngitis is excellent. Although a small group of patients have episodes of recurrent or prolonged symptoms, the majority have normal vocal function 7 to 10 days after the initial onset of symptoms. In patients with episodic, but troublesome, recurrent acute laryngitis symptoms, the interests of a knowledgeable laryngologist should be combined with the skills of a speech-language pathologist to seek out unusual causes of inflammation. In especially recalcitrant cases, other medical specialists from pulmonology, endocrinology, gynecology, and allergy may need to be consulted. In patients with long-standing inflammation and chronic changes of the vocal folds, normal voice qualities cannot be expected even with careful and aggressive management. Although considerable improvements may be made by interdisciplinary evaluation, medical intervention, rehabilitation, speech therapy, and occasionally surgery, the ultimate prognosis for the quality of the voice must be considered guarded. In patients afflicted with many years of chronic irritation to the larynx, the voice quality becomes feeble and loses its resonant timbre, the production of voice becomes tense and labored, and the sustainability of voice becomes difficult. The professional voice user who neglects proper voice care and mucosal hygiene is reduced to going from physician to physician to therapist with a woeful tale of reduced income and inability to perform up to expected standards, regretfully acknowledging that much of the sequelae of chronic laryngitis could have been prevented by a minimum of professional medical voice care.

Table 8-7. Role of the speech-language pathologist in chronic non-specific laryngitis.

1. Improve vocal hygiene
2. Assess respiratory support during phonation
3. Improve phonation range and loudness with existing disability
4. Reduce compensatory hyperfunction
5. Monitor compliance with ongoing treatment

REFERENCES

Bain, W. M., Harrington, J. W., Thomas, L. E., & Schafer, S. D. (1983). Head and neck manifestations of GER. *Laryngoscope, 93,* 175.

Baker, D. C., Jr. (1962). Laryngeal problems in singers. *Laryngoscope, 72,* 902.

Bloch, C. S., Gould, W. J., & Hirano, M. (1981). Effect of voice therapy on contact granuloma of the vocal fold. *Annals of Otology, Rhinology, and Laryngology, 90,* 98.

Brodnitz, F. (1961). Contact ulcers of the larynx. *Archives of Otology, Rhinology, and Laryngology, 74,* 70–78.

Charrow, A., Pass, F., & Ruken, R. (1971). Pemphigus of the upper respiratory tract. *Archives of Otolaryngology. 93,* 209–210.

Haar, J. H., Chandhry, A. P., Kaplan, H. M., & Milley, P. S. (1980). Granulamatous laryngitis of unknown etiology. *Laryngoscope, 90,* 1225.

Hughes, R. A., Paonessa, D. F., & Conway. W. F., Jr. (1984). Actinomycosis of the larynx. *Annals of Otology, Rhinology, and Laryngology, 93,* 520.

Kambic, V., Rodsel, Z., Zargi, M., & Acko, M. (1981). Vocal cord polyps: Incidence, histology, and pathogenesis. *Journal of Laryngology and Otology, 95,* 609.

Khz, J., Biebl, W., & Rauchegger, H. (1988). Functional aphonia: Psychosomatic aspects of diagnosis and therapy. *Folia Phoniatrica, 80,* 132–137.

Kleinsasser, O. (1990). *Microlaryngology and endolaryngeal microsurgery* (3rd ed.). St. Louis, MO: Mosby-Yearbook.

Levenson, M. J., Ingerman, M. Grimes, D., & Robett, W. F. (1984). Laryngeal Tuberculosis: A review of 20 cases. *Laryngoscope, 90,* 1225.

McGavran, M. H., Bauer, W. C., & Ogura, J. H. (1960). Isolated laryngeal keratosis: Its relation to cancer of the larynx based on clinical pathologic study of 87 consecutive cases with long term followup. *Laryngoscope, 70,* 932.

Punt, N. A. (1979). *The singer's and actor's throat.* (3rd ed.) London: William Heinemann Medical Books.

Rubin, H. J. (1967). Vocal intensity, subglottic pressure and air flow in relationship to singers. *Folia Phoniatrica, 19,* 393.

von Leden, H. (1960). Laryngeal physiology. *Journal of Laryngology, 74,* 705.

Ward, P. H., & Berci, G., (1982). Observations on the pathogenesis of chronic non-specific pharyngitis and laryngitis. *Laryngoscope, 92*(12), 1377–1382.

Wilson, J. A., White, A., Von Haache, N. P., Maran, A. E. et al. (1989). Gastroesophageal reflux and posterior laryngitis. *Annals of Otology, Rhinology, and Laryngology, 98*(6), 405–410.

Zhao, R., Cai Y., & Wang H. (1991). Pathological changes of hyperphonated cat vocal folds. *Auris-Nasis-Larynx, 18*(1), 559.

CHAPTER 9

NODULES AND POLYPS

FRANÇOISE CHAGNON, M.D.
R. E. (ED) STONE, JR., PH.D.

INTRODUCTION AND DEFINITIONS

Vocal fold polyps and nodules (VFPN) are distinct clinical entities unrelated to nodules and polyps arising elsewhere in the body. They are benign focal lesions of the vocal folds, thought to arise as a sequela to vocal abuse, and they present heterogeneous clinical and histological characteristics. Controversies and confusions as to their definition have persisted since their first description in the late 19th century. Nodules are referred to by a variety of synonyms: laryngeal nodes, teacher's nodes, screamer's nodes, Parson's nodes, corditis fibrosa, fibrous nodes, nodular laryngitis. Descriptive expressions for them abound: excrescence, swelling, protuberance, growth, callosity, and tumor. In this chapter we focus on polyps and nodules that present similarities in their appearance and clinical behavior and exclude from discussion pedunculated polyps and those of Reinke's edema.

Typically, VFPN occur at the junction of the middle and anterior third of the vocal folds. The clinical distinction between nodules and polyps has been based on their size and appearance. Nodules are said to be opaque, 1 to 5 mm in anterior-posterior dimension, firm, symmetrical, focal lesions on the free edge of the vocal folds. Polyps are fleshy, sessile, edematous, or hemorrhagic structures.

The distinction, however, between the nodule and the polyp on morphological appearance alone, is not always so evident. Arnold (1962) distinguishes polyps from nodules by a maturation process, from the early fleshy, edematous lesion to the hard, fibrotic more mature lesion. This suggests that polyps and nodules are different phases of the same pathological process (Härma, Sonninen, Vartiainen, Haveri, & Väisänen, 1975; Moore, 1971). Many clinicians and most histopathologists, however, use the terms interchangeably or use the term "nodule" in a generic way (Lancer, Syder, Jones, & Le Boutillier, 1988), and histopathological differentiation is not possible without clinical information (Fitz-Hugh, Smith, & Chiong, 1958).

Histologically, however, both lesions present anomalies of the epithelium and subepithelial space of Reinke. Loire, Bouchayer, Cornut, and Bastian (1988) found what they diagnosed in the clinic to be nodules were predominantly epithelial abnormalities whereas polyps presented histologic characteristics of submucosal fibrinous exudates. The epithelial abnormalities found in excised vocal nodules were dyskeratosis, and hyperkeratosis, and a thickened basement membrane (compare Figures 9–1B and 9–1C to 9–1A). Polypoid lesions involving the submucosa had moderate edema, cellular infiltrates, and hyaline sclerosis. In comparison, vocal polyps had atrophy of the epithelium, a thin basement membrane and more pronounced submucosal edema, with cellular infiltrates and fibrinous exudates (Figure 9–1A). Frenzel (1986) found similar histology for polyps, but he may have been considering pedunculated polyps.

Kotby, Nassar, Seif, Helal, and Saleh (1988b), studying ultrastructural features of nodules (Figure 9–2), noted gaping of intercellular junctions, disruption and duplication of the basement membrane, collagen fiber deposits in the submucosa, and keratinization of the epithelium. Polyps, however, had intact basement membranes, abundant stromal vascularity, and less collagen deposition than nodules. Disruption of the layered arrangement of fibers in the lamina propria was noted in both polyps and nodules. Kotby et al. (1988) suggested these lesions were variants in a group of related lesions called "minimal associated pathological lesions." Unfortunately, their comments are based

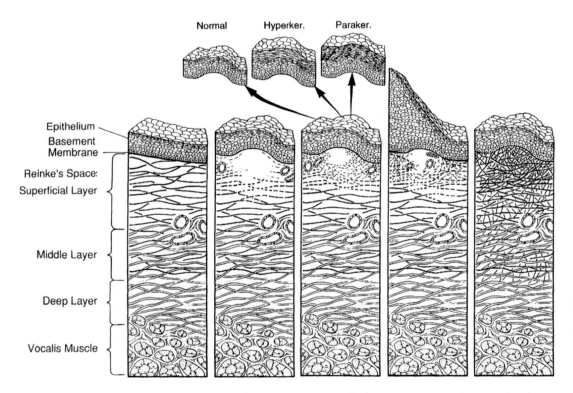

FIGURE 9–1. The vocal fold: spectrum of histopathological findings in vocal nodules and polyps. **A.** Normal vocal fold. **B.** Subepithelial edema. **C.** Subepithelial edema with fibrosis and normal epithelium or keratosis. Disorders of epithelial keratinization vary from hypertrophy of the horny layer of the epithelium (hyperkeratosis) to the retention of nuclei in the cells of the stratum corneum (parakeratosis). **D.** Subepithelial edema with fibrosis and epithelial hyperplasia. **E.** Subepithelial fibrosi.

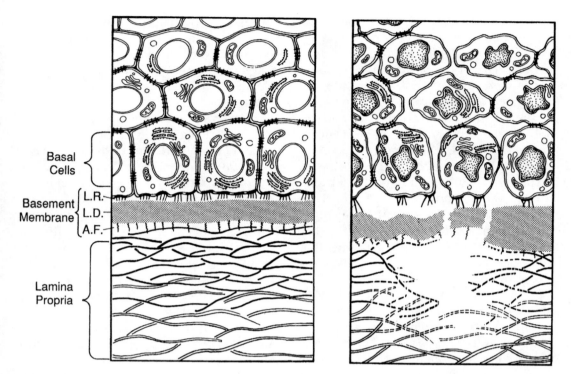

Basal
Cells

Basement
Membrane { L.R.-
L.D.-
A.F.-

Lamina
Propria

FIGURE 9–2. The vocal fold: ultrastructural changes in vocal nodules and polyps (LR: lamina rara, LD: lamina densa, AF: anchoring fibril). **A.** Normal vocal fold. **B.** Disordered vocal fold with epithelial loss, thickening and breakage of the basement membrane, intraepithelial and subepithelial edema.

only on surgically excised lesions, which do not represent all lesions seen clinically. Many lesions are not submitted to surgical excision but rather are treated behaviorally. Surgical selection criteria may favor lesions presenting more advanced tissue degeneration and fibrosis.

Interpretation of these histopathological findings based on the principles of wound repair would suggest that polyps and nodules are the result of vocal fold trauma showing varying phases of regeneration and repair. The phases of wound repair have been characterized as initial vasodilatation and edema, activation of fibroblast and histiocytes with phagocytosis of dead tissue components, growth of new blood vessels, collagen deposition, and, finally, remodeling of the tissues. It is likely

that VFPN are the result of "microtraumas" occurring at various phases of wound repair, thus accounting for the heterogeneity of histological and clinical manifestations (Ash & Schwartz, 1944). Such repeated microtrauma may impair wound healing and lead to scar formation.

PATHOGENESIS

Numerous theories have addressed the mechanisms by which polyps and nodules of the vocal folds develop. In a prevailing theory, vocal folds are mechanically traumatized in the process of phonation. Sonninen, Damsté, and Fokkens (1972), in discussing the various forces acting on the vibrating vocal folds, also considered frictional, compressional, longitudinal, and medial pulling forces.

Tarneaud (1935) hypothesized that hypotonicity of the vocal muscles would cause vibrations of great amplitude and increase compressional forces as folds strike against each other. This was not substantiated by subsequent electromyographic studies. The concept that nodules result from direct hammering or slapping effects is retained by Hirano, Kurita, Matsuo, and Nagata (1980). They suggest that nodules result from high-pitched phonation during falsetto patterns of vocal fold vibration, believing that vibratory movements are maximal at the edges of the vocal folds. Garde (1969) suggested that the mechanism of VFPN may be hernial rather than frictional, leading to focal subepithelial edema. Sonninen et al. (1972) postulate that strong negative pressures created by the Bernoulli effect exert a median pull and displace tissue fluid in the subepithelial space.

Until recently, lack of an animal model for laryngeal phonotrauma had prevented elucidation of the early tissue changes in response to injury. Furthermore, the use of the electron microscope and the study of the ultrastructural features of nodules and polyps has provided insight into the pathogenesis of vocal trauma not previously recognized by light microscopy. Gray, Titze, and Lusk (1987) and Gray and Titze (1988) observed hyperphonated canine vocal folds and found two levels of injury: the epithelium and the basement membrane. The early signs of injury are the loss of surface microvilli and superficial epithelial desquamation. In the deeper layers of the epithelium, there is intercellular edema and breakdown of desmosomes. More severe injury will detach basal cells from the basement membrane, creating space for fluid collection. Finally, there is disruption of the basement membrane attachment to the superficial layer of the lamina propria.

Similar ultrastructural features have been noted in human vocal nodules and polyps (Dikkers, Hulsteart, Oosterbaan & Cervera-Paz, 1993; Kotby, Nassar, Seif, Helal, & Saleh, 1988; Mossalam, Kotby, Ghaly, Nassar, & Barakah, 1986).

Factors stimulating collagen production have been proposed as links to the formation of VFPN. Hunt, Banda, and Silver (1985) demonstrated that periods of hypoxia stimulate collagen production by fibroblasts. Hirano et al. (1980) felt that vibratory and shearing forces could stimulate and activate subepithelial fibroblasts to produce collagen and eventual nodule formation. Despite the limitations of the canine experimental model, Gray and Titze (1988) support the role of these forces in nodule formation.

Many authors (Frenzel, 1986; Kleinsasser, 1982; Kotby et al., 1988) have emphasized the role of altered vascular permeability in the formation of microhematomas and subepithelial edema. Many factors can affect the permeability of the microcirculation: hypoxia, inflammation, local trauma, and heat. Frenzel (1986) noted ultrastructural features in the basement membrane of blood vessels in the lamina propria of the vocal fold, usually an indicator of high mechanical stress. Several reports have suggested that ischemic changes occur in the lamina propria and the vocalis muscle during phonation (Matsuo et al., 1987; Tomita, Matsuo, Maehara, Umezaki, & Shin, 1988). Although these investigators estimated blood flow from measurements of oxygen tension, a more sensitive technique directly measured regional blood flow and noted an increase in flow to the vocalis muscle and no change in the lamina propria (Arnstein, Trapp, Berke, & Natividad, 1989). Blood vessels in the free edge of the vascular network of the vocal fold are distinct from those in the vocalis muscle, and blood flows synchronously with inspiration. The vessels in the superficial layer are likely venous, and there is a reticulated vascular network especially at the lower surface of the free edge in the midportion of the vocal fold (Mishashi et al., 1981). The permeability of venules is selectively affected by inflammatory chemical mediators; capillary leakage may be affected by different factors, notably mechanical trauma (Joris, Cuenoud, Diern, Underwood, & Majno, 1991). Thus, with minimal phonotrauma, subepithelial blood vessel rupture may occur (Hirano et al., 1980). The anatomy of the microvasculature may explain the propensity for nodules and polyps to develop in the midportion of the vocal fold.

Further investigations are needed to determine the effects of prolonged phonation and muscular contraction on the microvasculature of the vocal fold. The effects of heat, frictional, tensional, and compressional forces on submucosal tissue alterations are not known. For nodules and polyps to occur, the vocal folds must be subjected to vibrational forces, yet the mechanisms by which this becomes traumatic are still the subjects of speculation.

From a clinical point of view, VFPN are said to result from vocal abuse and misuse. While vocal abuse refers to excessive use of the voice, vocal misuse refers to faulty vocal technique as resulting from the inappropriate use of laryngeal muscles. Common nonphonatory functions of the larynx, such as straining with a closed glottis, throat clearing, coughing, crying, or laughing, could be considered traumatic if they occur frequently or with excessive forces. The clinical observations of Roch, Cornut, and Bouchayer (1989) suggest that polyps can develop as a result of physical efforts with a closed glottis, because elevated subglottic pressures are followed by an abrupt release and subsequent strong closure of the folds during oscillation.

Misuse of the voice may be task-dependent. Vocal behaviors considered potentially damaging are straining to sing outside the comfortable vocal pitch range and the excessive use of the chest voice register in regions where the head register usually is advocated. The use of a loud voice may not be traumatic if it is achieved by proper respiratory contribution rather than increased glottic resistance, the latter method being common among untrained vocalists. However, for the untrained singer or speaker, a rise in vocal intensity is often accompanied by a rise in pitch and glottal resistance.

The development of VFPN results in increased vocal effort to correct for glottal inefficiencies. Such consequent compensatory effort is frequently maladaptive, promoting further trauma to the vocal folds and instituting a vicious cycle.

Clinical observations suggest that predisposing, precipitating, and aggravating factors may be involved in the pathogenesis of nodules and polyps. Arnold (1962) acknowledged the multifactorial etiologies, emphasizing general constitutional and psychological factors.

Nodule formation in children deserves special mention in view of the normative developmental changes occurring in the layered structure of the vocal fold. In the child, the vocal ligament is immature, and the ratio of the thickness of the vocal fold mucosa to the length of the membranous fold is greater than in adults (Hirano, Kurita, & Nakashima, 1983). Thus, the tissue reaction of a child's vocal fold during voice production may differ from that of an adult's. Children's vocal nodules appear soft and edematous and are seldom fibrose. In puberty, the lengthening of the membranous fold shifts the point of maximal vibration and may explain the tendency toward nodule resolution during this period (Strome, 1982).

The importance of psychological factors is emphasized by many authors (Arnold, 1962; Aronson, 1980; Rubin, & Lerhoff, 1962). In general, anxiety, stress, and emotional disturbances are often accompanied by hypercontraction of laryngeal muscles and poor vocal function (Moore, 1982). Persons with aggressive personalities (suffering from anxiety, depression, or interpersonal conflicts and confrontation) are said to have a higher incidence of nodules. Yano, Ichimura, Hoshino, and Nozue (1982) found a positive correlation between vocal nodules and polyps and extroverted personalities. Toohill (1975) found that anxiety may be a significant etiological factor in children's vocal abuse. Children may exhibit anxieties toward high expectations of performance at home, school, or sports, imposed by parents, teachers, or siblings. Le Huches (1987) argues that children may express their psychological suffering by the use of laryngeal hypertonicity. Green (1989) studied psychobehavioral characteristics of children with vocal nodules and noted a propensity for immature behaviors, acting out, distractibility, and disturbed peer relations.

Other factors may render the folds susceptible to VFPN. In general, factors that cause vocal fold edema, hypervascularity, and dehydration would render the fold more susceptible to the development of organic pathology in response to phonotrauma. Such factors include infection, endocrine imbalances, smoking and alcohol consumption, exposure to irritants and dehydrating agents.

Of clinical significance is the excessive or faulty use of the voice during an episode of infectious laryngitis. This has been recognized as a frequent triggering event in the development of vocal fold pathology. Infection alone, however, seems to play a less significant role. In children, the contribution of frequent upper respiratory tract infections may seem plausible, but it was not substantiated by Leeper, Leonard, and Iverson (1980).

In females, cyclical alterations in the levels of estrogen and progesterone cause laryngeal water retention, edema of the interstitial tissue, and venous dilatation (Abitbol et al., 1989). There is evidence of estrogen receptor sites on the membranes of epithelial cells of the human larynx (Fergusson, Hudson, & McCarty, 1987). Estrogen binding of these receptors could affect the histological characteristics of the epithelium (Beckford, Rood, & Schaid, 1985; Kahane, 1982). Progesterone stimulation, on the other hand, would act on Reinke's space. Silverman and Zimmer (1975, 1976, 1978) have documented the effects of the menstrual cycle on voice quality. We may conclude that the female larynx, being subject to hormone-mediated effects, is rendered more susceptible than the male larynx to the development of nodules and polyps.

A direct casual relation between smoking and nodule or polyp formation has not been the subject of formal studies. The presumed deleterious effects of heat transferred to vocal folds by inhaling the smoke of tobacco or illicit drugs would lead us to conclude that this is probably an aggravating factor. Smoking would also alter mucociliary flow, a factor to be further discussed. Cigarette smoking does impose a twofold risk of acute respiratory tract infection of protracted course and a cough of longer duration (Aronson, Weiss, Ben, & Komaroff, 1982). Chronic smoking induces tracheal hypersecretion and inflammation with resultant chronic cough and dyspnea (U.S. Department of Health and Human Services, 1990). In social situations, smoking is often accompanied by alcohol consumption and increased vocal abuse from lowered inhibitions.

Alterations in mucociliary flow, most commonly decreasing mucus production or increasing mucus viscosity secondary to dehydration, would expose the vocal fold cover to increased frictional forces. Factors affecting the lubrication of the vocal mechanism were emphasized by Punt (1974): emotional factors, smoking and alcohol, medications, environmental dryness, nose and sinus conditions. Experimental evidence derived from the excised human larynx (Hiroto, 1981) suggests that humid air is needed for vocal fold vibration and mucosal wave production. A canine model demonstrated the relation between increased vocal fold viscosity and an increased threshold of oscillation (Finkelhor, Titze, & Durham, 1988). Preliminary studies in human subjects also have indicated a direct relationship between phonation threshold pressure and vocal fold tissue viscosity (Verdolini-Marston, Titze, & Druker, 1990).

In Sjögren's syndrome, an auto-immune disorder affecting the salivary glands and leading to xerostomia, the secondary development of vocal nodules is known, although quite rare (Prytz, 1980).

The inhalation of airborne irritants (dust, oil fumes, chemical vapors, and steam), which occur in industrial work places and certain entertainment venues, may lead to vocal fold swelling and inflammation and act as predisposing or aggravating factors in the development of nodules and polyps.

Childs and Johnson (1991), in reviewing the multitude of factors that affect the human voice, acknowledge that there are individual susceptibilities and variabilities in responses. Thus, all factors may co-exist, but one factor alone may be sufficient. The cumulative effects of repeated injuries, whether factors act alone or in combination, and the ability of the vocal folds to heal themselves must be considered in the evaluation of a patient with vocal polyp or nodule.

DEMOGRAPHIC INFORMATION

Many factors diminish the accuracy of the incidence of VFPN reported to date. Reported prevalence of VFPN must be interpreted in light of controversial nomen-clature. Many studies fail to specify diagnostic criteria and methods of examination (i.e., clinical versus histopathological). Deriving frequency of occurrence figures is also handicapped by the existence of studies focusing only on specific cohort characteristics, such as age or symptomatology. In addition not all patients present themselves for identification, obscuring the prevalence of vocal nodules and polyps in the general population.

In otolaryngology populations, VFPN are the most commonly seen benign laryngeal pathologies. Nagata et al. (1983) reviewed their caseload and found that vocal polyps represented 1.5 to 2.6% and vocal nodules 0.5 to 1.3% of all their patients. Sellars (1979), reporting on the outcome of over 1,500 direct laryngoscopies, found a 20% incidence of nodules and polyps. The retrospective study of Herrington-Hall, Lee, Stemple, Niemi, and McHone (1988) reported a prevalence of nodules (21.6%) over polyps (11.4%).

General trends in the prevalence, according to age, gender, and occupation, are notable. In children, vocal nodules rank second to inflammatory conditions for causing hoarseness (Strome, 1982). The incidence of vocal nodules approaches 1% of all children identified by Toohill (1975). Boys between the ages of 5 and 10 years predominate over girls by a ratio of 3:1. Silverman and Zimmer (1975) reported a 23.4% incidence of chronic dysphonia among school-age children (kindergarten to grade 8), of which 77.7% had vocal nodules. A more conservative average of 6 to 9% incidence of chronic dysphonia is compatible with earlier studies (Baynes, 1966; Deal, McClain, & Sudderth, 1976; Leeper, 1976; Pannbacker, 1975; Senturia & Wilson, 1968), in which a majority probably reflect the presence of VFPN. Silverman and Zimmer (1977) noted that their screening was derived from children of an affluent Jewish community, suggesting that socio-ethnic background may be influential. Leeper, Leonard, and Iverson (1980) found a prevalence rate of 35% for vocal nodules and 28% for bilateral vocal fold thickening in children dysphonic for over 2 months.

In adults, nodules are frequent in females from their late teens until middle adulthood. Nodules can occur in adult males but are rare after the age of 40 (Herrington-Hall, Lee, Stemple, Niemi, & McHone, 1988). Most studies report a higher incidence of polyps (referring to pedunculated or sessile lesions larger than what our present definition of polyps encompasses) than nodules in males (Kleinsasser, 1982). Kambic, Radsel, Zargi, and Acko (1981), however, noted a slightly higher incidence for females than males, and attributed this to the presence of women factory workers in their sample, where exposure to dust, chemical fumes, and the noisy work place could explain this discrepancy. Herrington-Hall et al. (1988) suggested that the increasing occurrence of benign laryngeal lesions in women may be due to changing lifestyles, with more women having the dual responsibilities of the family and work place.

Vocally demanding occupations (teachers, singers, lawyers, salespeople, receptionists) experience an increased incidence of vocal pathology. The evidence of this is anecdotal, and Cooper (1973) and Herrington-Hall et al. (1988) found homemakers (noncareer women between the ages of 20 to 50 years) to have the greatest incidence of vocal nodules.

Other influences may be significant. Because profoundly hearing-impaired children have impaired auditory feedback for voice modulation (Monoson, 1979), they are more likely to develop vocal pathology. The findings of Dearkay, Thomsen, and Grundfast (1991), however, did not support this hypothesis.

Individuals with palatal clefts have a high occurrence of voice and laryngeal symptoms such as VFPN. D'Antonio, Muntz, Province, and Marsh (1988) found a 21% incidence of vocal fold nodules or thickening among patients referred for velopharyngeal dysfunction, possibly the compensatory result of elevated subglottal pressures being used in response to abnormal velopharyngeal valving.

Estimates of the prevalence of VFPN are still forthcoming and represent a need for mass screening or other assessments strategies (Stone, 1991).

ONSET AND COURSE OF THE DISORDER

Variations in the presenting symptomatology of VFPN depend on the position and size of these lesions on the vocal fold and their consequences on the vibratory cycle. Symptomatology is also dependent on the vocal needs of the individual. Singers may note vocal problems earlier than nonsingers, and the latter tend to be more tolerant of vocal dysfunction.

A patient's chief complaint of "hoarseness" is the most common presenting symptom, presumably referring to a change in voice quality, similar to the vocal deterioration experienced after prolonged yelling at an athletic event. Breathiness and pitch breaks can also occur. The fundamental pitch of the speaking voice may be lowered. The altered laryngeal biomechanics compound the execution of compensatory vocal behaviors; patients experience vocal fatigue and throat pain. In efforts to rid the airway of what they believe is mucus, patients will often attempt to clear their throats excessively.

The duration of symptoms may be longer for patients with nodules than those with polyps, because polyps may occur after only one episode of vocal abuse. In adults, the onset of the voice disorder often can be pinpointed in time. This is not necessarily so in children.

The dysphonia from VFPN may be present in the speaking voice or singing voice or both. The effect usually is first noticed in the middle or higher pitch range of the speaking voice but seems most obvious at the high frequencies during singing. Typically, the voice will be strong in the morning and deteriorate by midday, even with moderate voice use. Singers may find their voices unreliable, with a breathy middle register and voice "cracks" when approaching the head register.

MEDICAL CONSIDERATIONS

VFPN are primary laryngeal disorders and are not commonly the manifestation of systemic diseases. Presumably, identification and eventual treatment of coexistent medical disorders would benefit the patient's general well-being and, we postulate, influence vocal fold healing. A few medical disorders will be mentioned here, inasmuch as they are common in the general population and worth screening for.

Keeping in mind the proposed multifactorial etiologies to VFPN, the physician should establish the patient's general health status by a systemic inquiry.

Symptoms of altered bodily functions (fluctuations in body weight, gastrointestinal dysfunction, irregular menses, etc.) may warrant further endocrine investigations. Endocrine imbalances (particularly, thyroid hormone and gonadotropic hormones) are reported to cause diffuse "thickening" or "swelling" of the vocal folds (Boone, 1983). In Lawrence's (1978) experience, frank hypothyroidism with laryngeal myxedema seldom occurs. More commonly observed is a subtle edema of the superior aspect of the vocal folds in patients with borderline low values of thyroid hormones. Disorders of estrogen, progesterone, and testosterone hormones are known to affect vocal pitch, presumably by causing alterations in the consistency of the vocal fold cover (Abitbol et al., 1989). Their role in the pathogenesis of VFPN has been discussed.

The deterioration of vocal quality and intensity of a performer's voice may signal some deficiency of the respiratory system. Singing may provoke exercise-induced asthma and compensatory hyperfunction of the laryngeal muscles in response to the decreased expiratory airflow. Standard pulmonary function tests may fail to reveal the typical obstructive pattern of pulmonary function, and the methacholine bronchoprovocation test may be necessary to make this diagnosis. In the treatment of asthmatics, the use of inhaled steroids may cause dryness and fungal (Candida) overgrowth (Watkins & Ewanowsky, 1985) of the vocal folds. Other pulmonary disorders—bronchitis and chronic obstructive pulmonary disease—are associated with a chronic productive cough, and the use of cough-suppressant medication may help decrease laryngeal trauma.

The laryngological manifestations of gastroesophageal reflux include laryngitis, chronic cough, and asthma (Koufman, 1991). Whether this disorder contributes to the development of VFPN is unknown. Recent evidence suggests that gastroesophageal reflux may be occult and typical symptomatology absent, particularly in patients with the laryngeal complications of reflux (Koufman, 1991). Prolonged pH manometry testing is sensitive to the detection of this disorder, and dietary modification and treatment with systemic gastric acid inhibitors is recommended.

In Sjögren's syndrome, a lesser degree of vocal abuse than in healthy individuals may be involved in the pathogenesis of nodules (Prytz, 1980), possibly related to an associated sicca condition.

From a clinical and histopathological point of view, distinction must be made between VFPN and other pathologies. Autoimmune disorders, such as rheumatoid arthritis, systemic lupus erythematosus, dermatomyositis, and Hashimoto's thyroiditis, can be associated with "rheumatoid nodules." These lesions tend to be multicentric and have no site of predilection in the larynx, but if occurring in isolation on the vocal fold, could be indistinguishable from the typical nodule. A pathognomonic histopathology will differentiate them from the nodule (Schwartz, 1980).

Other vocal fold lesions may be mistaken for nodules or polyps: papilloma, cysts, amyloid deposits, benign granular cell tumors, and squamous cell carcinomas. The most commonly misdiagnosed are vocal fold cysts. In the absence of stroboscopy, distinguishing morphological features may not be recognized. Atypical location, multicentricity, or fluctuation in size may promote differing diagnoses and underline the importance of sequential examinations in the management of VFPN.

THE VOICE EVALUATION

Voice Characteristics

Hirano (1981a) suggests that the trained clinician can distinguish vocal pathologies based on psychoacoustic impressions and visual observation of the larynx. This implies that vocal nodules and polyps have peculiar acoustic characteristics. In accordance with Hirano's studies, polyps and nodules alter the mechanical properties of the folds by imparting mass and interfering with closure of the vibrating vocal folds.

Unfortunately, vocal fold lesions, particularly nodules and polyps, are not homogenous, and individual compensatory vocal behaviors vary accordingly. Perceptual, aerodynamic, and acoustic measurements should, therefore, show great variability between voices, and normative values are not well delineated.

Sampling of only sustained vowels may not be adequate for the evaluation of voice quality (Hammaberg, Fritzell, Gauffin, Sundberg, & Wedin, 1980). Connected speech samples may be required to provide the acoustic cues necessary to detect perceptual changes associated with vocal pathology. Perceptual measures may be subject to poor interjudge reliability, but they remain sensitive to abnormal voices not identified by acoustic measures such as jitter and shimmer or harmonic-to-noise ratio (Zyski, Bull, McDonald, & Johns, 1984).

Many perceptual rating scales are currently used clinically, with no consensus on the number of parameters to be evaluated or their reliability. The Japan Society of Logopedics and Phoniatrics (Hirano, 1981b) has proposed the "GRBAS" scale for evaluating hoarseness. This scale is based on a 4-point grading of five parameters: grade (G), rough (R), breathy (B), asthenic (A), strained (S). Voice disorders due to nodules and polyps typically elicit ratings of 0 (nonhoarse to normal) to 1 (slight) or 2 (moderate) in grade, roughness, breathiness, and strained qualities, but they are not usually asthenic.

In some cases, the speaking ability of an impaired voice is normal and the disorder is apparent only during singing. The disordered singing voice is said to be breathy, especially in the middle register, with pitch breaks and diplophonia occurring in the head register (Brodnitz, 1971). Lawrence (1991) relates a practical test which he uses to detect nodules: If a singer can achieve the highest pitch without excess breath pressure, he or she probably does not have nodules. However, if increased breath pressure is required to achieve a clear high note at mezzoforte or forte, it may suggest the presence of nodules interfering with glottal closure. Bastian, Keidar, and Verdolini-Marston et al. (1990), using simple vocal tasks such as a softly sung staccato on the vowel /i/ and a legato phrase, such as the opening phrase of "Happy Birthday to You" at high pitches in falsetto register, could detect the presence of vocal fold swellings such as nodules, particularly in singers.

Endoscopy

Laryngeal mirror examination is a valuable tool for observing the natural color and size of the larynx and giving an overview of pharyngeal structures. One pitfall of the laryngeal mirror examination is to mistake the presence of tenacious mucus on the surface of the vocal fold for pathological lesions, notably nodules and polyps. The patient may be asked to drink and clear the throat to see if the apparent excrescence remains, and phonation should be observed at various pitches. Nodules will appear as whitish, pimple-like lesions on the free edge of the vocal fold or as more fusiform, pale or pink swellings. Mirror examination cannot detect discrete lesions that appear only during certain phases of the vibratory cycle; these sometimes can be seen under stroboscopy during specific vocal activity.

Ideally, all patients with suspected vocal nodules or polyps should undergo video-laryngo-stroboscopy with the rigid scope (70° or 90°) or the flexible fiberoptic laryngoscope. Although the latter does not provide ideal illumination and magnification, it does allow evaluation of supraglottic activity, and it may be the only examination technique tolerated by the patient with an overactive gag reflex.

Nodules are classically located at the middle of the membranous vocal fold and are usually bilateral. Videoendoscopic examination has demonstrated considerable variation in their location, size, and texture (McFarlane & Waterson, 1990). Factors such as age, the practice of singing, and the sex of the speaker may account for the variations observed (McFarlane & Watterson, 1990; Peppard, Bless, & Milenkovic, 1988). Children's nodules may be situated slightly posterior to the middle of the membranous fold. In adults, nodules are usually bilateral, but patients' charts have reported instances of unilateral ones. Nodule location in adult singers also varies, sometimes near the lower lip of the vocal fold, and due to earlier diagnosis, the nodules tend to be smaller than in nonsingers.

As nodules and polyps are predominantly pathologies within Reinke's space, stroboscopy is particularly helpful in their evaluation. Lowered fundamental frequency and increased aperiodicity may be noted, but symmetry is usually not affected. Amplitude of vibration is usually normal. In such cases, pitch and loudness modification may allow better appreciation of the true amplitude of vibration. Most important, the status of the mucosal wave and the pattern of glottal closure are observed. At the site of the lesion, the mucosal wave may be decreased during vibratory cycle events. An edematous lesion will impair the mucosal wave less than will a fibrous lesion. The location of the lesions, usually on the free edge of the fold, upper or lower lip, can also be determined. The presence of a nonvibrating segment of the fold suggests more extensive pathology within Reinke's space than is implied by the present definition of nodules and polyps.

A typical hourglass pattern of incomplete glottic closure is associated with polyps and nodules. Patients with nodules may have a sizable glottal "chink" anterior to the vocal process (Morrison, Rammage, Belisle, Pullan, & Hamish, 1983). The degree of incomplete glottal closure may be influenced by the examination technique and the loudness of the patient's voice during examination (Söderston & Linstead, 1992). Use of the rigid telescope, in soft phonation, may not be representative of the patient's habitual phonation pattern but favors a greater degree of visualization of incomplete glottal closure.

Repeated videostroboscopic examinations are necessary to study fluctuations or progression of Reinke's space pathologies in response to vocal use and treatment. This is especially true in the case of nodules and polyps. Fluctuations in the appearance of nodules and polyps may occur in relation to the menstrual cycle, particularly if there are varicosities within Reinke's space. In some cases, it is difficult to differentiate nodules and polyps from other pathologies such as cysts, pseudocysts, or submucosal scarring, despite sequential videostroboscopic examinations. Cysts usually present on the superior surface of the fold as well as on the free edge. Submucosal scarring typically reduces the mucosal wave out of proportion to its size. In cases where definite vocal fold pathology is visualized but the clinical diagnosis is unclear, direct microlaryngoscopic examination under anesthesia is warranted.

Acoustic Evaluation

In 1971 Moore emphasized the need for standardized measurements of the voice; yet, clinicians and scientists still disagree about the description of voice quality and the objective voice parameters to be used. Their disagreement has been complicated by the persistence of different data acquisition techniques and methods of data analysis.

No single measurement has the sensitivity or specificity to detect vocal pathology (Baer, Sasaki, & Harris, 1987; Ludlow & Hart, 1981), and values within the normal range do not exclude laryngeal pathology (Zyski, Bull, McDonald, & Johns, 1984). Furthermore, tests relying on maximum performance tasks show tremendous intra- and intersubject variability and are affected by practice, motivation, and instructions (Kent, Kent & Rosenbek, 1987). Failing to distinguish singers from nonsingers may account for some discrepancies in the results obtained, because singers may present earlier symptomatology and smaller nodules (Peppard et al., 1988). Singers may also show greater

ability to compensate vocally (Sataloff, 1987); they often produce normal or superior profiles on tests such as maximum phonation time and maximum fricative ratio (Bastian, Keidar, & Verdolini-Matston, 1990).

The literature offers conflicting reports concerning the effects of nodules on speaking fundamental frequency and habitual loudness. Because these vocal fold lesions tend to increase the effective mass of the vocal folds (Hirano, 1981a), fundamental frequency would typically be lowered. This is not always so, and the frequency can increase or remain unaffected. Murry (1978) noted that the clinical impression of a lowered pitch in the pathological voice is due to the confounding perception of aberrant voice quality rather than perception of pitch alone. Peppard et al. (1988) reported that singers with nodules had lower fundamental frequency than normal singers. Coleman and Markham (1991) noted an 18% daily variation in the habitual pitch of normal voices. Habitual pitch seems stable in short-term sampling, but there is much intraspeaker variation over repeated samples and with the emotional content of speech. Assessment of maximum phonational pitch range may be more pertinent to phonatory capabilities and more revealing of disorders. Individuals with vocal nodules may demonstrate a restricted frequency range during connected speech and an increased frequency range during vowel phonation (Blalock, 1992). Fundamental frequency perturbations (jitter) are also expected to increase along with the severity of the hoarseness.

Hirano, Tanaka, Fujita, and Terasawa (1991) found the sound pressure level for habitual loudness to be elevated in males with vocal nodules. Hillman, Holmberg, Perkell, Walsh, and Vaughan (1990) recorded values for normal and loud voice phonation that were within the normal range. Bassich and Ludlow (1981) found a group of patients with vocal nodules to have reduced intensity range compared to age- and gender-matched controls.

Despite limitations in the clinical use of objective measures of voice, their use in assessing changes in the voice response to treatment is warranted. Many studies are reporting different pre- and post-therapy measurements, but not always. Ludlow, Bassich, Young, Connor, and Coulter (1984) did not find that the magnitude of jitter indicated changes in laryngeal pathology. Schneider (1993) reported the use of mean fundamental frequency, fundamental frequency range, and jitter in a patient with bilateral nodules in response to voice therapy. However, despite clinical resolution of the nodules and perceptual voice improvement, the acoustic parameters studied did not relate to the observed changes.

Few studies have used children as subjects in the determination of normative voice parameters; therefore, interpretation of the pathological significance of voice parameters in children with vocal nodules is doubtful. Nevertheless, Kane and Wellen (1985) found measures of jitter and shimmer in children with vocal nodules to correlate with clinical judgment of the severity of hoarseness.

Vocal nodules and polyps may alter the voice spectrogram. In Yanagihara's (1967) classification of four types of hoarseness based on spectrographic analysis, vocal nodules gave slight to severe dysphonia and were found to show all four spectrographic types, consistent with loss of harmonic components and a low harmonic-to-noise ratio.

Remacle and Trigaux (1991), in studying the characteristics of nodules, attended to peak fundamental frequency and the first harmonics and found that the 0 to 1000 Hz range was most sensitive in revealing small qualitative changes. Seventy-five percent of the cases in this study had normal fundamental frequency peaks and lower intensity harmonics that were slightly widened and notched. These findings, however, are not unique to nodules and polyps. Small cysts could result in the same findings.

Other parameters, such as voice-onset time, voice breaks, and pitch and intensity modulation are under study and may be more reliable for indicating vocal pathology.

Aerodynamic Evaluation

Most studies using aerodynamic measurements of vocal function in patients with vocal nodules have reported results that overlap the normal range. Such measurements must be interpreted in view of glottal closure patterns and supraglottic compensatory vocal behaviors. Vocal nodules and polyps typically yield excessive or highly variable airflow rates during sustained phonation because of incomplete vocal fold closure.

In keeping with the tremendous variability of airflow measurements and their variance due to age, gender, vocal effort, frequency, and register, Hirano, Koike, and von Leden (1968) reported that only 28% of females with vocal nodules had mean airflow rates outside of the normal range. Elevated average airflow rate as well as minimal flow rate due to incomplete glottic closure from nodules or polyps was reported by Hillman et al. (1989, 1990). Woo, Colton, and Shangold (1987) suggested that the measurement of phonatory airflow, using a constant hot wire anemometer, and the quantification of airflow characteristics (AC/DC ratio and frequency analysis of airflow waveform) may provide a reliable measure of vocal efficiency and a useful assessment of treatment efficacy. Vocal efficiency is reduced, and airflow rates are high, especially if the glottal chink is wide. Low vocal efficiency also can be associated with high airflow rates, and subglottic pressures result from the increased mass and stiffness of the vocal fold (Tanaka & Gould, 1985).

Eckel and Boone (1981) found the s/z ratio (maximum fricative duration) to reliably indicate vocal fold pathology and a reported mean ratio of 1:1.65 or greater obtained in the presence of nodules. The s/z ratio, however, may not be a sensitive indicator for vocal nodules (Fendler & Shearer, 1988). Two studies (Hufnagle & Hufnagle, 1988; Rastatter & Hyman, 1982) reported s/z ratios within the normal range (0.84 to 1.3). Yet, maximum duration of the individual fricatives, /s/ and /z/, was lower than the norms established by Tait, Michael, and Carpenter (1980). Maximum phonation times are quite variable and dependent on age and gender, pitch, vowel quality, number of trials, proper instruction, and patient effort (Schmidt, Kingholz, & Martin, 1988; Stone, 1983).

SOCIAL IMPLICATIONS

Emotional and Psychosocial

Dysphonia resulting from vocal nodules and polyps is not without emotional and psychological consequences. Individuals with dysphonia may develop a laissez-faire attitude, attributing their symptoms to a "cold" from which they expect spontaneous resolution. Dysphonia, however, does not go unnoticed; family members, peers, and clients, will inquire as to the presence of illness or fatigue. Dysphonia sufferers' gutteral throat clearing becomes habitual and annoying to themselves and to others who must endure it. Dysphonia becomes their identifiable trait, taking precedence over other personality or physical traits. Women with low-pitched voices will be mistakenly addressed as males on the telephone. Patients sensitive to the pejorative nature of their dysphonia begin to avoid socializing and verbal communication. Constant attempts to force vocal quality lead only to further vocal strain and throat discomfort. Their lack of insight into the nature of their dysphonia fosters anxiety and fear about the possible diagnosis. Finally, due to peer pressure and worsening vocal performance, dysphonia sufferers seek medical attention.

Educational

Confirming the diagnosis of vocal nodules or polyps can allay many of the patient's fears of a serious disease such as cancer. To the lay person, nodules and polyps are unknown disorders, and the viewing of one's videolaryngoscopy results enhances the understanding of the nature of the problem.

Children with voice disorders are adversely perceived by their peers. Lass, Ruscello, Stout, and Hoffman (1991) recommend early detection and intervention to reduce the potential psychological impact of voice disorders in children. Similar advice also is appropriate for adults; however, knowledge of the diagnosis does not always relieve patients' anxiety. Whereas the diagnosis may readily be accepted by the patient, the implications may be most traumatic. The consequences of therapy on lifestyle, work scheduling, and professional commitments will sometimes exacerbate the patient's fears about seeking treatment. Some of the patient's fears may be warranted. In general, treatment for vocal nodules and polyps demands long-term commitment to vocal behavior modification and repeated medical visits. The patient's first concerns may be financial in view of medical expenses incurred and loss of professional income from time off work to attend therapy sessions.

Vocational

Professional voice users tend to be hard-working, ambitious, and conscientious individuals, who have high expectations and demands on their vocal performance. Vocal polyps and nodules may be wrongly interpreted as faulty technique, if only to allay the fear that their symptoms may soon compel the end of a professional career. Such fear persists despite the advent of modern diagnostic and therapeutic modalities that, with early treatment, can often reverse the destructive potential of VFPN.

For employers and insurers, therapy for vocal dysfunction may not be deemed necessary or worthwhile. Professional voice users may wish to conceal the diagnosis from managers or promoters, for fear that they may be judged unworthy of future engagement. Patients must receive help from the voice care team in dealing with the multitude of exogenous factors imposing vocal demands that seemingly cannot be met. In many cases, the caregiver must convey medical orders directly to the individual's employer, manager, and insurance companies.

TREATMENT: OPTIONS AND OUTCOMES

When the voice care team determines the appropriate course of treatment for a particular patient, it is a consensus based on many factors: age, gender, occupation, relative disability from the dysphonia, and video-laryngo-stroboscopic findings. Some VFPN may be asymptomatic and detected incidentally during the course of an otolaryngological examination. If there is no doubt as to the diagnosis, VFPN can be safely followed by serial examinations; their mere presence does not mandate aggressive treatment. However, inasmuch as these lesions result from vocal abuse and misuse, all patients should be given appropriate counseling and offered vocal use management. However, the decision to proceed with benign or aggressive ther-

apy is based largely on the patient's motivation toward lifestyle changes, behavior, voice modification, and the importance of vocal function to the patient.

Some patients may not desire therapy. They interpret the presence of vocal fold lesions or dysphonia as inconsequential to their general well-being. For some, the resultant dysphonia is a distinguishable feature of their persona. In singers, VFPN may impart acoustic characteristics that become a kind of personal trademark, judged as desirable to certain music styles and contributing to their professional success. For patients who refuse therapy, guidelines should be agreed on as to when therapy may be warranted based on symptomatology or vocal demands. Professional voice users can be counseled as to the long-term consequences of continued voice abuse and misuse.

Treatment of VFPN begins with the identification and removal of precipitating (if still significant) and perpetuating or aggravating factors. General recommendations are made such as increased hydration, smoking cessation, and control of sinonasal allergies or infection, modification of techniques of voice production brought to the task of nonprofessional uses of voice, and then, as appropriate, professional use.

Stone (1982) has drawn attention to the need for proper laryngeal lubrication and considers this paramount in vocal abuse reduction. The decreased consumption of dehydrants such as caffeine and alcohol often is recommended along with increased intake of water and humidification of the inspired air. Phonation threshold pressures are lowest when vocal folds are exposed to humidified inspired air and when individuals are well hydrated (Verdolini-Marston, Titze, & Druker, 1990). The use of pharmacological mucolytics, indicated for the thinning of tenacious bronchial secretions, has not been the subject of scientific studies for laryngeal lubrication; however, they are frequently recommended (Lawrence, 1991a; Punt, 1974). Anecdotal experience suggests that they may decrease the tenacity of postnasal and laryngeal secretions, thus lessening the need for throat clearing.

Smoking cessation should be encouraged. The Surgeon General's report (1990) clearly outlines the benefit of smoking cessation on the risks of acute and chronic respiratory and cardiovascular diseases. Of direct beneficial consequence to voice production is the decrease in bronchial airway hyperactivity, improved pulmonary function, and decreased incidence of respiratory infections. The success rate of abstinence from smoking is greater if nicotine polacrilex (nicotine "gum") or nicotine transdermal patches are used in conjunction with participation in a smoking cessation program which deals with the psychological and behavioral consequences of addiction (Sachs & Leischow, 1991) and provides peer support.

The treatment of concurrent sinonasal disorders aims to improve the natural humidification properties of the nasal mucosa, allow nasal breathing, and lessen postnasal drip. Although the direct benefits for the resolution of VFPN are unknown, treatment of these conditions may be warranted prior to contemplated surgery on the vocal folds.

Total voice rest is commonly prescribed to patients presenting with VFPN despite the lack of consistent information as to its efficacy. Koufman and Blalock (1989) believe that voice rest is of no particular benefit in the nonsurgical or in the postoperative management of abuse-related vocal fold lesions. Nevertheless, many clinicians have observed resolution of VFPN with voice rest. Presumably, these lesions were relatively acute and the result of recent vocal abuse or misuse. For example, the occurrence of localized swellings on the margins of the vocal folds

subsequent to strenuous rehearsals or performances may warrant 2 to 3 days of voice rest. If there is no improvement, the voice rest may be extended for another week to 10 days (Miller, 1986). Prolonged voice rest (more than 2 weeks) may not be desirable for singers because it may be followed by sluggish laryngeal muscle coordination (Lawrence, 1991b) and adverse psychologic reactions.

Whispering (using the articulators to form words with rapid airflow but no phonation) could be considered an alternative to complete voice rest, because quiet whispering is not accompanied by vibratory movements of the vocal folds (Monoson & Zemlin, 1984). The recommendation should be made only after consideration that whispering may involve excessive expiratory muscle use and high glottal airflow rates but low subglottal pressure. Glottal configurations during different types of whispers show variability, and this may warrant visualization by fiberoptic laryngoscopy (Solomon, McCall, Trosset, & Gray, 1989) prior to recommending whispering as an alternative to, or in conjunction with, voice rest.

Patients find total voice rest difficult to implement and restrictive to their lifestyles. As an alternative, or as follow-up to voice rest, a "Vocal Abuse Reduction Program" (VARP) (Johnson, 1985) may be instituted under the guidance of a speech-language pathologist. The aim of VARP is to pinpoint the sources of vocal abuse and systematically decrease the probability of their occurrence during the most offensive time periods.

Vocal use management also implies a complete vocal use inventory which may warrant a field study. Patterns of vocal abuse must be highlighted to patients and pragmatic recommendations made. In many instances, communication with superiors at work or with the manager of the professional artist is required. Realistic scheduling of performances and recording sessions should allow for periods of voice rest and proper vocal warm-up and cool-down. Finally, attention should be given to the work or rehearsal and performance environment from the quality of inspired air to the use of appropriate amplification systems. VFPN that do not respond to vocal rest, at least with some reduction in size or symptoms, may be interpreted as evidence of more long-standing vocal trauma. Thus, voice rest that is not therapeutic may at least be diagnostic and have etiological implications. In addition, the sequential video-laryngo-stroboscopic examinations allow reconsideration of the diagnosis because features suggestive of a vocal cyst may be unmarked by removal of secondary pathology.

Singers may have to be convinced of the benefits of training with a vocal pedagogue. Correction of vocal technique, with particular attention to the use of appropriate vocal registers, is often needed. Modification of the vocal repertoire, at least temporarily, may also be in order in the form of performance in different "keys" or elimination of some members.

The most common medical treatment for VFPN involves systemic corticosteroids (Lawrence, 1991c; Miller, 1986c). Anti-inflammatory corticosteroids decrease edema as well as inflammation. Corticosteroids vary in their anti-inflammatory potency, onset time of effectiveness, and duration of action. Preferably, short-acting preparations, such as methylprednisolone are used. Some clinicians advocate the use of steroids only for the management of acute inflammatory laryngitis in professional voice users who must proceed with a vocal performance before they implement voice rest (Lawrence, 1991c; Sataloff, 1991). Inasmuch as inflammatory conditions and VFPN may coexist and the former may have brought these lesions into clinical evidence, short-term steroids may help manage the patient. Excessive, prolonged, or frequently repeated use of steroids is not advocated because it addresses the symptoms and not the cause of the problem.

Adjunctive measures to conventional vocal re-education, such as various biofeedback modalities (laryngeal imaging, acoustical, and tactile) are the subject of continuing evaluation. Laryngeal imaging biofeedback is said to be useful if an obvious abnormality of vocal fold posturing can be observed and behaviorally modified (Bastian, 1987). The patient's viewing of his or her own videostroboscopic examination during the course of therapy may encourage compliance and confidence in the therapeutic process (Lancer, Syder, Jones, & LeBoutillier, 1988; Murry & Woodson, 1992).

Clinical experience supports the efficacy of voice therapy in the treatment of VFPN, despite the paucity of objectively documented treatment results. Brodnitz (1963) found that patients' judgments were an important criterion for success. Yamaguchi, Yotsukura, Kondo, Hanyuu, Horiguchi, Imaizumi, and Hirose (1986), reporting on 20 adults with vocal nodules, noted that 65% of cases had disappearance or reduction in the size of the nodule after 3 to 4 months of voice therapy. Fox (1989) found that treatment time for vocal nodules varied from 6 to 18 hours for therapy, the average time being 6 to 8 hours. Recent studies (Lancer et al., 1988; Murry & Woodson, 1992) have compared various modalities of treatment, including voice therapy, surgery, or a combination of both. These studies support the generally accepted notion that voice improvement is possible with voice therapy alone, and that the greatest improvement can be achieved by joint, nonsurgical management by the speech-language pathologist and the otolaryngologist. Voice therapy, alone or in combination with surgery, does reduce the recurrence rate of nodules post-treatment. Unfortunately, most studies admit to a bias in the determination of study groups, because patients were not randomly assigned. Although many authors (Hirano, 1988; Sataloff, 1989; Vaughn, 1983) have recommended voice therapy as the initial treatment modality before surgery, surveys reveal that this may not always be practiced (Allen, Pettit, & Sherblom, 1991; Moran & Pentz, 1987) and that treatment may be based on the personal bias of the otolaryngologist. Some nodules may be arbitrarily judged too large for consideration of voice therapy, or patients judged a priori as unlikely candidates to pursue voice therapy.

In children, voice therapy is the cornerstone of management, with surgery having a limited role (Johnson 1985). On the other hand, Strome (1982) believes that once nodules are present in the child they will persist until puberty. Because the vocal folds elongate at puberty, there is a shift in the point of maximum vibration. In addition, the inner structure of the vocal fold (lamina propria) differentiates into distinct layers (Hirano, Kurita, & Nakashima, 1983). Presumably, these developmental changes are responsible for alterations in laryngeal biomechanics that favor VFPN resolution. Conservative therapy is advised because severely restricted vocalizations, whether during recreation or learning activities, may adversely affect children's psychological development and acquisition of verbal skills. Filter (1977) emphasizes the need for addressing the psychological component of this disorder. More detailed management of childhood dysphonias is discussed by Stone (1982) and Casteel and Stone (1982).

Surgery for vocal nodules should be considered only after a fair trial of voice therapy. If there is no improvement in the voice and the speech-language pathologist can attest to the patient's compliance in modifying vocal behavior, medical and/or surgical management becomes an option. Review of sequential video-stroboscopies helps in confirming that the dysphonia is indeed due to the presence of the vocal lesion and that it has stabilized. Finally, the patient must desire vocal improvement, be in good health, be free of active infection, understand the risks of proposed general anesthesia and surgery, and be capable of giving informed consent.

Assuming patient compliance, how long voice therapy must be conducted before surgery is considered can only be answered in relative time frames. Sataloff (1991) recommends a minimum of 6 to 12 weeks; others (von Leden, 1978) pursue voice therapy as long as there is improvement in the voice. Although the lesion may still be visible, it may have the potential to remodel itself and not affect the vibrational characteristics of the vocal fold or cause perceptible alterations in the voice. von Leden (1988) advises extreme caution in proposing surgery to the professional singer, especially one who may wish to hasten the resolution of his or her dysphonia by a "quick fix."

VFPN are excised according to the principles of laryngeal microsurgery: identification and preservation of the vocal ligament and vocalis muscle, selective removal of the pathology within Reinke's space, and a controlled epithelial excision, keeping the depth of the excision level within the vibratory margin (Sataloff, 1991). Surgical maneuvers, such as avulsing the lesion with cup forceps or "stripping" of the epithelial cover, are condemned because they may lead to the removal of normal mucosa (von Leden, 1988). Surgery is usually performed under general anesthesia using the microscope. Saito, Fukuda, and Kitahara (1975) described a technique for stroboscopic microsurgery under neuroleptanalgesia.

The use of the laser, particularly the carbon dioxide laser, to selectively "shave" the epithelial excrescence down to the desired level is of controversial benefit. Despite the benefits provided by its precise control, hemostatic properties, and improved visualization, concerns are expressed about the dissipation of heat into the lamina propria and its potential for delayed wound healing and fibrosis (Durkin, Duncavage, Toohill, Tieu, & Caya, 1986). Deleterious effects may be occurring on the nonepithelial components of the vocal folds (i.e., degeneration of neural elements) (Leonard, Gallia, & Charpied, 1992). The advent of improved laser micromanipulators allowing for smaller laser spot sizes and decreased laser power densities may prove valuable in refining the use of this surgical modality.

The use of voice rest in the postoperative period has not been the subject of scientific analysis. It is commonly prescribed, presumably to allow for undisturbed healing of the incision site and to prevent edema and hematoma formation in Reinke's space. The duration of voice rest is the decision of the surgeon, ranging from a minimum of just a few days to 10 to 14 days, depending on the extent of epithelial excision and the surgical tools used (laser versus scalpel). Koufman and Blalock (1989) believe that voice rest offers no significant benefit over vocal conservation techniques. Evidence gathered from experimental excisions on the vocal folds of cats suggests that epithelial and neural tissues may still be altered at 3 weeks postoperatively (Leonard, Gallia, Charpied, & Kelly, 1988).

Sequential videostroboscopic examinations at 2 and 4 weeks postoperatively will guide the course of treatment during the healing period. Progressive voice use and vocal rehabilitation can usually be resumed by the third postoperative week. Return of the vocal fold mucosal wave may take 3 to 6 months.

Persistent dysphonia following surgery may be due to the following: delayed wound healing with edema, hematoma, or granuloma; scarring of the vocal fold epithelium to the underlying vocal ligament; or loss of substance of the vocal fold (notching of the vibrating edge). Green (1972) has postulated that, although the vocal folds appear healed, lesions in the mucosal mechanoreceptors may persist and this could account for a disturbance in the tuning of the laryngeal musculature in phonation. Persistent hoarseness also may be due to the presence of dysplastic collagen fibrils in the vocal fold. Concomitant sinonasal disease (infection, allergies) may also be a significant factor. Incipient respiratory tract infection may impede the healing process (Andrews, 1970). This would substantiate the use of antibiotics in the postoperative period. The most likely cause for prolonged postoperative dysphonia is vocal abuse (Koufman & Blalock, 1989). A lower incidence of prolonged postoperative dysphonia can result from the use of preoperative voice therapy and postoperative voice conservation technique. Recurrence of VFPN is common and is likely related to the patient's inability to maintain vocal behavior modification and the continued presence of deleterious environmental factors. There are no studies to suggest that age, gender, or smoking affect recurrence of VFPN.

SUMMARY

In this chapter, we have acknowledged the lack of proper nomenclature for the different types of benign vocal fold lesions that occur in response to phonotrauma. An accurate clinical distinction between these lesions hopefully will be achieved as laryngeal stroboscopy becomes a common diagnostic tool. The lack of correlation between the clinical and histopathological diagnosis, noted 35 years ago, still prevails. With new laryngeal microsurgical techniques, the pathologist is asked to identify specimens arising from Reinke's space; knowledge of the clinical features is still needed.

There is a pressing need to pursue animal models of phonotrauma lesions. In particular, a definitive study of laryngeal mucosal blood flow during phonation is needed. Ischemia is likely to be an important determinant in vocal fold wound healing capabilities. If basement membrane damage is the earliest site of phonotrauma, then the composition, properties, and functions of the vocal fold basement membrane must also be further studied.

Finally, VFPN are largely preventable lesions. It is unfortunate that few speakers who depend on their voices professionally, other than some singers and actors, receive any instruction in the proper use of their voices or voice conservation. Everyone whose occupation makes excessive demands on voice use should have guidance during training in using his or her voice effectively to minimize unnecessary laryngeal tension.

In the future, treatment of VFPN will continue to rely on management of voice use therapy to reduce abuses, with stroboscopy playing a greater role in the determination of the nature of the lesion and surgical selection criteria.

REFERENCES

Abitbol, J., de Brux, J., Millot, G., Masson, M-F., Mimoun, O. L., Pau, H., & Abitbol, B. (1989). Does a hormonal vocal cord cycle exist in women? Study of vocal premenstrual syndrome in voice performers by videostroboscopy-glottography and cytology on 38 women. *Journal of Voice, 3,* 157–162.

Allen, S. A., Pettit, J. M., & Sherblom, J. C. (1991). Management of vocal nodules: A regional survey of otolaryngologists and speech-language pathologists. *Journal of Speech and Hearing Research, 34,* 229–235.

Andrews, A. H., Jr. (1970). Surgery for benign tumors of the larynx. *Otolaryngology Clinics of North America, 3,* 517–527.

Arnold, G. (1962). Vocal nodules and polyps: Laryngeal tissue reaction to habitual hyperki-netic dysphonia. *Journal of Speech and Hearing Disorders, 27,* 205–217.

Arnstein, D. P., Trapp, T. K., Berke, G. S., & Natividad, M. (1989). Regional blood flow to the canine vocal fold at rest and during phonation. *Annals of Otology, Rhinology, Laryngology, 98,* 796–802.

Aronson, A. E. (1980). *Clinical voice disorders.* New York: Thieme-Stratton.

Aronson, M. D., Weiss, S. T., Ben, R. L., & Komaroff, A. L. (1982). Association between cigarette smoking and acute respiratory tract illness in young adults. *Journal American Medical Association, 248,* 181–183.

Ash, J. E., & Schwartz, L. (1944). Laryngeal (vocal cord) node. Transactions of the *American Academy of Opthalmology and Otolaryngology, 48,* 330–332.

Baer, T., Sasaki, C., & Harris, K. (Eds.). (1987). *Laryngeal function in phonation and respiration.* Boston: College-Hill Press.

Baker, B. M., Fox, S. M., Baker, C. D., & McMurry, G. T. (1981). Persistent hoarseness after surgical removal of vocal cord lesions. *Archives of Otolaryngology, 107,* 148–151.

Bassich, C., & Ludlow, C. (1981, November). *Perceptual methods for assessing vocal pathology.* Paper presented at the annual meeting of the American Speech-Language-Hearing Association, Los Angeles.

Bastian, R. W. (1987). Laryngeal image biofeedback for voice disorder patients. *Journal of Voice, 3,* 279–282.

Bastian, R. W., Keidar, A., & Verdolini-Marston, K. (1990). Simple vocal tasks for detecting vocal fold swelling. *Journal of Voice, 4,* 172–183.

Baynes, R. (1966). An incidence study of chronic hoarseness among children. *Journal of Speech and Hearing Disorders, 31,* 172–176.

Beckford, N. S., Rood, S. R., & Schaid, D. (1985). Androgen stimulation and laryngeal development. *Annals of Otology, Rhinology, Laryngology, 94,* 634–640.

Blalock, P. D. (1992). Management of patients with vocal nodules. *The Visible Voice, 1,* 4–6.

Boone, D. R. (1983). *The voice and voice therapy* (3rd ed.). Englewood Cliffs, NJ: Prentice-Hall.

Brodnitz, F. S. (1963). Goals, results, and limitations of vocal rehabilitation. *Archives of Otolaryngology, 77,* 148–156.

Brodnitz, F. (1971). *Vocal rehabilitation.* Rochester, MN: American Academy of Ophthalmology and Otolaryngology.

Casteel, R. L., & Stone, R. E (1982). Intervention in childhood voice problems: Intervention thematics. In M. D. Filter (Ed.), *Phonatory voice disorders in children* (pp 166–180). Springfield, IL: Charles C Thomas.

Childs, D. R., & Johnson, T. S. (1991). Preventable and non-preventable causes of voice disorders. *Seminars in Speech and Language, 12,* 1–13.

Coleman, R. F., & Markham, I. W. (1991). Normal variations in habitual pitch. *Journal of Voice, 5,* 173–177.

Cooper, M. (1973) *Modern techniques of vocal rehabilitation.* Springfield, IL: Charles C Thomas.

D'Antonio, L. L., Muntz, H. R., Province, M. A., & Marsh, J. L. (1988). Laryngeal/voice findings in patients with velopharyngeal insufficiency. *Laryngoscope, 88,* 432–438.

Deal, R. E., McClain, B., & Sudderth, J. F. (1976). Identification, evaluation, therapy, and follow-up for children with vocal nodules in public school setting. *Journal of Speech and Hearing Disorders, 41,* 390–397.

Dearkay, C. S., Thomsen, J. R., & Grundfast, K. M. (1991). Laryngeal pathology in hearing-impaired children. *International Journal of Pediatric Otolaryngology, 21,* 163–168.

Dejonckere, P. H., & Lebacq, J. (1985). Electroglottography and vocal nodules. *Folia Phoniatrica, 37,* 195–200.

Dikkers, F. G., Hulsteart, C. E., Oosterbaan, J. A., & Cervera-Paz, F. J. (1993). Ultrastructural changes of the basement membrane zone in benign lesions of the vocal folds. *Acta Otolaryngologica* (Stockholm), *113,* 98–101.

Durkin, G. E., Duncavage, J. A., Toohill, R. J., Tieu, T. M., & Caya, J. G. (1986). Wound healing of true vocal cord squamous epithelium after CO_2 laser ablation and cup forceps stripping. *Otolaryngology—Head and Neck Surgery, 95,* 273–277.

Eckel, F. C., & Boone, D. R. (1981). The s/z ratio as an indicator of laryngeal pathology. *Journal of Speech and Hearing Disorders, 46,* 147–149.

Fendler, M., & Shearer, W. M. (1988). Reliability of the s/z ratio in normal children's voices. *Language, Speech, and Hearing Services in Schools, 19,* 2–4.

Fergusson, B. J., Hudson, W. R., & McCarty, K. S. (1987). Sex steroid receptor distribution in the human larynx and laryngeal carcinoma. *Archives of Otolaryngology—Head and Neck Surgery, 113,* 1311–1315.

Filter, M. D. (1977). *Communication disorders: A handbook for educators.* Springfield, IL: Charles C Thomas.

Finkelhor, B. K., Titze, I. R., & Durham, P. L. (1988). The effect of viscosity changes in the vocal folds on the range of oscillation. *Journal of Voice, 1,* 320–325.

Fitz-Hugh, G. S., Smith, D. E., & Chiong, A. T. (1958). Pathology of three-hundred clinically benign lesions of vocal cords. *Laryngoscope, 68,* 855–875.

Fox, D. R. (1989). Vocal nodules: Time, duration, and treatment protocol. In W. Singh (Ed.), *Proceedings of international voice symposium* (pp. 83–84). Livingston, Scotland: Waryam Singh.

Frenzel, H. (1986). Fine structural and immunohistochemical studies on polyps of human vocal folds. In J. R. Kirchner (Ed.), *Vocal fold histopathology. A symposium* (pp. 39–50). San Diego: College-Hill Press.

Garde, E. J. (1969). Nodules and polypi and the vocal cords: New considerations. *Annals Otolaryngology* (Paris), *78,* 378–398.

Gray, S. D., & Titze, I. (1988). Histologic investigation of hyperphonated canine vocal cords. *Annals of Otology, Rhinology, and Laryngology, 97*(4), 381–388.

Gray, S. D., & Titze, I. (1988). Histologic investigation of hyperphonated canine vocal cords. *Annals of Otology, Rhinology and Laryngology, 97,* 381–388.

Gray, S. D., Titze, I., & Lusk, R. P. (1987). Electron microscopy of hyperphonated canine vocal cords. *Journal of Voice, 1,* 109–115.

Green, G. (1989). Psycho-behavioral characteristics of children with vocal nodules: WPBIC ratings. *Journal of Speech and Hearing Disorders, 54,* 306–312.

Green, M. (1972). *The voice and its disorders.* Philadelphia, PA: J. B. Lippincott Company.

Hammaberg, B., Fritzell, B., Gauffin, J., Sundberg, J., & Wedin, L. (1980). Perceptual and acoustic correlates of abnormal voice qualities. *Acta Otolaryngologica, 90,* 441–451.

Härma, R., Soninnen, A., Vartiainen, E., Haveri, P., & Väisänen, A. (1975). Vocal polyps and nodules. *Folia Phoniatrica, 27,* 19–25.

Herrington-Hall, B., Lee, L., Stemple, J. C., Niemi, K. R., & McHone, M. M. (1988). Description of laryngeal pathologies by age, sex, and occupation in a treatment-seeking sample. *Journal of Speech and Hearing Disorders, 53,* 57–64.

Hillman, R. E., Holmberg, E. B., Perkell, J. S., Walsh, M., & Vaughan, C. (1989). Objective assessment of vocal hyperfunction: An experimental framework and initial results. *Journal of Speech and Hearing Research, 32,* 373–392.

Hillman, R. E. Holmberg, E. B., Perkell, J. S., Walsh, M., & Vaughn, C. (1990). Phonatory function associated with hyperfunctionally related vocal fold lesions. *Journal of Voice, 4,* 52–63.

Hirano, M. (1981a). Structure of the vocal fold in normal and disease states: Anatomical and physical studies. In C. L. Ludlow & M. O. Hart (Eds.), Proceedings of the conference on the assessment of vocal fold pathology. *ASHA Reports, 11,* 11–30.

Hirano, M. (1981b). Psycho-acoustic evaluation of voice. In G. E. Arnold, F. Winkel, & B. D. Wyke (Eds.), *Clinical examination of voice* (pp. 80–84). New York: Springer-Verlag.

Hirano, M. (1988). Endolaryngeal microsurgery. In G. M. English (Ed.), *Otolaryngology* (Vol. 3, pp. 1–22). Philadelphia: J. B. Lippincott.

Hirano, M., Koike, Y., & von Leden, H. (1968). Maximum phonation time and air usage during phonation. *Folia Phoniatrica, 20,* 185–201.

Hirano, H., Kurita, S., Matsuo, K., & Nagata, K. (1980). Laryngeal tissue reaction to stress. In V. Lawrence (Ed.), *Transcripts of the Ninth Symposium Care of the Professional Voice* (pp. 10–20). New York: The Voice Foundation.

Hirano, M., Kurita, S., & Nakashima, T. (1981). Growth, development, and aging of human vocal folds. In K. N. Stevens & M. Hirano (Eds.), *Vocal fold physiology.* Japan: University of Tokyo Press.

Hirano, M., Kurita, S., & Nakashima, T. (1983). Growth, development, and aging of the human vocal folds. In D. M. Bless & J. H. Abbs (Eds), *Vocal fold physiology: Contemporary research and clinical issues,* (pp. 22–43). San Diego: College-Hill Press.

Hirano, M., Tanaka, S., Fujita, M., & Terasawa, R. (1991). Fundamental frequency and sound pressure level of phonation in pathological states. *Journal of Voice, 5,* 120–127.

Hiroto, I. (1981). Introductory remarks. In K. N. Stevens & M. Hirano (Eds.), *Vocal fold physiology* (pp. 3–9). Tokyo: University of Tokyo Press.

Hufnagle, J., & Hufnagle, K. K. (1988). S/Z ratio in dysphonic children with and without vocal cord nodules. Language, *Speech, and Hearing Services in Schools, 19,* 418–422.

Hunt, T. K., Banda, M. J., & Silver, I. A. (1985). Cell interactions in post-traumatic fibrosis. In *Fibrosis. Ciba Foundation Symposium,* (Vol. 114, pp. 127–149). London: Pitman.

Johnson, T. S. (1985). *Vocal abuse reduction program.* Boston: College-Hill Press.

Joris, I., Cuenoud, H. F., Diern, G. V., Underwood, J. M., & Majno, G. (1991). Endothelial permeability in inflammation: The role of capillaries versus venules. In N. Simionescu & M. Simionescu (Eds.), *Endothelial cell dysfunctions* (pp. 233–242). New York: Plenum Press.

Kahane, J. C. (1982). Growth of the human prepubertal and pubertal larynx. *Journal of Speech and Hearing Research, 25,* 446–455.

Kambic, V., Radsel, Z., Zargi, M., & Acko, M. (1981). Vocal cord polyps: Incidence, histology and pathogenesis. *Journal of Laryngology and Otology, 95,* 609–618.

Kane, M., & Wellen, C. J. (1985). Acoustical measurements and clinical judgements of vocal quality in children with vocal nodules. *Folia Phoniatrica, 37,* 53–57.

Kent, R. D., Kent, J., & Rosenbek, J. (1987). Maximum performance tests of speech production. *Journal of Speech Hearing Research, 52,* 367–387.

Kleinsasser, O. (1982). Pathogenesis of vocal cord polyps. *Annals of Otology, Rhinology, Laryngology, 91,* 378–381.

Kotby, M. N., Nassar, A. M., Seif, E. I., Helal, E. H., & Saleh, M. M. (1988a). Ultrastructural changes of the basement membrane zone in benign lesions of the vocal folds. *Acta Otolaryngologica, 113,* 98–101.

Kotby, M. N., Nassar, A. M., Seif, E. I., Helal, E. H., & Saleh, M. M. (1988b). Ultrastructural features of vocal fold nodules and polyps. *Acta Otolaryngologica* (Stockholm), *105,* 477–482.

Koufman, J. A. (1991). The otolaryngologic manifestations of gastroesophageal reflux disease: A clinical investigation of 225 patients using ambulatory 24-hour pH monitoring and an experimental investigation of the role of acid and pepsin in the development of laryngeal injury. *Laryngoscope, 101*(Suppl. 53).

Koufman, J. A., & Blalock, P. D. (1989). Is voice rest never indicated? *Journal of Voice, 3,* 87–91.

Lancer, M., Syder, D., Jones, A. S., & Le Boutillier, A. (1988). The outcome of different management patterns for vocal cord nodules. *Journal of Laryngology and Otology, 102,* 423–427.

Lancer, J. M., Syder, D., Jones, A. S., & LeBoutillier, A. (1988). Vocal cord nodules: A review. *Clinical Otolaryngology, 13,* 43–51.

Lass, N. J., Ruscello, D. M., Stout, L. L., & Hoffman, F. M. (1991). Peer perceptions of normal and voice disordered children. *Folia Phoniatrica, 43,* 29–35.

Lawrence, V. (1978). Medical care/preventive therapy. Panel discussion. In V. Lawrence (Ed.), *Transcripts of the Seventh Symposium: Care of the Professional Voice* (pp. 71–91). New York: The Voice Foundation.

Lawrence, V. L. (1991a). Handy household hints: To sing or not to sing. In R. T. Sataloff & I. R. Titze (Eds.), *Vocal health and science* (pp. 30–36). Jacksonville, FL: The National Association of Teachers of Singing.

Lawrence, V. L. (1991b). Nodules and other things that go bump in the night. In R. T. Sataloff & I. R. Titze (Eds.), *Vocal health and science* (pp. 125–127). Jacksonville, FL: National Association of Teachers of Singing.

Lawrence, V. L. (1991c). What about cortisone? In R. T. Sataloff & I. R. Titze (Eds), *Vocal health and science* (pp. 11–13). Jacksonville, FL: National Association of Teachers of Singing.

Le Huches, F. (1987). Propos du nodule du pli vocal chez l'enfant. *Revue de Laryngologie, 108,* 287–295.

Leeper, H. A. (1976). Voice initiation characteristics of normal children and children with vocal nodules: A preliminary investigation. *Journal Communication Disorders, 9,* 82–94.

Leeper, H. A., Leonard, J. E., & Iverson, R. L. (1980). Otolaryngologic screening of children with vocal quality disturbances. *International Journal of Pediatric Otorhinolaryngology, 2,* 123–131.

Leonard, R. J., Gallia, L. J., Charpied, G., & Kelly, A. (1988). Effects of stripping and laser excision on vocal fold mucosa in cats. *Annals of Otology, Rhinology and Laryngology, 97,* 159–163.

Leonard, R. J., Gallia, L. J., & Charpied, G. (1992). Recovery of vocal fold mucosa from laser incision. *Journal of Voice, 6,* 286–291.

Loire, R., Bouchayer, M., Cornut, G., & Bastian, R. (1988). Pathology of benign vocal fold lesions. *Ear, Nose and Throat Journal, 67,* 357–362.

Ludlow, C. L., & Hart, M. O. (1981). *Proceedings of the conference on the assessment of vocal pathology* (ASHA Reports no. 11). Rockville, MD: American Speech-Language-Hearing Association.

Ludlow, C., Bassich, C. J., Young, J. L., Connor, N. P., & Coulter, D. C. (1984). The validity of using phonatory jitter to detect laryngeal pathology. *Journal of the Acoustical Society of America, 75,* S8(A).

Matsuo, K., Oda, M., Tomita, M., Maehara, N., Umezaki, T., & Shin, T. (1987). An experimental study of the circulation of the vocal fold on phonation. *Archives of Otolaryngology—Head and Neck Surgery, 113,* 414–417.

McFarlane, S. C., & Watterson, T. L. (1990). Vocal nodules: Endoscopic study of their variations and treatment. *Seminars in Speech and Language, 11,* 47–59.

Miller, R. (1986). *The structure of singing.* (pp. 229–230). New York: Schirmer Books.

Mishashi, S., Okada, M., Kurita, S., Nagata, K., Oda, M., Hirano, M., & Nakashima, T. (1981). Vascular network of the vocal fold. In K. N. Stevens & M. Hirano (Eds), *Vocal fold physiology* (pp. 45–59). Tokyo: University of Tokyo Press.

Monsen, R. B. Engebretson, A. M., & Venula, N. R. (1979). Some effects of deafness on the generation of voice. *Journal Acoustical Society of America, 66,* 1680–1690.

Moore, G. P. (1971). *Organic voice disorders.* Englewood Cliffs, NJ: Prentice-Hall.

Moore, P. (1982). Disorders of speech, voice and language. In G. H. Shames & E. H. Wiig (Eds.), *Human communication disorders: An introduction* (pp. 172–175). Columbus, OH: Charles E. Merrill.

Monoson, P., & Zemlin, W. R. (1984). A quantitative study of whisper. *Folia Phoniatrica, 36,* 53–65.

Moran, M. J., & Pentz, A. L. (1987). Otolaryngologists' opinions of voice therapy for vocal nodules in children. *Language, Speech, and Hearing Services in Schools, 18,* 172–178.

Morrison, M. D., Rammage, L. A., Belisle, G. M., Pullan, C. B., & Hamish, N. (1983). Muscular tension dysphonia. *Journal of Otolaryngology, 12,* 302–336.

Mossalam, I., Kotby, M. N., Ghaly, A. F., Nassar, A. M., & Barakah, M. A. (1986). In J. A. Kirchner (Ed.), *Vocal fold histopathology. A symposium* (pp. 65–80). San Diego: College-Hill Press.

Murry, T. (1978). Speaking fundamental frequency characteristics associated with voice pathologies. *Journal of Speech and Hearing Disorders, 43,* 374–379.

Murry, T., & Woodson, G. E. (1992). A comparison of three methods for the management of vocal fold nodules. *Journal of Voice, 6,* 271–276.

Nagata, K., Kurita, S., Yasumoto, S., Maeda, T., Kawasaki, H., & Hirano, M. (1983). A review of 1,156 patients. *Auris Nasus Larynx, 10*(Suppl.), 27–35.

Pannbacker, M. (1975). Comment concerning "Incidence of chronic hoarseness among school age children." *Journal of Speech and Hearing Disorders, 40,* 548–549.

Peppard, R. C., Bless, D. M., & Milenkovic, P. (1988). Comparison of young adult singers and nonsingers with vocal nodules. *Journal of Voice, 2,* 250–260.

Prytz, S. (1980). Vocal nodules in Sjögren's syndrome. *Journal of Laryngology and Otology, 94,* 197–203.

Punt, N. (1974). Lubrication of the vocal mechanism. *Folia Phoniatrica, 26,* 287–288.

Rastatter, M. P., & Hyman, M. (1982). Maximum phoneme duration of /s/ and /z/ by children with vocal nodules. *Language, Speech, and Hearing Services in Schools, 13,* 197–199.

Remacle, M., & Trigaux, I. (1991). Characteristics of nodules through the high resolution frequency analyzer. *Folia Phoniatrica, 43,* 53–59.

Roch, J. B., Cornut, G., & Bouchayer (1989). Mechanisms involved in the appearance of laryngeal polyps. *Revue de Laryngologie, 110,* 389–390.

Rubin, H. J., & Lerhoff, I. (1962). Pathogenesis and treatment of vocal nodules. *Journal of Speech and Hearing Disorders, 27,* 150–161.

Sachs, D. L., & Leischow, S. J. (1991). Pharmacological approaches to smoking cessation. In J. M. Samet & D. B. Coultas (Eds.), *Clinics in chest medicine* (Vol. 12, no. 4, pp. 769–791). Philadelphia: W. B. Saunders.

Saito, S., Fukuda, H., & Kitahara, S. (1975). Stroboscopic microsurgery of the larynx. *Archives of Otolaryngology, 101,* 196–201.

Sataloff, R. T. (1987). The professional voice: Common diagnosis and treatments. *Journal of Voice, 1,* 283–292.

Sataloff, R. T. (1989). The professional voice. In G. M. English (Ed.), *Otolaryngology* (Vol. 3, pp. 1–17). Philadelphia: J. B. Lippincott.

Sataloff, R. T. (1991). A "first aid kit" for singers. In R. T. Sataloff & I. R. Titze, (Eds.), *Vocal health and science,* (pp. 40–46). Jacksonville, FL: National Association of Teachers of Singing.

Schmidt, P., Kingholz, F., & Martin, F. (1988). Influence of pitch, voice sound pressure and vowel quality on maximum phonation time. *Journal of Voice, 1,* 245–249.

Schneider, P. (1993). Tracking change in dysphonia. A case study. *Journal of Voice, 7,* 179–188.

Schwartz, I. S. (1980). Rheumatoid nodules of the vocal cords as the initial manifestation of systemic lupus erythematosus. *Journal of the American Medical Association, 19,* 2751–2752.

Sellars, S. L. (1979). Benign tumors of the larynx. *South African Medicine Journal, 56,* 943–946.

Senturia, B., & Wilson, F. (1968). Otorhinolaryngic findings in children with voice deviations. *Annals of Otolaryngology, 77,* 1027–1041.

Silverman, E. M., & Zimmer, C. (1975). Incidence of chronic hoarseness among school age children. *Journal of Speech and Hearing Disorders, 40,* 211–215.

Silverman, E. M., & Zimmer, C. (1975b). Speech fluency fluctuations during the menstrual cycle. *Journal of Speech and Hearing Research, 18,* 202–206.

Silverman, E. M., & Zimmer, C. (1976). Replication of speech fluency fluctuations. *Perceptual Motor Skills, 42,* 1004–1006.

Silverman, E. M., & Zimmer, C. (1978). Effect of the menstrual cycle on voice quality. *Archives of Otolaryngology and Head—Neck Surgery, 104*, 7–10.

Södersten, M., & Lindestad, P. A. (1992). A comparison of vocal fold closure in rigid telescopic and flexible fiberoptic laryngoscopy. *Acta Otolaryngologica* (Stockholm), *112*, 144–150.

Solomon, N. P., McCall, G. N., Trosset, M. W., & Gray, W. C. (1989). Laryngeal configuration and constriction during 2 types of whispering. *Journal of Speech and Hearing Research, 32*, 161–174.

Sonninen, A., Damsté, P. H., & Fokkens, J. (1972). On vocal strain. *Folia Phoniatrica, 24*, 321–336.

Spiegel, J. R., Sataloff, R. T., Cohn, J. R., & Hawkshaw, M. (1988). Respiratory function in singers: Medical assessment, diagnosis, and treatments. *Journal of Voice, 2*, 40–50.

Staubesand, J., Lachner, J., & Beck, C H L. (1984). Dysplastic collagen fibrils in the human vocal fold. *Acta Otolaryngologica, 97*, 398–402.

Stone, R. E. (1982). Management of childhood dysphonias of organic bases. In M. D. Filter (Ed.), *Phonatory voice disorders in children*. Springfield, IL: Charles C Thomas.

Stone, R. E. (1983). Issues in clinical assessment of laryngeal function: Contra-indications for subscribing to maximum phonation time and optimal frequency. In D. M. Bless & J. H. Abbs (Eds.), *Vocal physiology: Contemporary research and clinical issues* (pp. 410–431). San Diego, College-Hill Press.

Stone, R. E. (1991) Toward models for national issues in the prevention of voice disorders. *Seminars in Speech and Language, 12*, 23–39.

Strome, M. (1982). Common laryngeal disorders in children. In M. D. Filter (Ed.), *Phonatory voice disorders in children* (pp. 3–20). Springfield, IL: Charles C Thomas.

Tait, N. A., Michael, J. F., & Carpenter, M. A.. (1980). Maximum duration of sustained /s/ and /z/ in children. *Journal of Speech and Hearing Disorders, 45*, 239–246.

Tanaka, S., & Gould, W. J. (1985). Vocal efficiency and aerodynamic aspects in voice disorders. *Annals of Otology, Rhinology, Laryngology, 94*, 29–33.

Tarneaud, J. (1935). *Le nodule de la corde vocale*. Paris: Maloine.

Tomita, M., Matsuo, K., Maehara, N., Umezaki, T., & Shin, T. (1988). Measurements of oxygen pressure in the vocal fold during laryngeal nerve stimulation. *Archives of Otolaryngology and Head and Neck Surgery, 114*, 308–312.

Toohill, R. J. (1975). The psychosomatic aspects of children with vocal nodules. *Archives of Otolaryngology, 101*, 591–595.

U.S. Department of Health and Human Services. (1990). *The health benefits of smoking cessation* (DHHS publication No. (CDC) 90-8416). Atlanta: U.S. Department of Health and Human Services, Centers for Disease Control, Center for Chronic Disease Prevention and Health Promotion, Office on Smoking and Health.

U.S. Department of Health and Human Services. (1996). *Reducing the consequences of smoking: 25 years of progress: A report of the Surgeon General* (DHHS publication NO (CDC) 89-8411). Atlanta: U.S. Department of Health and Human Services, Center for Disease Control, Center for Chronic Disease Prevention and Health Promotion, Office on Smoking and Health.

Vaughan, C. W. (1983). Benign lesions of the larynx. In G. M. English (Ed.), *Otolaryngology* (Vol. 3, pp. 1–29). Philadelphia: J. B. Lippincott.

Verdolini-Marston, K., Titze, I. R., & Druker, D. G. (1990). Changes in phonation threshold pressure with induced conditions of hydration. *Journal of Voice, 4*, 142–151.

von Leden, H. (1978, June). Surgical care of the professional voice. [Panel discussion]. *Transcripts of the Seventh Symposium on Care of the Professional Voice Part III. Medical/surgical therapy* (pp. 95–96). New York: The Voice Foundation.

von Leden, H. (1988). Legal pitfalls in laryngology. *Journal of Voice, 2*, 330–333.

Watkins, K. L., & Ewanowsky, S. J. (1985). Effects of aerosol beclomethasone depropionate. *Journal of Speech and Hearing Research, 28*, 301–304.

Woo, P., Colton, R. H., & Shangold, L. (1987). Phonatory airflow analysis in patients with laryngeal disease. *Annals of Otology, Rhinology, Laryngology, 96*, 549–555.

Yamaguchi, H., Yotsukura, Y., Kondo, R., Hanyuu, Y., Horiguchi, S., Imaizumi, S., & Hirose, H. (1986). Nonsurgical therapy for vocal nodules. *Folia Phoniatrica, 38*, 372–373.

Yanagihara, N. (1967). Significance of harmonic changes and noise components in hoarseness. *Journal of Speech and Hearing Research, 10,* 531–541.

Yano, J., Ichimura, K., Hoshino, T., & Nozue, M. (1982). Personality factors in the pathogenesis of polyps and nodules of the vocal cords. *Auris, Nasus, Larynx, 9,* 105110.

Zyski, B. J., Bull, G. L., McDonald, W. E., & Johns, M. E. (1984). Perturbation analysis of normal and pathologic larynges. *Folia Phoniatrica, 36,* 190–198.

CHAPTER 10

LESIONS OF THE LAMINA PROPRIA

MARK S. COUREY, M.D.
ROBERT H. OSSOFF, D.M.D., M.D.

INTRODUCTION AND DEFINITIONS

With the advent of cinematography and video-endostroboscopy, for the first time we have the ability to take pictures of the larynx, slow the motion, and review these films in slow motion sequence or real time. This affords us the opportunity to study the larynx and its pathology at leisure and repeatedly, without inconvenience or discomfort on the part of the patient. It also allows us the luxury of discussing our findings with as many consultants as necessary to arrive at a diagnosis. Nowhere is this more invaluable than for the identification of submucosal pathology.

Lesions of the lamina propria are located, by definition, between the mucosal cover and the body of the vocal ligament, that is, within Reinke's space. This includes, but is not limited to, true cysts, epidermoid or mucosal retention, submucosal scar tissue from years of misuse, sulcus vocalis, and Reinke's edema or polypoid corditis. Histologic examination of polyps and nodules has revealed that these lesions also involve the superficial layer of the lamina propria (Kotby, Nassar, Seif, Helal, & Saleh, 1988). As such, treatment of all surgical la-ryngeal lesions is predicated on the concept of mucosal preservation. Submucosal lesions should be removed with as little of the overlying normal mucosa and surrounding lamina propria as possible.

Absolute identification of a vocal fold cyst involves the identification of an epithelial lined sac within Reinke's space. True vocal fold cysts exist in two forms. First, mucoid- or serous-filled cysts are lined with a cuboidal or flattened columnar epithelium. Presumably this epithelium arises from a minor salivary gland within the larynx. As the mucoid or serous contents are trapped, the cyst enlarges. The epithelium is then flattened into a low columnar or cuboidal type epithelium (Figure 10–1). Second, true cysts may also be lined with squamous epithelium. These would then contain squamous debris or squamous elements (Figure 10–2).

Submucosal scar tissue, presumably derived from years of misuse or vocal abuse, results in pronounced submucosal edema with acellular infiltrates and fibrinous exudates. There is abundant stromal vascularity and collagen deposition.

Sulcus vocalis is a furrow which runs parallel to the free edge of the vocal fold.

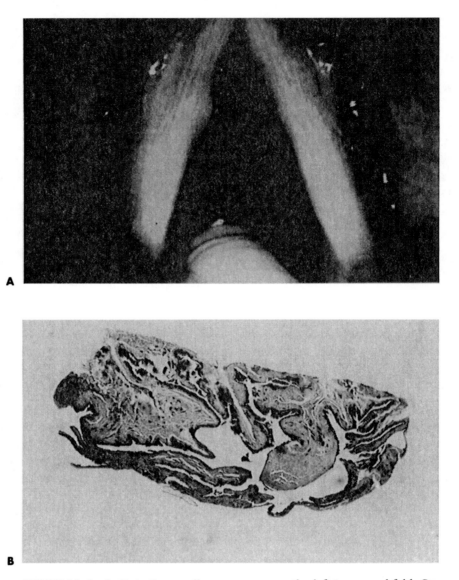

FIGURE 10–1. A. Note the small excrescence on the left true vocal fold. On preoperative videostroboscopy the mucosal wave was absent lateral to the lesion, vertical phase difference was impaired, and the amplitude of the vibration was reduced. These characteristics are common with submucosal lesions. **B.** Histologic examination revealed a lining epithelium consisting of a double layer of low columnar or cuboidal cells. This is consistent with a distended salivary gland acinus.

This is an infolding of the mucosal cover lined with basement membrane. The infolded mucosal cover forms a furrow which may dissect into the superficial layer of the lamina propria and may have intimate attachments to the intermediate or deeper layer (Nakayama, Ford, Brandenburg, & Bless, 1994) (see Figure 10–2).

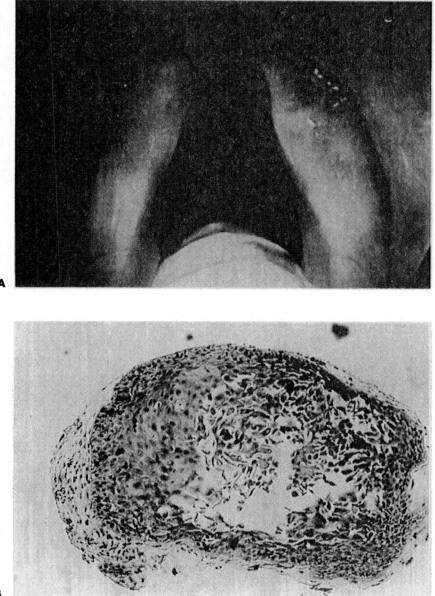

FIGURE 10–2. A. Compare the appearance of these lesions with the one in Figure 10–1. Note the fullness to the vocal folds which is more pronounced on the right. In addition, furrows or sulci can be seen bilaterally. Again, mucosal wave was absent on stroboscopy. **B.** Histologic examination revealed a cyst lined with a squamous epithelium. Clinically, this was adherent to the overlying mucosal cover.

Finally, Reinke's edema or polypoid corditis involves the full length of the membranous vocal fold. The mucosal membrane is redundant. Histologically, the superficial layer of the lamina propria is re-placed by a myxomatous stroma. There is, at times, a collection of serous fluid within the superficial layer of the lamina propria. In more mature polypoid changes, this serous fluid is replaced with acellular infiltrates (Figure 10–3).

The differentiation of lesions of the lamina propria from a classic nodule or polyp is aided by videoendostroboscopic examina-

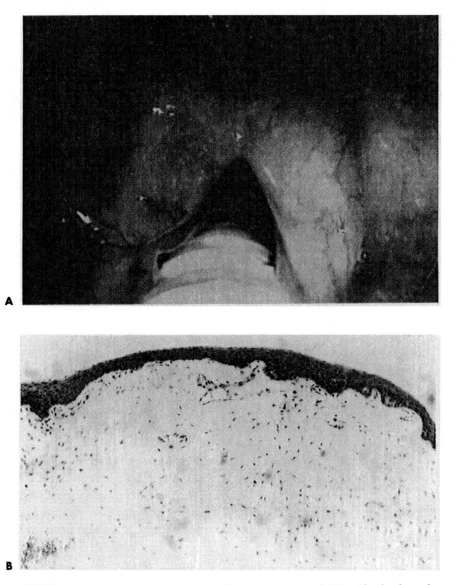

FIGURE 10–3. A. This patient was a female in her mid-60s. She had gradually developed vocal difficulties over the preceding 10-year period. On questioning, she noted dyspnea with moderate exertion. **B.** Histologic examination reveals an acellular material filling and enlarging the superficial layer of the lamina propria.

tion. Often, however, difficulty in distinction is encountered and direct manipulation is necessary for final confirmation. The characteristic finding of most submucosal lesions on videoendostroboscopy is a decreased mucosal wave. This results from adhesions, or scarring, of the vocal fold cover to the body by the pathology (Figure 10–4).

PATHOGENESIS

The etiology of intracordal lesions can be divided into two broad categories, congenital and acquired. Distinction is usually on the basis of history and not histology. Congenital lesions should, by definition, present in patients with a lifelong history of dysphonia. Presumably, as the cyst or sulcus enlarges, dysphonia would be aggravated. This theory of origin presupposes a congenital anomaly. By history, however, this appears to be rare. More commonly, patients complain of intermittent or continued vocal difficulties, beginning only during their adult years. The patient may complain of a new history of early vocal fatigue or loss of the upper range of the voice with recurrent increased roughness which develops after use. Physical examination may show the development of submucosal fullness or bowing of the vocal fold. This may represent the pathology. The development of such pathology within Reinke's space is as yet unclear and poorly understood.

Study of the anatomy of the vocal fold has revealed the normal absence of mucous glands on the true vocal folds. Therefore, mucoid filled cysts with a low columnar or cuboidal epithelium must arise from obstruction of a salivary gland within the adjacent sub- or supraglottis. Inflation of the obstructed acinus results in migration of the cyst into the area of the true vocal fold.

Sulcus vocalis, a furrow of vocal fold mucosa running the longitudinal length of the vocal fold, again may be of a congenital or acquired etiology. Repeated trauma could activate subepithelial fibroblasts to produce collagen (Hirano, Kurita, Matsuo, & Negata, 1980). This excess collagen could then result in tethering of the mucosal cover to the vocal ligament. Continued movement of the surrounding non-adherent mucosa over the vocal ligament would then result in the creation of a furrow.

Submucosal cysts filled with squamous debris, inclusion cysts, may arise from sulcus vocalis. Prolonged vocal fold vibration results in disruption of the basement membrane zone at its junction with the superficial layer of the lamina propria (Gray & Titze, 1988). Intuitively, the basement membrane zone surrounding the tethered portion of the mucosa in a sulcus would seem extremely susceptible to these shearing forces. Healing may result in formation of a new basement membrane over the top of the previous sulcus. This would then create a sac of squamous epithelium within the lamina propria, which could enlarge to form an inclusion cyst similar to those found in other areas of squamous epithelium. Sulcus vocalis may be associated with inclusion cysts. In these cases, the inclusion cyst is covered by a very atrophic area of vocal fold cover, which has the appearance of a sulcus in areas anterior and posterior to the cyst.

With regard to increased submucosal scar tissue formation, many authors (Frenzel, 1986; Kleinsasser, 1982; Kotby et al., 1988) have emphasized the role of altered vascular permeability in the formation of microhematomas and subepithelial edema. Again, Hirano et al. (1980) felt that the vibratory shearing forces could stimulate and activate subepithelial fibroblasts to produce collagen. These factors together may lead to excessive collagen deposition within the lamina propria. Years of repeated injury could then

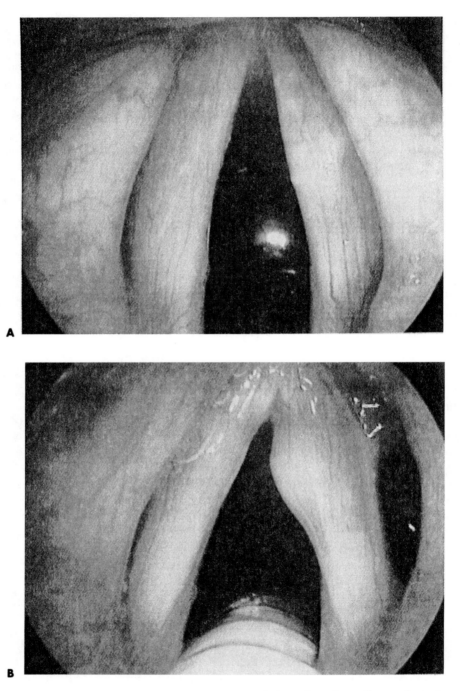

FIGURE 10–4. Compare the appearance of these histologically confirmed cysts with those shown in Figures 10–1 and 10–2. **A** shows minimal fullness on the mid portion of the right vocal fold. On stroboscopy, however, there was an adynamic segment of mucosal wave lateral to the fullness and a cyst was found at surgical exploration. **B** reveals a large fusiform swelling involving the anterior two thirds of the right vocal fold. Histologic examination revealed a low columnar epithelium lining the cyst.

result in tethering of the epithelium to the intermediate and deep layers of the lamina propria and prevent vocal fold vibration.

The origin of Reinke's edema may be linked to smoking, although a causal relationship has not been proven. Chronic smoking induces tracheal hypersecretion and inflammation which results in chronic cough (U.S. Department of Health and Human Services, 1990). Trauma from coughing could then result in altered vascular permeability (Kleinsasser, 1982; Kotby et al, 1988). Increased vascular permeability would lead to collections of subepithelial edema. Presumably on a chronic continued nature, massive polypoid corditis could develop.

Emotional and/or psychological factors do not appear to be significantly related to these types of vocal fold lesions as they are to classic vocal fold nodules or polyps. Studies such as those by Yano, Ichimura, Hoshino, and Nozue, (1982) demonstrating positive correlation between vocal nodules and polyps and extroverted personalities have not been performed in patients with submucosal, or intracordal, pathology. Rather, these lesions seem more common among vocal professionals, such as entertainers, ministers, lawyers, and teachers. These patients have excessive vocal demands. The appearance of these lesions in this group of patients favors the possibility of an acquired etiology over a congenital one. With the exception of polypoid changes, these lesions are more frequently unilateral. Often the opposite vocal fold may be normal in appearance or have minimal reactive edema. This suggests a minimal role of vocal hyperfunction in the etiology of these disorders.

DEMOGRAPHIC INFORMATION

The true incidence of vocal fold cysts is unknown. This stems from the difficulty in diagnosis and distinction of these lesions from classic vocal nodules or polyps. Whether the diagnosis is made on clinical grounds or actual histologic examination also affects the true incidence. An extensive review over 15 years by Kleinsasser (1990) seems to indicate that vocal fold cysts are half as common as nodules and/or polyps. In addition, they appear to be more common in males than females.

With regard to sulcus vocalis, no estimation of incidence is available. These lesions seem to be rare and occur more commonly in vocal professionals. However, it is possible that increased vocal performance demands by professionals stimulate greater identification in this population as opposed to the general population. Sulcus vocalis is presumed by many to be a congenital lesion (Bouchayer et al., 1985). In a 10-year study, they operated on 157 patients for either cysts or sulcus and found that 72 patients had sulci.

Polypoid corditis or Reinke's edema is certainly more prevalent in smokers than nonsmokers. Cigarette smoking, however, has not been shown to be a causative agent. With regard to distribution among the sexes, contradictory data have been reported. Review of the senior author's practice shows the disease to be more prevalent in females. This is in agreement with Lumpkin, Bishop, and Bennett (1987) and Yates and Dedo (1984). It is in direct contradiction to the experience of Kleinsasser (1990).

ONSET AND COURSE OF THE DISORDER

As the etiology of submucosal pathology is poorly understood, onset or presentation of symptoms may occur at any time during the life of an individual. For congenital disorders, presumably as the individual matures, dysphonia will become more problematic to the patient as his or her vocal demands increase. However, patients who present with newly diagnosed cysts or sulcus have not necessarily had a lifelong history of vocal difficulties. In many vocal professionals the disorder begins rather abruptly. Singers may note vocal problems earlier than nonsingers. In addition, nonsingers may be better able to tolerate the lesion than are singers.

Again, in all these lesions, with the exception of polypoid corditis, the patient's chief complaint is usually "hoarseness." On further questioning, this can be broken down into an increase in vocal roughness with breathiness. In addition, there may be loss of the upper singing and speaking registers. Patients complain of early onset of vocal fatigue and may note increased breathiness. An inciting event is usually not identifiable. The difficulty may have persisted in an intermittent nature for years or it may be of new onset. Often there is an intermittent nature to the symptoms, and dysphonia may be aggravated by excessive use.

Physical examination during symptomatic periods may reveal bilateral vocal fold fullness. Videostroboscopic analysis will demonstrate excessive mucosal wave on the reactive vocal fold, with a decreased or absent wave on the affected portion of the affected vocal fold. These findings are somewhat subtle. A period of voice rest may result in resolution of surrounding edema. Initially, on reinstitution of voice use, the patient's symptoms are greatly improved.

In the case of a vocal fold cyst, physical examination, again including videostroboscopy, often reveals a unilateral swelling. The affected portion of the vocal fold will have an absent or decreased mucosal wave on stroboscopy. Glottic closure on stroboscopic analysis often will be impaired anterior and/or posterior to the lesion. Repeated or interval examina-

tions are required to confirm the diagnosis. This may take place over weeks or months. It usually requires modification of voice use to help eliminate reactive surrounding edema. For males, interval examinations can be done at 2- to 4-week intervals after modification of voice use has been employed. In female patients, however, it is usually necessary to observe changes throughout different portions of the menstrual cycle to eliminate the effect that menstruation may have on the laryngeal appearance.

Once the diagnosis of submucosal cyst or scarring is strongly suspected and the patient is unable to continue the vocal requirements, the treatment is surgical excision. Confirmation of the diagnosis comes at histologic examination of the surgical specimen. The authors have found it necessary to change our preoperative diagnosis approximately 25% of the time after histologic examination of the surgical specimen (Shohet, Courey, & Ossoff, 1994). Even dedicated laryngologists often require surgical palpation and exploration with excision to be certain of the histologic diagnosis. It is imperative, however, that surgery not be performed unless the patient is absolutely aware of the potential risks to the existing voice, and we recommend not proceeding with surgery unless the patient can no longer perform his or her vocal duties to the required level.

With regard to polypoid corditis, the onset is insidious over years. Women usually complain of a prolonged period of a low vocal pitch. This is usually identified as a lowered fundamental frequency with increased roughness. Often these women are addressed as "Sir" over the telephone. When massive polypoid corditis exists, patients often complain of dyspnea on exertion. Physical examination reveals bilateral polypoid degeneration, usually filling the glottis and prolapsing in and out of the airway on respiration. In extreme cases, patients develop a compensatory plicae ventricularis mechanism to phonate. Polypoid corditis may or may not be associated with an increased risk of vocal fold carcinoma, although the two can present simultaneously in smokers.

MEDICAL CONSIDERATIONS

Diagnosis of submucosal lesions relies first on suspicion and awareness of existence. Patients present with dysphonia and a physical examination, including perceptual voice analysis and videostroboscopy, suggests the presence of submucosal pathology. It is usually difficult to distinguish this on the basis of one clinical examination. The patient is interviewed and a vocal inventory taken. Abuses and misuses are identified and vocal re-education is begun.

If necessary, a vocal abuse reduction program is undertaken (Johnson, 1985). In professional voice patients, it is usually not a matter of vocal abuse as much as vocal overuse. This readily defines itself in a vocal inventory. Patients are then asked to modify the amount of vocal use. Frequently, their expectations of vocal performance abilities are unrealistic. A marathon runner would not attempt to run 26 miles daily, particularly without proper warm-up or cool-down. Why, then, should we expect to use our vocal muscles at performance levels on a daily basis without using such precautions and without the insertion of recuperative periods? Vocal re-education under the direction of a speech-language pathologist is instituted. Attempts are made to train the singing or speaking voice into more efficient use patterns. Breath support, body alignment, and proper registration are emphasized.

This period of modified voice use through abuse reduction and vocal re-education is accompanied by interval glottic examination. The physical examination is reviewed periodically to assess how the lesion is being altered by vocal modification. Often vocal modification in this manner will result in resolution of the dysphonia. If the glottic examination returns to normal, then we realize that the dysfunction was secondary to incorrect use of the voice. Equally as common, however, is improvement in vocal capabilities but not a complete return to normal laryngeal appearance. In this instance, physical examination usually reveals the persistence of tethering of the vocal fold mucosa to the underlying vocal fold body. In addition, glottic closure also may be compromised.

Should vocal modification measures not result in elucidation of pathologies, then more drastic measures such as complete voice rest can be employed. Complete voice rest periods of up to 2 weeks can be helpful in allowing resolution of the pathology secondary to functional difficulties. In addition, if there is a physical abnormality and the patient continues to function with that abnormality in place, he or she may be damaging the uninvolved vocal fold by using hyperfunctional techniques in an attempt to compensate for reduced glottal efficiency. Complete voice rest eliminates any vocal hyperfunction. Contrary to some opinions (Koufman & Blalock, 1989), complete voice rest has not been shown to result in deleterious vocal fold atrophy. Emotionally, patients are usually distraught over the dysphonia and welcome a 2-week period of complete voice rest in hopes that it may further elucidate the cause of their dysphonia. If properly counselled, very few patients will refuse this critical step in diagnostic therapy.

The adjunctive use of pharmacologic agents to further reduce glottic edema, correct glottic lubrication problems, and reduce gastric hyperacidity, if present, can be helpful. Often corticosteroids will help eliminate the effects of allergic components on the vocal fold mucosa. High levels of corticosteroids are given in short 1- to 2-week rapid taper regimens. This allows maximum effect with minimal side effects. Mucolytic agents, such as guaifenesin and or iodine-based compounds, are useful to improve secretions in the aerodigestive tract. These substances help decrease the viscosity of aerodigestive secretions and result in increased lubrication which improves glottic vibration by lowering the phonation threshold pressure (Titze, 1994). Next, the use of H_2 blockers will significantly reduce gastric acid production. Previous history may have elucidated symptoms of esophageal reflux. If not, a short-term trial of an H_2 blocker may result in resolution of occult gastroesophageal reflux disease.

It should be noted that, during the period of vocal abuse reduction and vocal re-education, vocal hygiene measures are instituted. Specifically, dietary modifications are made to include an increase in free water consumption. Typically, 64 ounces of water per day is recommend. Substances high in fats, which tend to thicken glottic secretions, are eliminated. Diuretics, such as caffeine, are also to be avoided. These are commonly found in coffees, teas, colas, and chocolates. The patient is instructed on improved eating habits. He or she is asked to avoid greasy fried foods. In addition, the patient is instructed to avoid eating immediately prior to sleeping or lying down. Finally, the avoidance of alcohol or drug ingestion is stressed, particularly prior to vocal performances.

THE VOICE EVALUATION

Vocal Characteristics

Vocal characteristics of patients with mass lesions in the glottis show marked variability. Hirano (1981) suggests that the trained voice clinician can distinguish vocal pathologies based on psychoacoustic impressions and visual observations. However, all lesions that increase the mass and stiffness of the vocal fold will decrease vocal fold efficiency during vibration. This usually will result in an increase in vocal roughness and the perception of a lowered fundamental frequency. In addition, if the lesion is extremely large, it can inhibit glottic closure and result in an increased breathiness to the voice. Usually the timing of speech onset is not affected nor is the intensity of speech. The use of perceptual analysis is fraught with difficulty. Perceptual analysis is time consuming. For accurate assessment, multiple listeners are required. A listener's perception may be affected by external events, therefore, interjudge reliability measures are needed. Finally, although many grading scales exist, the acceptance and use of one universal scale has not been accomplished.

Endoscopy

Endoscopy is a valuable tool in assessing laryngeal physical characteristics. Multiple techniques exist. Indirect mirror examination allows the perception of depth of field. The color of glottic mucosa is unaltered by recording mechanisms. The ability to adequately visualize the larynx, however, is limited by the patient's tolerance of the mirror in the oropharynx. This may result in incomplete visualization secondary to an overhanging epiglottis and/or short periods of visualization secondary to gagging. The indirect rigid telescopic examination of the glottis is often better tolerated than the indirect mirror technique. The rod telescope can help depress the tongue posteriorly, thus improving visualization of the anterior commissure. In addition, magnification devices can be applied to the indirect rigid instrument, which then permit magnification of the glottic structures.

Finally, flexible laryngoscopes are available. These are usually well-tolerated by most patients; however, lighting and a relatively narrow field of visualization limit its usefulness, particularly under stroboscopic examination.

Submucosal lesions, such as cysts or submucosal scar tissue, will usually appear as a convexity on the involved vocal fold on still light examination. Sulcus vocalis often appears normal on still light or a slight bowing of the vocal fold may be noted. Patients with polypoid corditis show full-length vocal fold changes of an irregular appearance. On inspiration, these irregular areas can prolapse in and out of the glottic airway.

Videostroboscopic examination of submucosal lesions, including cysts, scar tissue, and sulcus vocalis, will show a reduction in upper and lower mass formation on the involved vocal fold. In addition, there is usually an absent or significantly reduced mucosal wave (Shohet et al.,1994). Glottic closure on stroboscopy also is impaired in a significant percentage of patients. The mass lesion usually prevents anterior closure and results in an anterior phonation gap. With regard to polypoid degeneration, the mass of tissue in Reinke's space does not allow enough periodic vibration to trigger the stroboscopic device.

Acoustic Analysis

Acoustic analysis in the evaluation of these patients may be useful as a research tool. No single or combined group of measurements has the sensitivity or specificity to detect and diagnose vocal fold lesions. Many patients with lesions of the lamina propria may fall within the normal range of accepted values. Also, as in perceptual analysis, a standardized test battery for acoustic analysis has not been accepted for universal use.

Aerodynamics

It can be presumed that aerodynamic evaluations of patients with submucosal lesions of the true vocal folds will have similar results to aerodynamic evaluations of patients with vocal fold polyps or nodules. Specifically, measures of mean airflow rate would be either in the normal range or slightly elevated (Hirano, Koike, & von Leden, 1968). As glottal efficiency is decreased, airflow rates should be high, particularly if glottic closure is impaired. As in polyps or nodules, subglottic pressures would be increased as a result of the increased stiffness of the vocal fold (Tanaka & Gould, 1985).

SOCIAL IMPLICATIONS

The development of dysphonia is a frightening event in any patient's life. Whether a vocal professional or a nonprofessional, a patient's first fears include thoughts of cancer. Vocal professionals who rely on their voices to earn a living develop anxiety about their potential to continue work. Indeed, their livelihood depends on the use of their voice, and its loss threatens the livelihood of those who are emotionally and economically dependent on them. In the case of a professional singer, this includes family members, secretaries, band members, employers, promoters, and agents. The singer is suddenly caused to doubt his or her ability to continue to work and anxiety may aggravate the symptoms. There is a fear that someone else may notice or no longer enjoy the quality of his or her vocal performance. As the dysphonia progresses, the singer's fears are realized and loss of time from work compounds the physical, emotional, and financial problems. This translates into immediate loss of earnings and potential loss of supporters.

It is at this point that the patient often seeks medical attention. Initial examination usually alleviates the fear of potential glottic carcinoma, although vocal professionals who abuse their voices and use tobacco and alcohol often have erytho-leukoplakic changes. Before the patient is overburdened with the potential risk of carcinoma, it is best to observe him for a short 2-week period on complete voice rest, with or without steroids and antibiotic therapy, and then re-evaluate the examination findings in light of these changes. Often, severe erythema and the appearance of leukoplakia will resolve significantly in this short period if vocal abuse is abruptly halted. The potential risks can then be discussed with the patient in view of the new examination so that the physician's recommendations are based on a more stable physical appearance of the glottis, as opposed to the appearance in the acute phases of trauma. In any case, visualization of a lesion of the vocal fold in patients who depend on their voices for livelihood creates great anxiety and the fear of a potential premature end to their careers. It is imperative at this point that vocal re-education and vocal hygiene measures be instituted promptly to allow potential improved functioning. This will require reduction in vocal use, with decreased productivity and potential disruption in income. When the diagnosis of submucosal pathology is more firm, surgery becomes the treatment option of choice if the patient can no longer perform his or her job-related duties.

Surgical intervention is offered only if the dysphonia causes the patient an inability to maintain daily voice use. If vocal re-education, regardless of the lesion, allows the patient to return to a state of improved functioning, then surgery can and should be delayed. Surgical therapy results in immediate hospital and medical expenses. In addition, patients are usually asked to observe periods of voice rest and then undergo extensive vocal rehabilitation which can take from 2 to 6 months.

During this time, we ask the patients to refrain from professional vocal activity for a minimum of 3 months. The patient must decide whether to continue paying the people in his or her employ or face the possibility of losing band members or support staff to more lucrative positions. In addition, the down time from performances may result in the loss of crowd support or fans (short for fanatics). If vocal performances have been scheduled, they will need to be canceled and this may result in direct out-of-pocket expenses without potential income.

It is often imperative that the surgeon, at this time, make telephone calls or write letters to employers regarding the nature of the patient's illness. This can help in the reduction of financial liabilities on the patient's part. It is, however, a double-edged sword. While imparting credibility to the patient's dysphonia, it also has the potential to label the patient as ill or having a weakness. This may, then, have long reaching career effects.

Insurance carriers often need to be contacted, as they will initially refuse to support vocal re-education or rehabilitation efforts. These therapy services are not covered in many insurance policies, and their costs are shifted to the patient.

TREATMENT: OPTIONS AND OUTCOMES

Speech Pathology

To establish the diagnosis of submucosal pathology and to distinguish it from vocal fold polyps or nodules, the patient usually undergoes a period of modified voice use and vocal re-education. This initial behavior therapy is imperative. Patients may continue to function at an acceptable level with vocal modifications. This then obviates the need for further treatment, if the glottic examination remains stable.

As discussed previously, vocal modification includes the use of improved vocal hygiene, vocal abuse reduction strategies, and vocal coaching for both the singing and speaking voice. Improved vocal hygiene includes the elimination of dietary substances that are high in fat and may therefore thicken glottal secretions. These include fried foods and dairy products. Patients usually are asked to increase their free water consumption, so that an intake of 64 ounces of water a day is completed. Mucolytic agents, such as guaifenesin or iodine-based compounds, are also beneficial in reducing the viscosity of the laryngeal secretions. If necessary, vocal abuse reduction measures are instituted and a standard vocal abuse reduction program outlined.

Vocal re-education stresses body alignment, breath management, and proper registration. These sessions are accomplished with a qualified speech-language pathologist and/or vocal pedagogue if the singing voice is a consideration. Therapy sessions can take place as frequently as necessary. Often, weekly intervals are slowly lengthened to every other week, then monthly. If vocal modification is successful at achieving a stable voice and glottic appearance, then reminder sessions can take place at 2-, 3-, or 4-month intervals as necessary.

Surgical Management

If the patient is unable to perform or continue voice use to his or her expected or desired level or the lesion continues to change in appearance despite behavior modification, surgical therapy is recommended. For treatment of submucosal cysts or scarring, the preferred technique of surgical correction involves elevation of a microflap, with excision of the submucosal pathology (Courey, Gardner, Stone, & Ossoff, 1995). The larynx is exposed through an operating binocular microlaryngoscope. It is then viewed through the binocular microscope at 10 to 25 times life size magnification. Microlaryngeal instrumentation, including microcup forceps, micro-knives and micro-scissors, are then used as appropriate to remove the pathology while the mucosal cover is preserved. It is usually best to avoid laser use in these cases, as the laser imparts heat to the surrounding normal structures and may have a tendency to result in increased scarring. Initially, a sickle knife is used to make an incision on the superior surface of the vocal fold laterally towards the ventricle. A blunt-angled probe termed a flap elevator is then inserted and used to elevate a flap of tissue consisting of the mucosal cover and superficial layers of Reinke's space. The pathology is elevated with the cover while the vocal ligament is identified and preserved laterally. Sharp and blunt dissection are then required to separate the lesion from the mucosal cover. The operative field is inspected for secondary areas of pathology. A corticosteroid preparation is then injected under the mucosal flap and the flap redraped into position. This type of mucosal preservation surgery has been studied over a 3-year period at Vanderbilt University Medical Center. It has been shown to allow the excision of pathology. In the majority of patients with submucosal lesions, the mucosal wave is absent preoperatively. In patients with the diagnosis of submucosal cyst or polyp, who had absent mucosal waves preoperatively, postoperatively the mucosal wave returned in 74% of the patients (Courey et al., 1995).

Treatment of polypoid corditis or Reinke's edema is also best performed by a microflap excision technique. This allows simultaneous surgery of both vocal folds and results in earlier return of sustained phonation (Lumpkin et al., 1987). Again, the larynx is exposed with the binocular operating microlaryngoscope.

It is then viewed through the binocular operating microscope at 10 to 25 times magnification. An incision is made laterally on the superior surface of the polypoid degeneration. A flap of tissue, consisting of the mucosal cover of the vocal fold, is elevated with a blunt elevator. The submucosal tissue is then removed with blunt dissection. The vocal ligament is identified and preserved. The remainder of the microflap is then redraped over the superior surface of the vocal fold and trimmed to fit the mucosal defect.

Postoperatively, these patients note improved breathing and improved vocal capabilities. Video examination shows straight vocal folds. Stroboscopic examination, however, does not reveal return of the normal mucosal wave. This is not surprising as the disease process involves the majority of Reinke's space. Surgical treatment results in removal of the majority of the tissue from this space and disruption of the normal vocal fold laminar structure. Regeneration of the tissue within the superficial lamina propria does not occur, thus, the vocal fold remains stiff and without the normal vibratory characteristics. This does not permit the movement of the mucosa over the vocal ligament.

Sulcus vocalis is a very rare condition in which a furrow running the length of the vocal fold causes tethering of the mucosal cover to the underlying ligament. This results in decreased mucosal wave with impaired glottic closure and dysphonia. If surgical excision is to be performed on an isolated sulcus, the furrowed mucosa needs to be excised. This is best approached by a microsurgical technique. The larynx is exposed with an operating binocular microlaryngoscope and the operating microscope at 10 to 25 times life-size magnification used to visualize the glottis. A straight sickle knife is used to make an incision along the superior margin of the sulcus vocalis. The blunt eleva-

tor is then used to elevate a flap of mucosa from the incision laterally toward the superior surface of the vocal fold. Tissue forceps are used to grasp the edge of the furrowed mucosa and the flap elevator used to elevate a small flap of mucosa consisting of the furrow and infraglottal portion of the mucosal cover. The furrowed mucosa is then removed with upbiting micro-scissors. The remaining edges of the mucosa are brought together to promote primary healing. If the mucosal defect is large, a bipedicaled flap can be created with the mucosa from the superior surface of the vocal fold to primarily resurface the free edge. This is done by making an incision laterally on the superior surface of the vocal fold. The mucosa is elevated with a flap elevator and then advanced to cover the medial/vibratory surface of the vocal fold. The superior surface mucosal defect is left to heal by secondary intention.

Patients require extensive postoperative therapy. This can be conveniently divided into four phases. Phase one consists of 2 weeks of complete voice rest. This is a controversial issue. Some phoniatricians do not believe there is particular benefit in voice rest and, further, that it may be harmful, leading to muscle atrophy (Koufman & Blalock, 1989; Lawrence, 1991). In addition, complete voice rest is associated with psychologic stress and may produce adverse reactions on the part of the patient. On the other hand, premature use of the postoperative vocal fold, which is at first edematous and then quickly becomes indurated, can result in the development of hyperfunctional techniques. The indurated vocal fold does not have normal vibratory characteristics, and patients may, therefore, hyperfunction to overcome this undue stiffness. Study of wound healing indicates successive collagen deposition and healing occur at 10 to 14 days postoperatively. Prior to this time, tensile strength of the wound is decreased. Therefore, secondary to induration and wound healing characteristics, 2 weeks of postoperative voice rest seem ideal.

Postoperative phase two consists of the resumption of vocal activity. If stroboscopic examination reveals reformation of upper and lower masses during phonation and the possible partial return of mucosal wave, the patient is ready to begin phonating on a limited basis. Patients are instructed to begin phonating for 5 minutes the first day following voice rest. This is doubled to 10 minutes the second day, 20 minutes the third, 45 minutes the fourth, 1.5 hours the fifth, 3 hours the sixth, 6 hours the seventh, and 12 hours the eighth. The patient is asked to observe limited voice use during this time. If increased anterior neck pain or irritation of the pharynx develops, vocal use is reduced. The use of biofeedback is important in avoiding vocal overuse during the postoperative period.

Repeat examination at postoperative week 5 usually shows improvement in the upper and lower lip formation with partial return of mucosal wave. More extensive speech therapy and singing lessons are then begun, if appropriate. During these phases, continuance of vocal hygiene measures, such as the dietary restrictions of high fat foods and diuretics, as well as the increased intake of water and potential mucolytic agents, are encouraged. Patients are advised and strongly urged to refrain from smoking.

During phase three, rehabilitation consists of measures that improve body alignment, breath support, and breath management. Phase three occurs during postoperative months 2 and 3 and is culminated in phase four, which is the return to an active normal vocal schedule. The patient is then followed at bimonthly intervals for the remainder of the first postoperative year to assess the laryngeal condition.

SUMMARY

The human vocal fold is a complex layered structure composed of muscle, connective tissue, and epidermis. It is unlike other animal vocal folds in that the connective tissue layer, between the epidermis and muscle layer, has evolved into a three-layered system which, in some as yet poorly understood manner, allows movement of the vocal fold cover over the vocal fold body during phonation. It is this movement, along with periodic vibrations of the vocal fold, that seems to create adequate phonation.

Lesions can arise within this connective tissue layer. When they do, they interfere with normal mucosal wave, normal vocal fold vibration, and, consequently, normal phonation. Understanding these concepts is crucial to proper identification and management of a vocal fold lesion. Videoendostroboscopy allows us to visualize a representative image of vibrating vocal folds. Study of these patterns of vibration and mucosal wave formation can enhance the identification of submucosal lesions.

Once pathology is identified, vocal modification can be used. Changing the vocal behavior may help the patient to improve phonation while leaving the lesion in place. If this is not possible, surgical excision of the pathology is appropriate if the patient desires a more normal voice. Surgery is directed at removing the pathology with as little disruption to the surrounding normal structures as possible. Surgical techniques have been improved with newer instrumentation and better understanding of vocal fold histology and physiology. However, surgery is not without risks and should be relied on as a last resort in the management of these patients.

REFERENCES

Bouchayer, M., Cornut, G., Loire, R., Witzig, E., Roch, J. B., & Bastian, R. W. (1985).

Epidermoid cysts, sulci, and mucosal bridges of the true vocal cord: A report of 157 cases. *Laryngoscope, 95,* 1087–1094.

Courey, M. S., Gardner, G. M., Stone, R. E., & Ossoff, R. H. (1995). The endoscopic vocal fold microflap: A three year experience. *Annals of Otology, Rhinology, and Laryngology, 104,* 4, 267–273.

Frenzel, H. (1986). Fine structural and immunohistochemical studies on polyps of human vocal folds. In J. Kirshner (Ed.), *Vocal fold histology: A symposium.* San Diego: College-Hill Press.

Gray, S. D., & Titze, I. (1988). Histologic investigation of hyperphonated canine vocal cords. *Annals of Otology, Rhinology, and Laryngology, 97,* 381–388.

Hirano, M. (1981). Structure of the vocal fold in normal and disease states: Anatomical and physical studies. In C. L. Ludlow & M. L. Hard (Eds.), Proceedings of the conference on the assessment of vocal fold pathology. *ASHA Reports, 11,* 11–30.

Hirano, M., Koike, Y., & von Leden, H. (1968). Maximum phonation time and air usage during phonation. *Folia Phoniatrica, 20,* 185–201.

Hirano, M., Kurita, S., Matsuo, K., & Nagata, K., (1980). In V. Lawrence (Ed.), *Transcripts of the Ninth Symposium on Care of the Professional Voice.* New York: The Voice Foundation.

Johnson, S. T. (1985). *Vocal abuse reduction program (VARP).* Boston, MA: College-Hill Press.

Kleinsasser, O. (1982). Pathogenesis of vocal cord polyps. *Annals of Otology, Rhinology, Laryngology, 91,* 378–381.

Kleinsasser, O. (1990). *Microlaryngoscopy and endolaryngeal microsurgery: Technique and typical findings.* Philadelphia, PA: Hanley and Belfus.

Kotby, M. N., Nassar, A. M., Seif, E. I., Helal, E. H., & Saleh, M. (1988). Ultrasound changes of the basement membrane zone in benign lesions of the vocal folds. *Acta Otolaryngologica, 113,* 99–101.

Koufman, J. A., & Blalock, P. D. (1989). Is voice rest never indicated? *Journal of Voice, 3,* 87–91.

Laurence, V. L. (1991). Nodules and other things that go bump in the night. In R. T. Sataloff & I. E. Titze (Eds.), *Vocal health and science* (pp. 125–127). Jacksonville, FL: The National Association of Teachers of Singing.

Lumpkin, S. M., Bishop, S. G., & Bennett, S. (1987). Comparison of surgical techniques in the treatment of laryngeal polypoid degeneration. *Annals of Otology, Rhinology, and Laryngology, 96,* 254–257.

Nakayama, M., Ford, C. N., Brandenburg, J. H., & Bless, D. M. (1994). Sulcus vocalis in laryngeal cancer: a histopathologic study. *Laryngoscope, 104,* 16–24.

Shohet, J. A., Courey, M. S., & Ossoff, R. H. (1994). The value of videostroboscopic parameters in differentiating benign true vocal fold cysts, nodules, and polyps. *Laryngoscope, 106,* 19–26.

Tanaka, S., & Gould, W. J. (1985). Vocal efficiency and aerodynamic aspects in voice disorders. *Annals of Otology, Rhinology, and Laryngology, 94,* 29–33.

Titze, I. R. (1994). *Principles of voice production.* Englewood Cliffs, NJ: Prentice-Hall.

United States Department of Health and Human Services. (1990). *Reducing the consequences of smoking: 25 years of progress.* A report of the Surgeon General (DHHS publication No. (CDC) 9-8411). Atlanta: U.S. Department of Health and Human Services, Center for Disease Control, Center for Chronic Disease Prevention and Health Promotion, Office on Smoking and Health.

Yano, J., Ichimura, K., Hoshino, T., & Nozue, M. (1982). Personality factor in the pathogenesis of polyps and nodules of the vocal cords. *Auris, Nasus, Larynx, 9,* 105–110.

Yates, A., & Dedo, H. H. (1984). Carbon dioxide laser enucleation of polypoid vocal cords. *Laryngoscope, 97,* 731–736.

CHAPTER 11

LARYNGEAL PAPILLOMA

CHARLES N. FORD, M.D.

INTRODUCTION AND DEFINITIONS

Laryngeal papilloma is a problematic benign neoplasm that affects the voice and compromises the airway. Florid growth in the upper respiratory tract, rapid recurrence following surgical ablation, and the potential for malignant transformation make papilloma a pernicious disease. The most common site of occurrence is on the true vocal fold, so hoarseness is an early symptom. In children, airway compromise is also an early symptom because the airway dimensions are relatively small. Attempts to classify papilloma into juvenile and adult onset are based on clinical course and epidemiological differences; histologically, both forms are identical. (Michaels, 1984). The separation is also made difficult because there are cases of juvenile-onset papilloma that persist into adulthood. Both adults and children risk permanent dysphonia from repeated surgical ablations that can produce scarring and web formation. Although a viral etiology has been demonstrated, effective therapy remains primarily laser-assisted surgical ablation. Antiviral and immunotherapy have not proven totally effective, but they are useful adjunctive measures.

ETIOLOGY/PATHOGENESIS

Laryngeal papillomatosis is one in a spectrum of epithelial lesions ranging from warts to carcinoma caused by human papillomaviruses (HPV). More than 60 different types of HPV have been identified, all associated with either cutaneous or mucosal diseases. Although HPV is difficult to propagate in tissue culture, a number of techniques have been employed to gather information about HPV in respiratory papillomatosis. In situ hybridization and biotinylated DNA probes provide a sensitive technique that has been successfully used to identify and type HPV in papillomas (Dickens et al., 1991; Duggan et al., 1990; Kashima et al., 1992b; Lindeberg & Johansen, 1990; Pignatari et al., 1992; Rimell et al., 1992). In a group of 20 patients (9 adult-onset and 11 juvenile-onset), Rimell et al. (1992) found that all tested positive for HPV type 6/11. Using similar techniques to type HPV in patients with papilloma during initial clinical presentation and after recurrence of the disease, Duggan et al. (1990) demonstrated the presence of type 6 and/or 11 in a 10-year study of 53 biopsies in nine patients. No change in HPV type was observed despite laser surgery or adjunctive interferon treatment. Amount of HPV DNA varied greatly even when only HPV types 6 and 11 were present and there was no evidence of types 16 and 18. Because these are the same HPV types (6/11) found in the more aggressive-acting papilloma cases, their study concluded that variation in clinical course is more likely due to host rather than viral factors. Other attempts to identify oncogenic HPV types 16/18 or 31/33/35 in laryngeal papilloma have been unsuccessful (Pignatari et al., 1992; Rimell et al., 1992).

HPV tends to replicate at a low copy number in basal cells, and it is difficult to eradicate (Cripe, 1990). Subclinical infections occur and prolonged latent periods are common. Tissues adjacent to obvious lesions may appear normal but have been found to contain HPV DNA. Even tissues as remote from the vocal folds as the nasopharynx, posterior tonsillar pillar, trachea, and bronchi may appear normal and yet harbor HPV infection in patients with laryngeal papilloma. Pignatari et al. (1992) identified HPV types 6 and 11 in obvious laryngeal lesions, and in 40% (4/10) of those patients found HPV in normal-appearing, remote, nondiseased sites. Patients with multiple papillomatous lesions, not those with solitary isolated papillomas, had HPV DNA in the nondiseased sites. These findings support the concept that HPV exists in clinically negative sites in the aerodigestive tract of patients with laryngeal papilloma; furthermore, clinically nondiseased site involvement may be a prognostic indicator of the real extent of the disease and the likelihood of recurrence.

DEMOGRAPHIC INFORMATION

Papilloma is considered the most benign laryngeal neoplasm, accounting for up to 92% of benign tumors of the larynx (Holinger & Johnson, 1951). To keep this in perspective, it must be noted that laryngeal papillomatosis is relatively uncommon, with an incidence rate of approximately seven cases per million/year in the United States. There is not significant difference in incidence by sex or race, but socioeconomic factors have been implicated (Seid & Cotton, 1983).

In Denmark, a comparatively lower incidence of laryngeal papillomatosis has been reported. With a population of 2.8 million, Denmark has 3.6 cases per million for juvenile-onset papillomas and 3.9 for adult-onset papillomas (Lindeberg & Elbrønd, 1990). The Danish study found no significant difference in incidence between two time intervals (1956–1968 and 1968–1984). These data were interesting because they did not reflect any increased incidence of laryngeal papilloma during a time when there was a documented increase of cervical HPV infections in women of child-bearing age in that country.

Peng, Searle, Shah, Repke, and Johnson (1990) studied the prevalence of HPV infections in the lower genital tracts of pregnant and nonpregnant women. Using exfoliated cervicovaginal cells, they identified HPV type 6/11 in 2% of the women, with no significant differences between the two groups; most of the women were asymptomatic and had negative Papanicolaou smears. In a related work, Smith, Johnson, Cripe, Pignatari, and Turek (1991) studied not only the mother's exfoliated cells, but also cells from the oropharynx and vulva (or foreskin) of the newborn. Eighteen percent of the mothers (13/72) were HPV positive, and 2.8% of the neonates tested positive. This study supports the hypothesis that respiratory tract papillomatosis can develop secondary to perinatal vertical transmission of HPV.

In a recent epidemiological study, Kashima, Shah, Lyles, and Glackin (1992a) compared risk factors for adult- and juvenile-onset recurrent respiratory papillomatosis. Using age-matched controls, they found that juvenile-onset respiratory papilloma patients were more often first-born ($p<.05$), delivered vaginally ($p<.05$), and born to a teenage mother ($p<.01$). Adult-onset patients reported more lifetime sex partners ($p<.01$) and a higher frequency of oral sex ($p<.05$). These data suggest that, whereas there may be similarities in the histopathology and responsible pathogenic organisms in the two conditions, juvenile- and adult-onset respiratory papillomatosis probably have different modes of transmission. Data were less compelling in a study done to assess the prevalence of upper respiratory tract papillomatosis in a group of 53 patients with genital warts and their sexual partners (Clarke et al., 1991). Although 70% of the group indulged in orogenital contact, only two patients (3.8%) had pharyngeal lesions (one laryngeal) attributable to HPV infection.

ONSET AND CLINICAL COURSE

The onset of symptoms is insidious. The first symptom is usually hoarseness, which is typically ascribed to chronic laryngitis in adults and often mistaken for nodules in children. Progressive hoarseness, dyspnea, and certainly stridor prompt medical attention. Once the diagnosis is confirmed, initial surgical treatment is successful in nearly two of every three patients (Jones, Myers, & Barnes, 1984). Most of the patients seen at the Clinical Science Center at the University of Wisconsin, however, have required multiple procedures.

Clinically, laryngeal papillomas can be classified as juvenile-onset (females predominate 2:1) and adult-onset (males predominate 2:1). Lindeberg and Elbrønd (1989) reviewed 231 patients with laryngeal papilloma and divided them into four clinical groups: (1) juvenile solitary, (2) juvenile multiple, (3) adult solitary, and (4) adult multiple papillomas. They concluded that it was impossible to predict the clinical course of any individual case but that solitary papilloma in adults tended to be cured with a single procedure. Quiney, Hall, and Croft (1989) reached a similar conclusion using multivariate analysis of 113 patients with laryngeal papillomatosis. They found that single-site lesions in adults had the best prognosis and female children with confluent lesions had the worst. In newborns, the disease is rare, but the prognosis appears particularly poor. One study reports 100% mortality in a group of four premature and term infants who developed symptoms during the first 6 months of life (Chipps, McClurg, Friedman, & Adams, 1990). Aggressive laser surgery, medical, and immune therapy failed to control progression of the disease in this group.

The most disturbing aspect of laryngeal papillomatosis is that it is unpredictable and capable of capricious transformation. In the short term, it may recur shortly after gross surgical ablation. It is impossible to consider a patient cured, even after several years. Recurrences as late as 42 years after remission have been reported (Lindeberg & Elbrønd, 1989). Activation during pregnancy led to death of a woman at 20 weeks of gestation (Helmrich, Stubbs, & Stoerker, 1992). Malignant transformation of laryngeal papillomatosis is an infrequent event but one of grave concern. Although the probability of malignant change is greater in smokers and in patients previously irradiated, there have been reports of laryngeal papillomatosis progressing to invasive carcinoma in nonsmoking and nonirradiated patients (Gaylis & Hayden, 1991; Guillou et al., 1991). In an in situ hybridization study of lung cancer patients, HPV DNA was found in 6 of 20 cases of squamous cell carcinoma and in 1 of 6 cases of large cell undifferentiated carcinoma (Yousem, Ohori, & Sonmez-Alpan, 1992). No HPV

DNA was identified in 32 other lung cancer cases that included adenocarcinoma, bronchioalveolar carcinoma, and small-cell carcinoma.

MEDICAL CONSIDERATIONS: EXAMINATION AND DIAGNOSIS

Although extralaryngeal papillomas can be found anywhere in the upper aerodigestive tract, the physical examination, except for laryngoscopy, is usually negative. Indirect laryngoscopy, when tolerated, gives an excellent view of the larynx with good illumination and color resolution. Flexible fiberoptic nasolaryngoscopy is helpful in examining the entire upper respiratory tract; this is important in ruling out multifocal disease. Rigid fiberoptic systems permit magnification and laryngeal videostroboscopy that can be helpful in defining an isolated lesion and distinguishing benign papilloma from invasive carcinoma. Papillomata are superficial lesions that do not disturb vibratory activity and mucosal wave to the extent of invasive cancer. Repeated surgical intervention, however, can cause scarring that will lead to stiffness and abnormalities that are evident on stroboscopic examination.

Laryngeal papillomas appear as granular reddish to whitish lesions. The anterior half of the vocal fold is most commonly affected, but the false vocal fold, subglottis, and vestibule are often secondarily involved. It is particularly important to identify lesions in these sites during surgery to avoid leaving gross reservoirs of disease. The epiglottis, trachea, and bronchi are rarely involved, but lesions can be found anywhere in the respiratory tract. Papilloma may exist as a solitary lesion, multiple distinct lesions, or multiple contiguous lesions. Invariably, respiratory papilloma occur at the junction of respiratory and squamous epithelium (Kashima, personal communication,

May 1992). In the larynx, such a juncture exists at the true vocal fold, perhaps explaining the predilection of papilloma for that site.

VOICE EVALUATION

Voice Characteristics

The voice is affected early in most patients with laryngeal papilloma because the vocal folds are the usual site of origin. Papillomatous involvement of the vocal folds and adjacent supraglottic and subglottic sites will alter vocal fold vibration and transglottic airflow. Impairment of voice might vary from mild hoarseness to severe dysphonia or aphonia (Aronson, 1980). With progressive airway compromise, stridulous breathing and a croupy cough can occur. Repeated surgical excisions or laser ablations of papilloma can cause secondary scarring of the vocal fold, web formation, and reduced excursion that aggravates the dysphonia. Almost any parameter of vocal quality can be affected. Pitch is commonly altered and frequency range reduced. Harmonics-to-noise ratio is decreased, and the patient may have great difficulty producing a sufficiently loud voice. These factors often lead to harmful compensatory strategies.

Although laryngeal papilloma is the most common neoplastic laryngeal lesion in children, diagnosis often is delayed because vocal nodules are suspected. Unlike nodules, papillomas should be initially managed with direct laryngoscopy and biopsy rather than voice therapy (Cohen, Thompson, Geller, & Birns, 1983).

When the lesions are addressed surgically, voice therapy can play an important role in vocal rehabilitation. Patients with scarred larynges following surgery can benefit from laryngeal stretching and relaxing exercises. Therapy to decrease supraglottic hyperfunction can result in a stronger and perceptually more pleasant voice. A videolaryngoscopy system is helpful in allowing the patient to observe his or her laryngeal activity; the stroboscopy permits identification of adynamic segments and vibratory mucosa that can be utilized through visual feedback to assist in voice therapy. The patient can be helped to reduce effort, strain, and fatigue. Vocal hygiene measures are always helpful; in some cases, rehabilitation is facilitated through the use of amplification devices. Adjunctive hypnotherapy has also been proposed as a method of increasing the speed of acquisition of vocal skills in patients with severe recurrent disease. Increased motivation for change and actual prolongation of remission have been ascribed to the use of hypnotherapy (Gildston & Gildston, 1992).

Psychosocial and Other Considerations

Respiratory papilloma can severely affect patients. The area of involvement, extent of disease, and pattern of recurrence are the key factors. In severe cases, the disease compromises the airway and threatens life. Often the voice is sufficiently dysphonic to interfere with communication. Even with minimal disease, the hoarse voice alters communication and suggests illness or distress. The emotional strain can be great, as the patient may be unable to relate appropriately to family, friends, and co-workers. During the formative years, a young persons's self-image and self-confidence can be adversely affected. In adults, papilloma can be a source of anxiety and great frustration. Repeated trips to the hospital for laryngoscopic surgery extracts an emotional as well as economic toll. In our current health-care climate, individuals may be overwhelmed by the medical expenses incurred, and third-party payers often are reluctant to meet the needs of the patient or to reimburse surgeons appropriately for the skills and effort required to adequately manage these difficult problems.

TREATMENT: OPTIONS AND OUTCOMES

Historical

Treatment options have been refined, but there still is no curative therapy offering predictable success. Historically, many types of therapy have been tried (Seid & Cotton, 1983), including topical caustics, podophyllin, and cryotherapy. Systemic heavy metals, potassium iodide, bismuth, antibiotics, and hormones have been used empirically. Bovine wart vaccines as well as autogenous papilloma vaccines have been tried with very limited success; chemotherapeutic agents including methotrexate and alkylating agents may play a limited role in selected recalcitrant cases.

Radiation therapy was used for over 30 years to treat patients, especially children, with multiple and recurrent laryngeal papillomatosis. This practice stopped when a number of these patients later developed laryngeal cancers. Subsequent reports revealed an increased incidence of laryngeal and bronchial carcinoma in both irradiated and nonirradiated patients with a history of laryngeal papillomatosis. In a careful analysis of 113 patients with laryngeal papillomas, Lindeberg and Elbrønd (1991) demonstrated in previously irradiated papilloma patients a 16-fold increased risk of developing subsequent carcinoma of the respiratory system.

Surgical management has been the mainstay of treatment. Atraumatic removal of the lesion with minimal disturbance of surrounding tissues has remained the essential goal. Endoscopic removal of papilloma with cupped forceps has largely been replaced by the CO_2 laser to improve accuracy, avoid bleeding, and decrease trauma to surrounding tissues.

At one time, tracheotomy was a common adjunct to surgical management to secure an airway and facilitate subsequent administration of anesthesia. This practice was abandoned when it became apparent that many tracheotomized patients develop endotracheal papilloma. Cole, Myer, and Cotton (1989) studied a group of 58 children with papilloma, 12 of whom underwent tracheotomy. Six of the 12 (50%) developed endotracheal papillomas in the peristomal and subsequently more distal tracheal sites. Risk factors included subglottic disease at the time of tracheotomy and prolonged cannulation. Current data suggest that the risk of complications from tracheotomy in papilloma patients has been overstated and the procedure should certainly be performed when indicated (Shapiro, Rimell, Shoemaker, Pou, & Stool, 1996). Generally, tracheotomy is avoided if feasible; however, when necessary, it should be done as atraumatically as possible and cannulation should be brief.

Contemporary Surgical Treatment

The CO_2 laser has been the greatest advance in the surgical management of laryngeal papilloma. Careful microdissection of very small focal lesions is a useful technique. For larger lesions, microcup forceps are used for debulking and biopsy purposes, but the laser is used for the definitive ablation of the lesion at the interface with normal laryngeal tissues. Although use of the CO_2 laser for many benign laryngeal lesions has been challenged, it remains the preferred approach for treating papilloma (Shapshay, Rebeiz, Bohigian, & Hybels, 1990).

Several precautions are in order. It is important to obtain a biopsy for histologic confirmation prior to vaporizing the lesion. Anesthesia should be administered with the least trauma to the lesion to avoid bleeding or direct spread. In adults, we use a small laser-safe endotracheal tube; in children we prefer a spontaneous breathing technique without the use of a tube. Apneic techniques generally fail to provide sufficient time, and jet-ventilation poses physical risks (damage to vocal folds, subcutaneous emphysema, and pneumothorax) in addition to the risk of insufflating viral particles to distant tracheal sites. In treating lesions of the vocal fold, the goal should be to remove the lesion but to avoid extensive damage to the underlying vocal ligament and vocalis muscle. It is important to look carefully for occult sites such as the laryngeal ventricle that might serve as a reservoir for reseeding papilloma.

Great care must be taken to avoid complications with the laser. Meticulous technique is essential to avoid adjacent thermal damage to normal tissues and yet perform a comprehensive removal of the lesion. Nonoperative sites should be protected with wet cottonoids and towels. Oxygen concentration should be kept below 30% and nitrous oxide avoided to reduce the risk of combustion during laser use. It is seldom necessary to use settings over 10 watts, and we prefer the repeat mode with small spot size, varying depending on the area treated to achieve vaporization and hemostasis without deep penetration. With the microspot laser, deep penetration is possible even at low wattage and care must be taken to limit the plane of vaporization to the diseased tissues.

At the anterior commissure, it is important to preserve intact mucosa on one side to avoid web formation. Careful incremental vaporization from lateral to medial might avoid damage to the medial mucosal surface and yet allow for complete removal of anterior commissure lesions. Such an approach was suggested by Kashima (personal communication, May 1992) and has proven helpful in avoiding staged surgical procedures. Errant laser beams can damage mucosa away from the lesion, which might predispose these distant sites to active papilloma growth, given the assumption that papilloma arise at junctional areas of respiratory and squamous epithelium (Kashima, personal communication, May 1992). The intraoperative soft-tissue complications can be minimized using proper technique. Ossoff, Werkhaven, and Dere (1991) reported having no intraoperative complications in 105 procedures, although two patients developed some scarring and one patient formed a laryngeal web.

Precautions must be taken to effectively evacuate the laser plume because HPV DNA has been detected in the plume from vaporization of papilloma (Abramson, Dilorinzo, & Steinberg, 1990; Kashima Kessis, Mounts, & Shah, 1991). Concern has been heightened by a recent report of a 44-year-old laser surgeon who appeared to develop laryngeal papillomatosis from multiple exposures to anogenital condylomas during laser surgery. Specially designated high-filtration surgical laser masks offer additional protection to the surgeon and operating room personnel.

Failure of the CO_2 laser to consistently eradicate papillomas and the tendency for occult disease to seed recurrences have led to recent interest in photodynamic therapy. The intravenous administration of a photosensitizing agent such as hematoporphyrin (or the newly purified form, dihematoporphyrin) 2 or 3 days prior to photoactivation with an argon pump dye laser has had mixed results in limited trials (Basheda et al., 1991; Kavuru, Mehta, & Eliachar, 1990). In a series of 33 patients with moderate to severe recurrent papillomatosis, Abramson and his co-workers (1992) demonstrated a 50% reduction in the average rate of regrowth after treatment. Interestingly, the response seemed greater in patients with the most aggressive disease. Concerns with the argon pump dye laser (notably, cost, size, special cooling-water requirements, and

amount of electrical power necessary to yield limited power output) led Shikowitz (1992) to try a different activating light source. He found the gold vapor laser to be more efficient, offering a pulsed output of greater power with less electrical input. Although the gold vapor laser produced a greater initial rate of tumor response, the overall cure rates were no different from those with the argon pump dye laser.

Adjunctive Medical Measures (Pharmacologic Management)

Efforts to eradicate HPV infection and laryngeal papillomatosis have been frustrated by the inability to localize the infection and destroy the viral agent. A theoretical basis suggests that retinoids might be used to prevent and treat laryngeal papillomatosis. In vitro studies have demonstrated modulation of human laryngeal papilloma cell differentiation with retinoic acid (Reppucci, Dilorenzo, Abramson, & Steinberg, 1991). Increased concentration of retinoic acid caused a decrease in the HPV DNA content of the papilloma cells. Some reports claim regression of papillomatosis in patients treated with 13 cis-retinoic acid (acutane) (Alberts, Coulthard, & Meyskens, 1986). The antiviral agent acyclovir also has been used for laryngeal papillomas with some short-term success reported in a small series (Lopez Aguado et al., 1991). It is probable that the improvement noted was due to control of co-infection viruses and not HPV. The authors are currently studying the possible efficacy of indole-3-carbinol, a food supplement, as an adjunctive treatment. However, at this time, the most widely studied adjunctive medical treatment has been interferon.

The parenteral administration of interferon is one approach to enhance the immune response. Interferons (alpha, beta, and gamma) comprise one of the body's natural defenses to tumors, viruses, and other foreign proteins. Preliminary results have shown alpha interferon to be effective in moderating the growth of laryngeal papillomatosis (Baron et al., 1991). Several clinical trials have been reported with successful regression noted in many patients but concern was raised when some of the same patients developed recurrent disease after discontinuation of interferon. Leventhall, Kashima, Mounts, and Thurmond (1991) reported favorable long-term results in a large series that was carefully studied. Patients in that study were treated with 2-4 MU per square meter of body surface area every other day for 6 months and then off for 6 months before being treated on a PRN (per requested need) basis. Twenty-two of 60 treated patients were in complete remission; 25 had partial remissions. Only 13 patients had no apparent response. The median duration of follow-up was 550 days in the complete remission group and 400 days in the partial group. Interferon is expensive, requires repeated injections, high doses, and prolonged treatment (at least six months), and has serious potential side-effects. It should not be used in patients with cardiac disease, renal disease, liver failure, or active central nervous system disorders. Patients should be monitored for leukopenia, elevated hepatic enzymes, thrombocytopenia, and proteinuria. There has been an isolated report of systemic lupus erythematosus developing in a 10½-year-old boy treated with interferon alpha-N1 for 7 years (Tolaymat, Leventhal, Sakarcan, Kashima, & Monteiro, 1992). This patient recovered after drug withdrawal but it raises concern that interferon administration might induce autoimmune diseases. Because of the enormous problems posed by severe recurrent papillomatosis, these risks are often offset by the potential benefits. Interferon is indicated for severe recurrent papillomatosis where it can be a useful adjunct to laser ablation in suppressing recurrence and prolonging periods of remission.

SUMMARY

Great strides have been made in defining the pathology and viral etiology of laryngeal papillomatosis. Epidemiological studies have provided some insight into factors associated with the disease. Further research efforts are needed in the broad area of control and prevention of viral infections in humans. Although behavioral changes might play a role in prevention of HPV infection, work is needed to explore chemopreventive measures. Immunotherapy appears to be an important avenue of research. Current studies on interferon have been largely empirical, and further work is needed to define the proper role for this agent. Other lymphokines might be explored. Antiviral agents such as acyclovir have had limited trials and newer agents might be more effective.

The mainstay of surgical management has been the CO_2 laser, but what is needed is a "smart" laser that can selectively destroy the lesion but preserve the delicate laryngeal tissues. Photodynamic therapy using different photosensitizing agents and different activating light sources probably deserves further study. Overall, the most cost-effective strategies will be to prevent the disease from occurring and to modify host resistance through immunotherapy.

REFERENCES

Abramson, A. L., Dilorenzo, T. P., & Steinberg, B. M. (1990). Is papillomavirus detectable in the plume of laser-treated laryngeal papilloma? *Archives of Otolaryngology, Head and Neck Surgery, 116*, 604–607.

Abramson, A. L., Shikowitz, M. J., Mullooly, V. M., Steinberg, B. M., Amella, C. A., & Rothstein, H. R. (1992). Clinical effects of photodynamic therapy on recurrent laryngeal papillomas. *Archives of Otolaryngology, Head and Neck Surgery, 118,* 25–29.

Alberts, D. S., Coulthard, S. W., & Meyskens, F. L. (1986). Regression of aggressive laryngeal papillomatosis with 13-cis-retinoic acid (Acutane). *Journal of Biological Response Modifiers, 5,* 124–128.

Aronson, A. E. (1980). *Clinical voice disorders: An interdisciplinary approach.* New York: Thieme-Stratton.

Baron, S., Tyring, S. K., Fleischmann, W. R., Jr., Coppenhaver, D. H., Niesel, D. W., Klimpel, G. R., Stanton, G. J., & Hughes, T. K. (1991). The interferons. Mechanisms of action and clinical applications. *Journal of the American Medical Association, 266,* 1375–1383.

Basheda, S. G., Mehta, A. C., De Boer, G., & Orlowski, J. P. (1991). Endobronchial and parenchymal juvenile laryngotracheobronchial papillomatosis. Effect of photodynamic therapy. *Chest, 100,* 1458–1461.

Chipps, B. E., McClurg, F. L., Jr., Freidman, E. M., & Adams, G. L. (1990). Respiratory papillomas: presentation before six months. *Pediatric Pulmonology, 9,* 125–130.

Clarke, J., Terry, R. M., & Lacey, C. J. (1991). A study to estimate the prevalence of upper respiratory tract papillomatosis in patients with genital warts. *International Journal of STD AIDS, 2,* 114–115.

Cohen, S. R., Thompson, J. W., Geller, K. A., & Birns, J. W. (1983). Voice change in the pediatric patient: A differential diagnosis. *Annals of Otology, Rhinology, and Laryngology, 92,* 437–443.

Cole, R. R., Myer, C. M., III, & Cotton, R. T. (1989). Tracheotomy in children with recurrent respiratory papillomatosis. *Head and Neck, 11,* 226–230.

Cripe, T. P. (1990). Human papillomaviruses: Pediatric perspectives on a family of mutifaceted tumorigenic pathogens. *Pediatric Infections Diseases Journal, 9,* 836–844.

Dickens, P., Srivastava, G., Loke, S. L., & Larkin, S. (1991). Human papillomavirus 6, 11, and 16 in laryngeal papillomas. *Journal of Pathology, 165,* 243–246.

Duggan, M. A., Lim, M., Gill, M. J., & Inoue, M. (1990). HPV DNA typing of adult onset respiratory papillomatosis. *Laryngoscope, 100,* 639–642.

Gaylis, B., & Hayden, R. E. (1991). Recurrent respiratory papillomatosis: Progression to invasion and malignancy. *American Journal of Otolaryngology, 12,* 104–112.

Gildston, P., & Gildston, H. (1992). Hypnotherapeutic intervention for voice disorders related to recurring juvenile laryngeal papillomatosis. International *Journal of Clinical Experience in Hypnotherapy, 40,* 74–87.

Guillou, L., Sahli, R., Chaubert, P., Monnier, P., Cuttat, J. F., & Costa, J. (1991). Squamous cell carcinoma of the lung in a nonsmoking, nonirradiated patient with juvenile laryngotracheal papillomatosis. Evidence of human papillomavirus–11 DNA in both carcinoma and papillomas. American *Journal of Surgical Pathology, 15,* 891–898.

Helmrich, G., Stubbs, T. M., & Stoerker, J. (1992). Fatal maternal laryngeal papillomatosis in pregnancy: A case report [corrected] [published erratum appears in American Journal of Obstetrics and Gynecology, 1992, 166(4), 1313]. *American Journal of Obstetrics and Gynecology, 166,* 524–525.

Holinger, P., & Johnston, K. (1951). Benign tumors of the larynx. *Annals of Otology, Rhinology, and Laryngology, 60,* 496–509.

Jones, S. R., Myers, E. N., & Barnes, L. (1984). Benign neoplasms of the larynx. *Otolaryngological Clinics of North America, 17,* 151–178.

Kashima, H. K., Kessis, T., Mounts, P., & Shah, K. (1991). Polymerase chain reaction identification of human papillomavirus DNA in CO2 laser plume from recurrent respiratory papillomatosis. *Otolaryngology Head and Neck Surgery, 104,* 191–195.

Kashima, H. K., Shah, F., Lyles, A., & Glackin, R. (1992a). A comparison of risk factors in juvenile-onset and adult-onset recurrent respiratory papillomatosis. *Laryngoscope, 102,* 9–13.

Kashima, H. K., Kessis, T., Hruban, R. H., Wu, T. C., Zinreich, S. J., & Shah, K. V. (1992b). Human papillomavirus in sinonasal papillomas and squamous cell carcinoma. *Laryngoscope, 102,* 973–976.

Kavura, M. S., Mehta, A. C., & Eliachar, I. (1990). Effect of photodynamic therapy and external beam radiation therapy on juvenile laryngotracheobronchial papillomatosis. *American Review of Respiratory Diseases, 141,* 509–510.

Leventhal, B. G., Kashima, H. K., Mounts, P., & Thurmond, L. (1991). Long-term response of recurrent respiratory papillomatosis to treatment with lymphoblastoid interferon alpha-N1. *New England Journal of Medicine, 325,* 613–617.

Lindeberg, H., & Elbrønd, O. (1989). Laryngeal papillomas: Clinical aspects in a series of 231 patients. *Clinical Otolaryngology, 14,* 333–342.

Lindeberg, H., & Elbrønd, O. (1990). Laryngeal papillomas: The epidemiology in a Danish subpopulation 1965–1984. *Clinical Otolaryngology, 15,* 125–131.

Lindeberg, H., & Elbrønd, O. (1991). Malignant tumors in patients with a history of multiple laryngeal papillomas: The significance of irradiation. *Clinical Otolaryngology, 16,* 149–151.

Lindeberg, H., & Johansen, L. (1990). The presence of human papillomavirus (HPV) in solitary adult laryngeal papillomas demonstrated by in situ DNA hybridization with sulphonated probes. *Clinical Otolaryngology, 15,* 367–371.

Lopez Aguado, D., Perez Pinero, B., Betancor, L., Mendez, A., & Campos Banales, E. (1991). Acyclovir in the treatment of laryngeal papillomatosis. *International Journal of Pediatric Otorhinolaryngology, 21,* 269–274.

Michaels, L. (1984). *Pathology of the larynx.* Berlin: Springer-Verlag.

Ossoff, R. H., Werkhaven, J. A., & Dere, H. (1991). Soft-tissue complications of laser surgery for recurrent respiratory papillomatosis. *Laryngoscope, 101,* 1162–1166.

Peng, T. C., Searle, C. P., III, Shah, K. V., Repke, J. T., & Johnson, T. R. (1990). Prevalence of human papillomavirus in term pregnancy. *American Journal of Perinatology, 7,* 189–192.

Pignatari, S., Smith, E. M., Gray, S. D., Shive, C., & Turek, L. P. (1992). Detection of human papillomavirus infection in diseased and non-diseased sites of the respiratory tract in recurrent respiratory papillomatosis patients by DNA hybridization. *Annals of Otology, Rhinology, and Laryngology, 101,* 405–412.

Quiney, R. E., Hall, D., & Croft, C. B. (1989). Laryngeal papillomatosis: Analysis of 113 patients. *Clinical Otolaryngology, 14,* 217–225.

Reppucci, A. D., Dilorenzo, T. P., Abramson, A. L., & Steinberg, B. M. (1991). In vitro modulation of human laryngeal papilloma cell differentiation by retinoic acid. *Otolaryngology—Head and Neck Surgery, 105,* 528–532.

Rimell, F., Maisel, R., & Dayton, V. (1992). In situ hybridization and laryngeal papillomas. *Annals of Otology, Rhinology, and Laryngology, 101,* 119–126.

Seid, A. B., & Cotton, R. (1983). Tumors of the larynx, trachea, and bronchi. In C. D. Bluestone & S. E. Stool (Eds.), *Pediatric otolaryngology.* Philadelphia: W. B. Saunders.

Shapiro, A. M., Rimell, F. L., Shoemaker, D., Pou, A., & Stool, S. E. (1996). Tracheotomy in children with juvenile-onset recurrent respiratory papillomatosis: The Children's Hospital of Pittsburgh experience. *Annals of Otology–Rhinology and Laryngology, 105,* 1–5.

Shapshay, S. M., Rebeiz, E. E., Bohigian, R. K., & Hybels, R. L. (1990). Benign lesions of the larynx: should the laser be used? *Laryngoscope, 100,* 953–957.

Shikowitz, M. J. (1992). Comparison of pulsed and continuous wave light in photodynamic therapy of papillomas: An experimental study. *Laryngoscope, 102,* 300–310.

Smith, E. M., Johnson, S. R., Cripe, T. P., Pignatari, S., & Turek, L. (1991). Perinatal vertical transmission of human papillomavirus and subsequent development of respiratory tract papillomatosis. *Annals of Otology, Rhinology, and Laryngology, 100,* 479–483.

Tolaymat, A., Leventhal, B., Sakarcan, A., Kashima, H., & Monteiro, C. (1992). Systemic lupus erythematosus in a child receiving long-term interferon therapy. *Journal of Pediatrics, 120,* 429–432.

Yousem, S. A., Ohori, N. P., & Sonmez-Alpan, E. (1992). Occurrence of human papillomavirus DNA in primary lung neoplasms. *Cancer, 69,* 693–697.

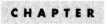

LARYNGEAL ULCERS

THOMAS R. PASIC, M.D.

INTRODUCTION AND DEFINITION

Laryngeal contact ulcers are erosions of the respiratory epithelium over the vocal processes of the arytenoid cartilages. They are often found in association with adjacent reactive granulation tissue. These benign inflammatory lesions were described by Virchow in 1858 as well as others (reviewed by Brodnitz, 1961). However, it was Chevalier Jackson who coined the term "contact ulcer" in 1928 and defined it as a distinct clinical entity. He described a contact ulcer as a "superficial ulceration occurring on one or both sides of the larynx posteriorly, the ulcerated surface coming in contact on phonation with that of its fellow of the opposite side." The characteristic location of contact ulcers on the posterior one-third of the true vocal folds makes hoarseness an early symptom. Airway compromise is uncommon but, when present, is caused by the formation of abundant granulation tissue. Treatment is aimed at reversing the underlying etiologic process (e.g., speech therapy for ulcers caused by laryngeal hyperfunction). The history of the treatment of contact ulcers shows that a successful outcome depends on treatment of the underlying pathology. Furthermore, a team approach including the physician and speech-language pathologist greatly facilitates achieving this goal (Bloch, Gould, & Hirano, 1981; Cooper & Nahum, 1967).

PATHOGENESIS

Contact ulcers usually are found in three clinical conditions: voice abuse, prolonged endotracheal intubation, and gastroesophageal reflux. These situations are similar in that they provide a source of repeated mechanical or chemical trauma to the mucosa overlying the arytenoid cartilages. These distinctly independent risk factors also can interact with each other. Thus, contact ulcers caused by voice abuse may be less likely to improve when gastroesophageal reflux also is present. Similarly, reflux may worsen the laryngeal injury associated with endotracheal intubation. As a result, some cases might require treatment directed against more than one risk factor before a clinical response is obtained.

Voice Abuse

In early studies of contact ulcers, the name and anatomic descriptions of the disorder emphasized the role of trauma as an etiologic factor (Baker, 1961; Brodnitz, 1961; Holinger & Johnston, 1960). Jackson (1928) described the vocal processes as a "hammer and anvil" violently striking and grinding upon each other during speech production. This mechanical trauma is especially marked at low speech frequencies, high speech intensities, and during nonlinguistic activities such as throat clearing (von Leden & Moore, 1960). The effect of low speech frequency on traumatic arytenoid injury is consistent with findings by Peacher and Holinger (1947) who described the abnormal vocal production of 16 patients with contact ulcers. They found a forced pitch far below the optimum and proposed that vocal abuse was the chief factor perpetuating contact ulcers.

However, several investigators have observed that chronic voice abuse alone could not fully account for the development of contact ulcers since voice abuse is common and ulcers are uncommon (Brodnitz, 1961; von Leden & Moore, 1960). Holinger and Johnston (1960) found that approximately 30% of their patients with contact ulcers had an upper respiratory infection that preceded the onset of persistent hoarseness. Baker (1961) also noted an occasional history of a severe cold before onset of symptoms. Other authors have noted that emotional stress and vocal abuse act together to cause contact ulcers and that symptomatic exacerbations are often associated with periods of severe personal or professional stress (Brodnitz, 1961; Peacher, 1961). Similarly, investigators have made a more general observation that contact ulcers tend to occur in "ambitious" and "anxious" individuals (Baker, 1961). Thus, although voice abuse is a major etiologic factor, the development of ulcers is likely multifactorial and might depend on the synergistic effects of several predisposing events.

Gastroesophageal Reflux

It is interesting to note that Jackson (1928) wrote that many of his patients complained of waking with a "choking, strangling cough at night." Although he attributed these symptoms to aspiration of oral secretions, he may well have been describing gastroesophageal reflux (GER). The reflux of acidic gastric contents through the lower esophageal sphincter (LES) into the esophagus occurs in all individuals (Demeester et al., 1976; Johnson, 1981). This "normal" reflux is relatively brief, infrequent, and asymptomatic. In contrast, up to 7% of the general population has daily symptoms of GER and another 36% of the population has symptoms on at least a monthly basis (Nebel, Fornes, & Castell, 1976). This type of reflux is more severe than in "normal" persons, is associated with a pathologically incompetent lower esophageal sphincter (LES) and has been associated with the development of symptomatic esophageal inflammation and ulceration.

Cherry and Margulies (1968) demonstrated GER in three patients whose contact ulcers failed to respond to voice therapy. Delahunty and Cherry (1968) went on to show that gastric acid applied to the laryngeal mucosa in experimental animals could lead to the development of laryngeal ulcers. Over the ensuing years, others also have noted a close relationship between esophageal dysfunction and the development of laryngeal contact ulcers (Goldberg, Noyek, & Pritzler, 1978; Miko, 1989; Nebel, Tibbling, Olofsson, & Ericsson, 1983).

Further evidence of the etiologic role of GER is provided by the improvement of symptoms of contact ulcers following treatment with antireflux therapy. Briefly, antireflux therapy consists of pharmacological, dietary, and positional interventions whose goals are to decrease gastric acidity, decrease gastric acid production, increase LES tone, and improve esophageal clearance of refluxed gastric contents. Toward these ends, antacids are given to decrease the pH of gastric contents, histamine receptor blockers (e.g., ranitidine) are given to decrease gastric acid production, and medications or foods that lower LES tone are avoided (e.g., theophylline, calcium channel blockers, tobacco, and alcohol) (Richter & Castell, 1981, 1982). In addition, elevation of the head of the bed by at least 6 inches has been found to improve clearance of refluxed acid. Institution of this therapy in patients with contact ulcers has been found to decrease the signs and symptoms of ulceration (Olson, 1983; Ward, Zwitman, Hanson, & Berci, 1980). Several authors have noted the development of laryngeal carcinoma in some of their patients with contact ulcers (Jackson, 1928; Peacher, 1961). Gastroesophageal reflux has also been associated with the development of squamous cell carcinoma in the posterior half of the larynx (Olson, 1986; Ward & Hanson, 1988). The relationship between reflux, contact ulcers, and laryngeal carcinoma highlights the importance of recognizing and treating reflux-induced laryngeal disease. Laryngeal ulcers and the associated granulation tissue, even those typical in location for contact lesions, should be followed closely and biopsied to evaluate for possible malignancy.

Endotracheal Intubation

Endotracheal tubes are believed to cause laryngeal ulcers by two mechanisms. First, the endotracheal tube can cause repeated abrasions of the laryngeal mucosa if the head is moved. On average, an endotracheal tube moves 3.8 cm when the head is moved from flexion to extension (Conrardy, Goodman, Lainge, & Singer, 1976). Second, the endotracheal tube exerts pressure posteriorly and laterally on the laryngeal mucosa. This pressure greatly exceeds the capillary perfusion pressure (Weymuller, Bishop, Fink, Bibbard, & Spelman, 1983) and can result in ischemic necrosis of the mucosa over the arytenoid cartilages. Loss of epithelium can occur after only 1 to 2 hours of intubation (Donnelly, 1969; Klainer, Turndorf, Wu, Maewal, & Allender, 1975).

Factors that increase the risk of ulceration and granuloma formation include the duration of intubation and the size of the endotracheal tube. An increased incidence of laryngeal injury has been associated with an increased duration of intubation in both clinical and laboratory studies (Bishop, 1989; Donnelly, 1969; Whited, 1984). The use of larger endotracheal tubes is also more likely to be associated with laryngeal injuries than is the use of smaller tubes (Santos, Afrassiabi, & Weymuller, 1989). Furthermore, the use of a nasogastric tube at the same time as an endotracheal tube increases the risk of laryngeal injury (Santos et al., 1989; Sofferman & Hubbell, 1981). The nasogastric tube traps the posterior larynx against the endotracheal tube and can worsen ischemic necrosis. Alternatively, the nasogastric tube may stent the LES and cause gastroesophageal reflux. Indeed, Gaynor (1988) has found that reflux is an etiologic factor in laryngeal complications of intubation.

DEMOGRAPHIC INFORMATION

Laryngeal hyperfunction and GER are both common in the general population. Contact ulcers, however, are clearly uncommon (Baker, 1961; Brodnitz, 1961). Similarly, the incidence of postintubation laryngeal ulcers and granulomas is low relative to the number of persons undergoing endotracheal intubation (Balestrieri & Watson, 1982). The disparity between the incidence of risk factors and the incidence of the disorder raises the possibility that risk factors are not by themselves sufficient to cause contact ulcers. It is likely that events superimposed on the risk factor (e.g., an upper respiratory infection or nasogastric intubation) are required to establish an ulcer. Once established, it is possible that constant mechanical or chemical irritation caused by hyperfunction, acid reflux, or endotracheal tube trauma acts to prevent healing of the ulcer. It has been observed that contact ulcers due to laryngeal hyperfunction or GER are more common in men than in women (Cooper & Nahum, 1967; Feder & Mitchell, 1984; Holinger & Johnston, 1960). The reasons for this difference are not clear. In contrast, ulcers due to prolonged intubation have been noted more commonly in women than in men by most (Balestrieri & Watson, 1982), but not by all, investigators (Donnelly, 1969). The difference in incidence between sexes could be a result of a larger size of endotracheal tubes used in women relative to the smaller size of the larynx.

ONSET AND COURSE OF THE DISORDER

The most common symptoms of laryngeal contact ulcers are hoarseness and throat pain. The severity of the hoarseness varies widely among affected individuals, but is frequently worse after voice use. Also, severity is associated with a sense of vocal fatigue (Cooper & Nahum, 1967; Feder & Mitchell, 1984; Peacher, 1961). The throat pain is described as a "sharp, sticking pain," may become worse on swallowing and is often associated with otalgia (Jackson, 1928; Feder & Mitchell, 1984). Other patients have described a "foreign body" sensation in the throat, a sense of fullness, and a constant urge to clear the throat (Brodnitz, 1961).

For contact ulcers resulting from vocal abuse or GER, the natural history, in the absence of therapy, is characterized by frequent exacerbations and slow improvements. The exacerbation of symptoms often coincides with worsening predisposing factors such as increased emotional stress, recurrent voice abuse, or worsening GER. Often, medical attention is sought only after symptoms persist or worsen and the diagnosis of contact ulcers is made.

In contrast, the vast majority of contact ulcers following endotracheal intubation heal spontaneously after extubation and no specific intervention is required (Alessi, Hanson, & Berci, 1989; Colice, 1992; Klainer et al., 975). This is understandable because the risk factor for development of contact ulcers has been removed. When postintubation ulcers do not resolve spontaneously, previously unsuspected laryngeal hyperfunction or GER could be implicated.

MEDICAL CONSIDERATIONS

Laryngeal contact ulcers have a characteristic appearance on clinical examination: shallow mucosal erosions with surrounding erythema along the posterior third of the true vocal folds. These findings, in association with the typical history of hoarseness and throat pain of longstanding duration, make the diagnosis of contact ulcers very likely. The clinician should seek an additional history of voice use patterns and symptoms of possible reflux esophagitis. A biopsy of the lesion during a direct laryngoscopic examination is essential to evaluate for other possible diagnoses, such as a malignancy, primary infectious disorder, or granulomatous disorder (Jackson, 1928; Ward et al., 1980). Histopathological examination in the case of contact ulcers should show nonspecific chronic inflammation (Donnelly, 1969). If there are findings of posterior laryngitis or if voice therapy alone provides limited clinical improvement, testing or empiric treatment for GER might be indicated.

VOICE EVALUATION

Vocal Characteristics

The voice is affected early in the natural history of contact ulcers. Hoarseness and vocal fatigue are noted by almost all affected individuals. Other characteristic abnormalities of voice production include speech musculature hypertension, an explosive speech pattern with confined pitch range, glottic plosive attack, and a forcing of the pitch below the optimum pitch (Peacher & Holinger, 1947). Limitation of intensity range is also frequent (Peacher, 1961).

Endoscopy

Endoscopic evaluation, whether indirect, fiberoptic, or direct, shows ulceration over the vocal processes of the arytenoid cartilages (Alessi et al., 1989). Cooper and Nahum (1967) have suggested three phases in contact ulcer formation that can be detected on endoscopic examination. The first phase is characterized by erythema and edema in the posterior larynx. The second phase shows evidence of mucosal loss in the typical location, and the third phase is characterized by granuloma formation around the rim of the ulcer. It should be noted, however, that a clear progression from one phase to the next in a longitudinal study has not been demonstrated.

Acoustic Analysis

Priebe, Henke, and Hedley-White (1988) studied acoustic characteristics of the voice following endotracheal intubation and noted an abnormally wide spread of speech energy across the frequency range. They often observed a bimodal or trimodal frequency pattern. These changes reversed with time, which is consistent with the expected course of contact ulcers following extubation.

TREATMENT: OPTIONS AND OUTCOMES

The historic treatment of contact ulcers consisted of several months of complete voice rest (Jackson, 1928). Not only was compliance with the recommended therapy difficult, but ulcers that improved with voice rest tended to recur as soon as voice use was resumed (Baker, 1961; Brodnitz, 1961).

Speech Pathology

The high recurrence rate and association with voice abuse led Peacher and Holinger (1947) to attempt voice reeducation for patients with contact ulcers. Their success in six patients treated by voice therapy initiated a widespread change in clinical practice that, in large part, has persisted to this today. Results of voice therapy for contact ulcers have continued to be encouraging. In a subsequent article, Peacher (1961) reported that 65 of 70 patients (93%) had a consistently clear voice after speech therapy. No recurrences of contact ulcer formation were noted. Bloch and co-workers (1981) achieved a response rate of 71% following speech therapy on an evaluation by a laryngologist, speech pathologist, and the patient. They noted, however, that only 4 of 17 patients noted a complete relief of symptoms and another 10 patients noted symptomatic improvement. Thus, not all patients improve with voice therapy alone, and improvement is not always complete.

Pharmacologic Management

It was findings such as these that led Cherry and Margulies (1968) to investigate gastroesophageal reflux as an etiologic factor, especially in those patients who failed speech therapy. Findings by others have confirmed both the role of reflux in contact ulcer formation and the benefit of anti-reflux therapy (Goldberg et al., 1978; Ward et al., 1980). Current treatment recommendations should include speech therapy (hyperfunction is usually present even when GER is the prime etiologic factor) and antireflux therapy when GER is present. Intralesional injection of steroids can be a helpful adjunctive measure (Crary, Sapienza, Cassisi, & Moore, 1995).

Surgical Management

Surgery is more useful in the diagnosis of contact ulcers than in its treatment. Early investigators quickly found that removal of ulcerations and granulation tissue only increased the amount of traumatized tissue and did not result in sustained symptomatic improvement (Baker, 1961; Jackson, 1928). Surgical removal is indicated, however, if granulation tissue is bulky or compromises the airway. In the case of granulation tissue that does not spontaneously resolve after endotracheal intubation, endoscopic removal may be required. Injection of the base of the lesions with steroids also can help prevent recurrence in these cases (Weymuller, 1992).

SUMMARY

A rational treatment strategy based on the pathogenesis of contact ulcers has emerged over the past 60 years. A significant improvement in the response to treatment has accompanied these changes

in management. However, several areas are yet to be explored. First, the relationship between the development of ulcers and formation of granulation tissue is unclear. Benjamin and Croxson (1985) have suggested that laryngeal ulcers and granuloma may not represent manifestations of the same pathological process, as has been assumed. Perhaps elucidation of separate host factors or risk factors that predispose to granulation tissue formation can be elucidated and the formation of obstructing granulation tissue avoided.

Second, endotracheal tube trauma is clearly related to contact ulcer formation. Modifications of endotracheal tube design and evaluation of biocompatible materials used in the manufacture of endotracheal tubes could help diminish laryngeal trauma (Weymuller, 1992). An endotracheal tube with a foam cuff at the level of the glottis has been developed and might help reduce the incidence of laryngeal ulcers (Santos et al., 1989).

Finally, the anecdotal reports of laryngeal carcinoma developing in patients with contact ulcers deserves additional study. Contact ulcers and carcinoma might share a common risk factor of gastroesophageal reflux. This association, in light of the endemic nature of GER, should be evaluated further .

REFERENCES

Alessi, D. M., Hanson, D. G., & Berci, G. (1989). Bedside videolaryngoscopic assessment of intubation trauma. *Annals of Otology, Rhinology, and Laryngology, 98,* 568–590.

Baker, D. C. (1961). Contact ulcers of the larynx. *Laryngoscope, 64,* 73–78.

Balestrieri, F., & Watson, C. B. (1982). Intubation granuloma. *Otology Clinics of North America, 15,* 567–579.

Benjamin, B., & Croxson, G. (1985). Vocal cord granulomas. *Annals of Otology, Rhinology, and Laryngology, 94,* 538–541.

Bishop, M. J. (1989). Mechanisms of laryngo-tracheal injury following prolonged tracheal intubation. *Chest, 96*, 185–186.

Bloch, C. S., Gould, W. J., & Hirano, M. (1981). Effect of voice therapy on contact granuloma of the vocal fold. *Annals of Otology, 90*, 48–52.

Brodnitz, F. S. (1961). Contact ulcer of the larynx. *Archives of Otolaryngology, 74*, 70–80.

Cherry, J., & Margulies, S. I. (1968). Contact ulcer of the larynx. *Laryngoscope, 73*, 1937–1940.

Colice, G. L. (1992). Resolution of otolaryngeal injury following translaryngeal intubation. *American Review of Respiratory Diseases, 145*, 361–364.

Conrardy, P. A., Goodman, L. R., Lainge, F., & Singer, M. M. (1976). Alteration of endotracheal tube position. *Critical Care Medicine, 4*, 8–12.

Cooper, M., & Nahum, A. M. (1967). Vocal rehabilitation for contact ulcer of the larynx. *Archives of Otolaryngology, 85*, 41–46.

Crary, M. A., Sapienza, C., Cassisi, N. J., Moore, G. P. (1995, October). *Treatment of contact granuloma with steroid injections*. Paper presented at the Pacific Voice Conference, San Francisco.

Delahunty, J. E., & Cherry, J. (1968). Experimentally produced vocal cord granulomas. *Laryngoscope, 78*, 1941–1948.

Demeester, T. R., Johnson, L. F., Joseph, G. J., Toscano, M. S., Hall, A. W., & Skinner, D. B. (1976). Patterns of gastroesophageal reflux in health and disease.

Donnelly, W. H. (1969). Histopathology of endotracheal intubation: an autopsy study of 99 cases. *Archives of Pathology, 88*, 511–520.

Feder, R. J., & Mitchell, M. J. (1984). Hyperfunctional, hyperacidic and intubation granulomas. *Archives of Otolaryngology, 110*, 582–584.

Gaynor, E. B. (1988). Gastroesophageal reflux as an etiologic factor in laryngeal compli-cations of intubation. *Laryngoscope, 98*, 972–979.

Goldberg, M., Noyek, A. M., & Pritzler, K. P. H. (1978). Laryngeal granuloma secondary to gastro-oesophageal reflux. *Journal of Otolaryngology, 7*, 196–202.

Holinger, P. J., & Johnston, K. C. (1960). Contact ulcer of the larynx. *Journal of the American Medical Association, 172*, 511–515.

Jackson, C. (1928). Contact ulcer of the larynx. *Annals of Otology, Rhinology, and Laryngology, 37*, 227–230.

Johnson, L. F. (1981). New concepts and methods in the study and treatment of gastroesophageal reflux. *Medical Clinics of North America, 65*, 1195–1221.

Klainer, A. S., Turndorf, H., Wu, W. H., Maewal, H., & Allender, P. (1975). Surface alterations due to endotracheal intubation. *American Journal of Medicine, 58*, 674–683.

Miko, T. L. (1989). Peptic (contact ulcer) granuloma of the larynx. *Journal of Clinical Pathology, 42*, 800–804.

Nebel, O. T., Fornes, M. F., & Castell, D. O. (1976). Symptomatic gastroesophageal reflex: Incidence and predisposing factors. *American Journal of Digestive Disorders, 21*, 953–956.

Nebel, O. T., Tibbling, L., Olofsson, J., & Ericsson, G. (1983). Esophageal dysfunction in patients with contact ulcers of the larynx. *Annals of Otology, Rhinology, and Laryngology, 92*, 228–230.

Olson, N. R. (1983). Effects of stomach acid on the larynx. *Proceedings of the American Laryngology Association, 104*, 108–112.

Olson, N. R. (1986). The problem of gastroesophageal reflux. *Otolaryngology Clinics of North America, 19*, 119–133.

Peacher, G. M. (1961). Vocal therapy for contact ulcer of the larynx: a follow-up of 70 patients. *Laryngoscope, 71*, 37–47.

Peacher, G. M., & Holinger, P. (1947). Contact ulcer of the larynx II. The role of vocal re-education. *Archives of Otolaryngology, 36*, 617–623.

Priebe, H. J., Henke, W., & Hedley-White, J. (1988). Effects of tracheal intubation on laryngeal acoustic waveforms. *Anesthesia and Analgesia, 67*, 219–227.

Richter, J. E., & Castell, D. O. (1981). Drugs, foods, and other substances in the cause and treatment of reflux esophagitis. *Medical Clinics of North America, 65*, 1223–1233.

Richter, J. E., & Castell, D. O. (1982). Gastroesophageal reflux: Pathogenesis, diagnosis, and therapy. *Annals of Internal Medicine, 97*, 93–103.

Santos, P. M., Afrassiabi, A., & Weymuller, E. A. (1989). Prospective studies evaluating the standard endotracheal tube and a prototype endotracheal tube. *Annals of Otology, Rhinology, and Laryngology, 98,* 935–940.

Sofferman, R. A., & Hubbell, R. N. (1981). Laryngeal complications of nasogastric tubes. *Annals of Otology, 90,* 465–468.

von Leden, J., & Moore, G. P. (1960). Contact ulcers of the larynx: experimental observations. *Archives of Otolaryngology, 72,* 746–751.

Ward, P. H., & Hanson, D. G. (1988). Reflux as an etiological factor of carcinoma of the laryn-gopharynx. *Laryngoscope, 98,* 1195–1198.

Ward, P. W., Zwitman, D., Hanson, D., & Berci, G. (1980). Contact ulcers and granulomas of the larynx: New insights into their etiology as a basis for more rational treatment. *Otoloaryngology—Head and Neck Surgery, 88,* 262–269.

Weymuller, E. A., Bishop, M. J., Fink, B. R., Bib-bard, A. W., & Spelman, F. A. (1983). Quantification of intralaryngeal pressure exerted by endotracheal tubes. *Annals of Otology, Rhinology, and Laryngology, 92,* 444–447.

Weymuller, E. A. (1992). Prevention and management of intubation injury of the larynx and trachea. *American Journal of Otology, 13,* 139–144.

Whited, R. E. (1984). A prospective study of laryngotracheal sequelae in long-term intubation. *Laryngoscope, 94,* 367–377.

CHAPTER 13

MALIGNANT LESIONS OF THE LARYNX

NICHOLAS J. CASSISI, D.D.S., M.D.
CHRISTINE SAPIENZA, Ph.D.
BETSY P. VINSON, M.M.S.

INTRODUCTION AND DEFINITIONS

Persons who are faced with the diagnosis of laryngeal cancer have many concerns and fears which need to be addressed by the patient and his or her family with the assistance of the medical team involved in his or her care. Typically, patients with laryngeal cancer have the same fears as those who face any cancer. Their concerns include the recurrence of cancer and the possibility of death, as well as concern about their ability to continue to work and maintain the lifestyle they enjoyed prior to being diagnosed with cancer. In addition, those with laryngeal cancer face the possible loss of oral communication and fear their ability to maintain an active role in their usual lifestyle. Naturally, there is fear about the possibility of social isolation due to the use of nonstandard communication methods. Therefore, to effectively meet the many needs of the patient and his or her family, a team approach which involves the surgeon, the speech-language pathologist, social workers, counselors, and nurses is critical (Reed, 1988).

PATHOGENESIS

Smoking tobacco is the etiologic agent primarily related to cancer of the larynx. Abstention from the use of tobacco for 5 years results in a decline in tobacco-related cancers of the alimentary and respiratory tracts, and after 10 years of nonuse, the risk approaches that of non-smokers (Wynder, 1978). It is not known whether smoking cigarettes that are low in tar and nicotine decreases the risk of laryngeal cancer (Hammond, Garfinkel, Seidman, & Lew, 1976). It is interesting to note that, in spite of preoperative counseling regarding the role of smoking as a cause of laryngeal cancer, many of the male patients and their wives will not acknowledge the relationship. In one study, 98% of the male patients with laryngeal cancer smoked at least one pack of cigarettes per day, and 36% smoked two or more packs per day. However, 42% of their wives denied that smoking was related to the laryngeal cancer (Kommers, Sullivan, & Yonkers, 1977).

Other agents also appear to play a role in the etiology of laryngeal cancer. The excessive use of marijuana (greater than 10 marijuana cigarettes per day) also appears to cause an increase in laryngeal cancer, particularly in young adults. Alcohol as an etiologic agent in head and neck cancer is also well established. Its importance in the etiology of laryngeal cancer is unclear (Wagenfield, Harwood, Bryce, Van Nostrand, & De Boerg, 1980), although individuals who combine heavy smoking and daily drinking are 15.5% more likely to develop laryngeal malignancy than the general population (McKenna, Fornataro-Clerici, McMeamin, & Leonard, 1991).

DEMOGRAPHIC INFORMATION

Cancer of the larynx is the most common head and neck cancer, representing approximately 2–5% of all cancer. In the United States in 1993, it was estimated that approximately 12,600 new cases of laryngeal cancer were diagnosed, with 3,800 deaths due to the cancer (Boring, Squires, & Tong, 1993).

Cancer of the larynx has increased by 33% in white men but was three-and-one-half times greater in nonwhite men from 1935–1970. In women, however, the incidence has increased only slightly, even though lung cancer in women has quadrupled in the same period of time (Devesa & Silverman, 1978). Statistics for 1993 indicated a 5:1 ratio of laryngeal cancer in men versus women. In men, laryngeal cancer is found most frequently between 50 and 70 years of age (McKenna et al., 1991). Less data are available for the female population.

The incidence of laryngeal cancer appears to be highest in the northeastern portion of the United States, with northern New Jersey, New York City, and the area along the Hudson River having the greatest incidence of laryngeal cancer. It is not known what role the air environment contributes to the increased incidence of laryngeal cancer in this highly industrialized area of the country.

ONSET AND COURSE OF THE DISORDER

Anatomically, the larynx is divided into the supraglottic, glottic, and subglottic larynx. The symptoms and course of the disease will vary depending on the anatomic site in which the cancer occurs.

Supraglottic Cancer

The supraglottic larynx consists of the epiglottis, false vocal folds, ventricles, aryepiglottic folds, and arytenoids; therefore, hoarseness is not a prominent symptom of cancer of the supraglottic larynx unless the lesion becomes quite large. Pain while swallowing, which is most often described as mild and persistent, is the most frequent initial symptom. Often with lesions of the supraglottic larynx, patients complain of a sensation of a "lump in the throat," otherwise known as a globus sensation. Referred pain to the ear by way of Arnold's nerve, a branch of the vagus nerve, may occur with lesions of the epiglottis. Although an asymptomatic neck mass may be the first sign of a supraglottic cancer, late symptoms include weight loss and dysphagia.

Glottic Cancer

Hoarseness is typically the initial symptom of carcinoma of the true vocal folds. Airway obstruction can occur resulting in inspiratory and expiratory stridor. Pain and coughing may also occur (Casper & Colton, 1993).

Tumors of the true vocal folds can range in size and often take on an irregular shape. Ninety-five percent of the tumors are localized to the mid-membranous portion of the true vocal fold and are whitish in color (Aronson, 1990).

Subglottic Cancer

Hoarseness is the most common symptom followed by airway obstruction with larger lesions. Frequently the patient is asymptomatic with early lesions.

MEDICAL CONSIDERATIONS

Fiberoptic examination of the larynx should be used routinely to complement mirror examination of the larynx. Lesions of the epiglottis should be designated as suprahyoid or infrahyoid epiglottic lesions. A lesion of the true vocal folds should be described in terms of the extent of the lesion, that is, whether the opposite vocal fold and/or the arytenoids are involved. Finally, the mobility of the true vocal folds should be addressed. This should be performed prior to doing direct laryngoscopy and biopsy.

The work-up of lesions of the larynx should include indirect laryngoscopy, CT scanning with contrast, MRI in selected cases, chest x-ray, and direct laryngoscopy with biopsy. All imaging should be performed prior to direct laryngoscopy and biopsy.

The American Joint Committee on Cancer (AJCC) developed a classification system which stages cancer of the larynx based on the tumor, node, and metastasis (TNM) (see Table 13–1) (McKenna et al., 1991).

THE VOICE EXAMINATION

The voice examination is part of the comprehensive medical care provided to a pa-

tient who presents symptoms of laryngeal cancer. Clinical protocols are often developed by an interdisciplinary team to act as a guideline for what type of procedures will be completed during the diagnostic work-up. The diagnostic process usually begins with the patient's completing a written case-history questionnaire or answering questions directly to a physician, physician assistant, nurse, or speech-language pathologist. Information gained from a case history provides the medical team with an array of factors that may be related to the symptoms of the patient's presenting disorder. The case history typically includes questions that are related to psychological and physiological factors of the disorder. During the case history, the examiner gains specific information about the disorder, such as the onset of the disorder, description of the symptoms, related illnesses, previous treatments, social and occupation considerations, and overall functionality of the patient in daily living (Case, 1991).

During the voice examination the phonatory characteristics of the disorder are often recorded. An audio recording allows the team member to evaluate certain parameters of the patient's phonation, either perceptually or objectively. Perceptual examination of patients who present symptoms of laryngeal cancer might include rating the degree of hoarseness and the pitch and loudness level of the voice. Because perceptual rating scales can be unreliable, particularly with inexperienced clinicians (Baken, 1987), a combination of objective indices and perceptual judgments are advocated in the clinical evaluation of voice.

Objective measures can be extracted from many types of instrumentation. They are beneficial in the assessment of voice because they provide a means for numerically documenting the status of the voice prior to intervention. Gould (1988) reviewed the types of instrumentation that

Table 13–1. American Joint Commission on Cancer Staging of Laryngeal Lesions.

I. Tumor
    A. Supraglottis
        T1   Tumor limited to one subsite of supraglottis with normal vocal fold mobility.
        T2   Tumor invades more than one subsite of supraglottis or glottis with normal vocal fold mobility.
        T3   Tumor limited to larynx with vocal fold fixation and/or invades postcricoid area, medial wall of piriform sinus or pre-epiglottic spaces.
        T4   Tumor invades through thyroid cartilage, and/or extends to other tissues beyond the larynx (e.g., to the oropharynx, soft tissues of the neck).
    B. Glottis
        T1   Tumor limited to vocal folds (may involve anterior or posterior commissure with normal mobility).
        T1a Tumor limited to one vocal fold.
        T1b Tumor involves both vocal folds.
        T2   Tumor extends to supraglottis and/or subglottis with impaired vocal fold mobility.
        T3   Tumor limited to the larynx with vocal fold fixation.
        T4   Tumor invades through thyroid cartilage and/or extends to other tissues beyond the larynx (e.g., oropharynx, soft tissues of neck).
    C. Subglottis
        T1   Tumor limited to the subglottis.
        T2   Tumor extends to vocal folds with normal or impaired mobility.
        T3   Tumor limited to larynx with vocal fold fixation.
        T4   Tumor invades through cricoid or thyroid cartilage and/or extends to other tissues beyond the larynx (e.g., oropharynx, soft tissues of neck).

II. Cervical Lymph Node Classification
    N0   No clinically positive nodes
    N1   Single clinically positive ipsilateral node less than 3 cm in diameter.
    N2a Single clinically positive ipsilateral node, 3–6 cm in diameter.
    N2b Multiple clinically positive ipsilateral nodes, none over 6 cm in diameter.
    N3   Massive ipsilateral node(s), bilateral nodes, or contralateral node(s)
    N3a Clinically positive ipsilateral node(s), none over 6 cm in diameter.
    N3b Bilateral clinically positive nodes (in this situation, each side of the neck should be staged separately; that is N3b:right, N3a:left, N1)
    N3c Contralateral clinically positive node(s) only

III. Distant Metastasis
    M0   No (known) distant metastasis
    M1   Distant metastasis present
            Specify sites according to the following notation:
                Pulmonary - PUL
                Osseous - OSS
                Hepatic - HEP
                Brain - BRA
                Bone Marrow - MAR
                Lymph Nodes - LYM
                Pleura - PLE
                Skin - SKI
                Eye - EYE
                Other - OTH

(continued)

Table 13-1. *(continued)*

IV. 5.0 Stage Grouping
    Stage I   T1N0M0
    Stage II   T2N0M0
    Stage III T3N0M0
               T1 or T2 or T3N1M0
    Stage IV   T4N0 or N1M0
               Any T1N2 or N3M0
               Any T1, Any N; M1

Source: From *Manual for Staging of Cancer* (3rd ed.) by American Joint Committee on Cancer, 1988. Philadelphia: J. B. Lippincott. Reprinted with permission.

are often used in the clinical voice laboratory. Generally, these measures can be divided into two categories, acoustic and aerodynamic. Acoustic measures assess the frequency, intensity, and duration of the phonatory segment. Aerodynamic measures quantify the amount of airflow and air pressure during phonation. Other objective measures exist and may be pertinent. However, each measure must be evaluated as to what information it will provide to the team members and how the information will enhance the care of the patient.

Visual examination is a critical part of the voice examination. Typically, if a patient comes to the voice clinic with a complaint of hoarseness and a positive history for other etiological factors of laryngeal cancer such as smoking or alcohol abuse, the team of examiners will initially observe the laryngeal structures using either indirect examination or endoscopic procedures. If a lesion is observed, its size can be documented. Indirect examination procedures and endoscopic procedures (rigid and fiberoptic) were described in detail in Chapter 6. With the transnasal fiberoptic endoscopic techniques (see Chapter 6), the examiner can approach the vocal fold structure fairly closely, which assists in identifying and describing the lesion, although the light source is not as powerful as that used with rigid endoscopy. Finally, as part of the

visual examination, videostroboscopy can be completed which aids in visualizing the vibration of the vocal folds. By using a stroboscopic light source, the motion of the vocal folds is slowed down, allowing the examiner to assess the vibratory characteristics of the vocal folds. See Chapter 6 for more details of this technique.

SOCIAL IMPLICATIONS

Emotional

Depression, anxiety, nervousness, denial, isolationism, irritability, and difficulty adjusting to the physical changes that have been incurred by the patient have all been listed as emotional states that are present in survivors of laryngeal cancer (Blood, Luther, & Stemple, 1992). Thirty percent of the spouses of laryngectomees indicated that the period of postoperative adjustment was more difficult than they had anticipated. The presence of strain and burden, and the resultant stress in spouses of laryngectomized patients has been well-documented by Blood, Simpson, Dineen, Kauffman, and Raimondi (1994). Yet, according to Gardner (1961), "success or failure in rehabilitation often depends on the attitude of the spouse toward the laryngectomee's handicap and his/her effort to talk." This points out the need for spousal support groups that are separate from those for the laryngectomee early in the rehabilitation process because this is when the spouse typically experiences the most psychological stress and strain.

It is not uncommon for an individual who has been diagnosed with a catastrophic illness to go through a grief process. A laryngectomized person may mourn the "death" of the "old" self as he moves toward acceptance of the "new self" which is redefined by the illness and recovery process. Consequently, the laryngectomized patient often will become self-focused, even selfish, as he or she passes through the stages of grief. While focusing on his or her own needs, the laryngectomee becomes less able to recognize the anxieties felt by family members, and is frequently unavailable to them as they work through their own set of worries and concerns.

It is important for all team members to recognize that the grieving process is a normal response to a life-altering illness. Likewise, the spouse needs to be assured that grieving is a normal part of accepting the illness and the changes that will occur as a result of it. Even though the patient and his or her family may have some of the same concerns and fears, their desire to protect each other creates a need to provide counseling for the spouse separate from the laryngectomee. However, as the patient and his or her family move into the acceptance stage of the grief process, the feelings related to the cancer and its effects on the family can be more readily shared with each other. Perhaps the self-study that occurs as patients and their families progress through the grief process is what results in the statement by many cancer survivors that he or she is a stronger and better person as a result of the cancer.

Kommers and Sullivan (1979) found that, during the preoperative stage, older wives tended to be less optimistic, expressing concerns about spreading of the cancer and their husband's mortality. Conversely, during this stage, younger wives were more optimistic, often assuming the attitude that the surgery would end the threat of the cancer and that they could proceed as a couple through the rehabilitation, eventually returning to a normal lifestyle. However, during the postoperative period, the levels of optimism reversed, with more of the older wives feeling optimistic (primarily due to relief that the spouse survived the surgery) and the younger wives being less optimistic as they felt the impact of the consequences of the surgery. Many of the younger wives, in retrospect, indicated that the post-operative period immediately following surgery was the time when they were the least optimistic. All of this information again supports the need for separate counseling pre- and postoperatively for the spouses of individuals with laryngeal cancer (Kommers et al., 1977).

Forty-four percent of the wives in Kommers and Sullivan's study indicated that they had decreased communication with their spouses. Furthermore, 68% of the wives reported that their husbands became upset if the wife did not understand their speech. These wives reported that their husbands refused to repeat their utterance, and would become angry, nervous, frustrated, and/or irritated by the lack of intelligibility. In the same study, 31% of the wives indicated that the adjustment to the absence of speech by their spouse was more difficult than they had anticipated.

Psychosocial

To many individuals, the loss of the larynx equates to never being able to communicate normally again. Kommers and Sullivan (1979) found that 58% of 45 wives reported an increase in their husband's irritability and/or nervousness.

Eighteen percent of the husbands had mentioned suicide postoperatively. In the same group, 51% of the wives reported that their own irritability and nervousness also increased during the postoperative period.

Another emotional and psychosocial barrier that a patient who has undergone a total laryngectomy must overcome is the fact that he or she now has some deformities which can have a debilitating effect. The anatomical and physiological changes that occur as part of a total laryngectomy interfere with not only speech, but also vision, hearing, balance, smell, and taste (Mathieson, Stam, & Scott, 1990). Furthermore, many patients express frustration that, even though they understood that they would not be able to use voice to speak postoperatively, it was not made clear that their laughter and crying would also be nonvocal. Additionally, the patient must overcome the fact that he or she must have a permanent stoma. Concern is expressed over the aesthetics of the stoma, as well as the ever-present danger of aspiration of a foreign body into the trachea. However, once a patient has either seen the various methods of covering the stoma, as well as some of the various devices available, such as the one that allow the individual to take showers, these fears and concerns are gradually overcome.

Finally, some patients have complained of loss of libido after laryngectomy. Mathieson, Stam, and Scott (1990) found that "maintaining satisfactory sexual relationships was significant in predicting spouses' quality of life and psychological state." When spouses have been asked to list problems they face due to the laryngectomy, maintenance of sexual relationships is often cited (Blood et al., 1994). In a survey of 45 wives of laryngectomees, 20% reported that the surgery had "robbed their husband of his manhood," and 31% of the husbands complained about what the surgery "had done" to them (Kommers & Sullivan, 1979). This problem appears to resolve with time and proper counseling.

Vocational

Many laryngectomees are able to return to the jobs they held prior to the diagnosis of laryngeal cancer. Seventy-five percent of the individuals who were employed at the time of the diagnosis and surgery were able to return to their previous job at least part-time. Of these 75%, 70% returned to their original job within 3 months postoperatively. One-fourth of the patients returned to work in a different employment setting than the one they had prior to the diagnosis of laryngeal cancer (Kommers & Sullivan, 1979).

In some instances (11%), the wife began to work to support the family and pay the medical bills (Kommers & Sullivan, 1979). Eleven percent of the families borrowed money to pay the medical bills. For 78% of the patients, the family (private) insurance helped to pay anywhere from 10–100% of the costs. Medicare and other public forms of assistance contributed to the payment of medical costs for 38% of the patients in their survey.

For the laryngectomized patient and his or her spouse or caregiver, management does not end with the surgical procedure. Psychosocial issues often need to be addressed effectively by the team members before proceeding with other areas of management.

TREATMENT: OPTIONS AND OUTCOMES

Surgical Management

Vocal Fold Carcinoma

Treatment for vocal fold carcinoma will depend largely on whether the treatment occurs in an early or late stage of the disease. Early disease usually results in some sort of voice-sparing treatment. However, late disease often results in total laryngectomy, although a trial of radiation treatment is an option (Million, Cassisi, & Mancuso, 1994).

For early vocal fold carcinoma, irradiation is the initial form of treatment offered at most centers. Surgery is reserved for radiation therapy failures. Hemilaryngectomy, cordectomy, and laser incision all are viable alternatives for treatment of early vocal fold carcinoma. However, the voice is likely to be better with radiation therapy than with surgical therapy. For early lesions, the cure rates for all of these modalities are comparable.

In comparing the voice after treatment for early vocal fold carcinoma, the voice after successful irradiation is usually better than before therapy. Occasionally, there may be no improvement in the voice after radiation therapy, and even less commonly, the quality of the voice may worsen. After hemilaryngectomy, the quality of the voice remains hoarse, or it may worsen with loss of vocal loudness and breathiness often occurring.

Moderately advanced vocal fold cancers usually include lesions that demonstrate vocal fold fixation. These lesions can be further classified into favorable and unfavorable lesions, with the latter usually having extensive bilateral disease with a compromised airway. Favorable T3 lesions are mainly confined to one side of the larynx; the patient has a good airway and the larynx is easy to examine. Classically, the majority of patients with a T3 lesion were treated by total laryngectomy; however, patients deemed as having favorable lesions now are offered the option of radiation therapy and surgical salvage if the radiation therapy fails. The alternative is to offer total laryngectomy as the initial form of treatment. Most patients initially choose the option of radiation therapy with surgical salvage over total laryngectomy. The patient is advised that there may be a 5–10% reduction in the 5-year survival rate compared to immediate laryngectomy. They are also advised that the complication rate may increase slightly if surgical salvage is required. The patients are also advised that they must return for close follow-up. Using this philosophic approach for these moderately advanced vocal fold cancers, the local control rate with voice preservation is 50–70%. Of the ones that fail, 50–70% are cured with surgical salvage. The major problem with this approach is that, with more advanced lesions, it is sometimes difficult to distinguish between radiation edema and local recurrence. Often the recurrence is submucosal, and deep biopsies may be required to diagnose the recurrence.

Advanced vocal fold carcinoma is most often treated with a total laryngectomy and neck dissection. Postoperative radiation therapy is often added. The base of the tongue, cervical lymph nodes, and tracheal stoma are the most common sites of failure.

Supraglottic Laryngeal Carcinoma

Early lesions can readily be treated with either external beam irradiation or subtotal supraglottic laryngectomy. Supraglottic laryngectomy is the treatment of choice if the lesion is bulky and infiltrative and if the patient has good pulmonary reserve. Radiation therapy is often the treatment of choice for these early lesions either because of medical reasons (e.g., poor pulmonary reserve, systemic disease, etc.) or because the patient refuses surgery early. Supraglottic lesions that would require a total laryngectomy are generally given radiation and surgery is reserved for salvage. Generally, it is preferable to use only one modality of treatment for early lesions;

therefore, some type of neck dissection on the most involved side of the lesion is typically done. If there are close margins or multiple nodal metastasis, postoperative radiation therapy is added. If the patient has a small supraglottic primary tumor and advanced neck disease, radiation therapy to the primary tumor and the neck followed by a neck dissection for residual disease is frequently recommended. The voice is usually good with either radiation therapy or supraglottic laryngectomy. Advanced supraglottic lesions are treated with combined therapy. If the cervical lymph nodes are resectable, postoperative radiation therapy is used. If nonresectable, preoperative irradiation is used followed by laryngectomy and neck dissection.

SPEECH PATHOLOGY

Alternative Modes of Communication

Following total laryngectomy, the typical mode of speech cannot be used. The pulmonary air has been diverted to the stoma and the vibratory source or vocal folds have been removed (see Figure 13–1). An alternative source of phonation must be provided for the patient to be able to effectively communicate. Two general methods of communication have been used by laryngectomized persons. The first method is referred to as an external method, such as artificial speech aids (electronic and pneumatic). The second method is referred to as an internal method, which includes esophageal speech or surgical-prosthetic devices (Christensen & Dwyer, 1990). Each method of communication has advantages and disadvantages which need to be realized by the surgeon treating the patient, the speech-language pathologist involved in rehabilitating the patient, and the laryngectomized patient.

The External Methods: Pneumatic Devices

A comparison of alaryngeal speech methods reveals that, although external methods can be the easiest to use and learn, the sound quality is the poorest. Two main mechanical devices used to produce alaryngeal phonation include the pneumatic device and electronic device. The pneumatic device relies on the expiratory air from the lungs. The expiratory air drives an artificial vibrating source within the device that is fitted over the stoma by the patient. Tubing leads from the stoma source to the patient's mouth, where the airflow is shaped into specific speech sounds (see Figure 13–2). The advantage of the pneumatic device is that it is very easy to learn how to use. Intelligible speech can be produced very soon after the laryngectomy (Casper & Colton, 1993), which is certainly a benefit to the patient and the caregivers. The main disadvantage of the pneumatic device is that the patient must ensure an adequate seal is made between the pneumatic unit and the stoma to provide enough pulmonary airflow to the mouth. Finally, manipulating a pneumatic device is an obvious disability to the user as one hand is needed to hold the device to the stoma. Specific types of pneumatic devices include the Dutch Speech DSP8 speech aid and the Tokyo Speech Aid.

The External Methods: Electrolaryngeal Devices

Speech produced by electronic devices employs electric power (battery) to provide an artificial sound source. Three main types of electronic devices are available: the neck type, intraoral type, and dental appliance-type. All of these techniques are easy to learn and provide a fairly immediate way in which to communicate with caregivers following laryngectomy.

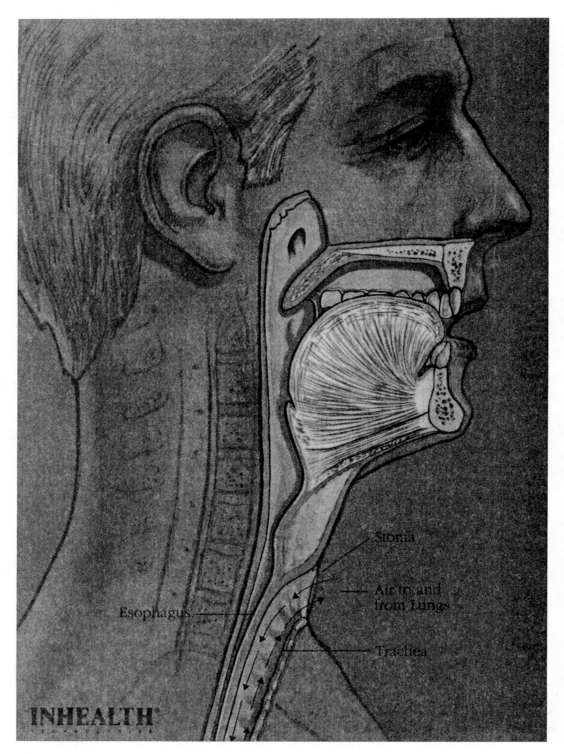

Stoma

Air to and
from Lungs

Esophagus

Trachea

INHEALTH

FIGURE 13-1. Depiction of neck anatomy following total laryngectomy. (Reprinted with permission of Inhealth Technologies. Inc.. 1995.)

288

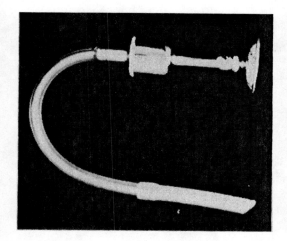

FIGURE 13–2. Picture of pneumatic device, the Tokyo Speech Aid. (Reprinted with permission of Clyde Welch.)

There are a variety of neck type electronic devices, which vary in their ability to produce a quality sound. Figure 13–3 shows one such model. Casper and Colton (1993) provide an excellent review of the specific types of electronic neck speech aids providing a description of the device, its price, and manufacturer of the device. Additionally, Casper and Colton provide an overview of the pros and cons of each of the particular devices. The main disadvantage of neck-type devices is the quality of the sound they produce. Recall that electrolaryngeal devices are mechanical devices and therefore produce a mechanical sound that is monotone in quality. Pitch variations are minimal. Furthermore, the sound transmission to the oral cavity can be poor in certain circumstances (e.g., poor placement, scarring), resulting in unintelligible speech.

Internal Methods: The Esophageal Speech Method

Esophageal speech is another alternative method for producing speech. The support for esophageal speech comes from moving air into the upper esophagus. The source of vibration is the PE segment. The PE segment is located approximately between cervical vertebrae C3–C6 during esophageal speech (Isman & Obrien, 1992). The segment is formed by the inferior pharyngeal constrictor muscle and the cricopharyngeous muscles (lower portion of the inferior constrictor muscle), and the segment is narrowed or constricted during vocalization. With narrowing, air can be driven out of the esophagus under pressure to produce a vibratory air source.

Esophageal speech is considered a more natural way to produce speech because the patient is generally able to control the air that is used in the vibration of the voice source and is unrestricted during communication. No device needs to be held or inserted into the mouth to produce vocalization. Another advantage of esophageal speech, which is appealing for many laryngectomees, is that no additional surgeries are needed to produce vocalization (McKenna, et al., 1991). However, not all laryngectomees can successfully use or learn esophageal speech. Lack of success with esophageal speech may be due to physiological reasons, such as poor vibratory characteristics of the PE segment, or poor motivational and compliance factors. Another disadvantage of the esophageal speech technique is that the physiological drive or esophageal air capacity is very small compared to the total lung capacity. As a result, the duration of speech is limited. Air must be replenished often or a disruption to ongoing speech will result (McKenna et al., 1991). For those who can be successful with esophageal speech there are a number of techniques that can be used to inject or pump the air into the esophagus. Some will be briefly described here.

The two main techniques for providing an air source to vibrate the esophageal segment are the injection and inhalation techniques. The injection technique relies on being able to inject air from the mouth

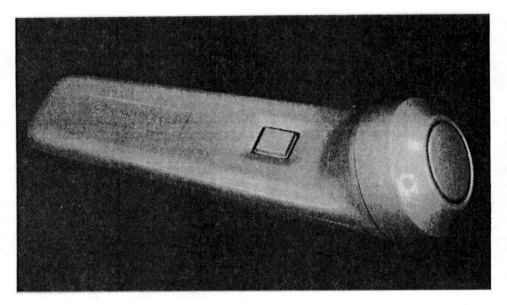

FIGURE 13-3. Photo of an electrolaryngeal device.

into the esophagus through the coordinated movements of the tongue and the pharynx. As illustrated in Figure 13–4, the glossal press is the first phase of the injection technique whereby air is trapped behind the tongue and moved backward into the oral cavity. The second phase includes tongue movement farther back toward the pharyngeal wall to drive the air down into the esophagus.

The second technique is referred to as the inhalation method. With this method, air is inhaled into the lungs. If the PE segment can be relaxed, the air pressure within the esophagus will become substantially lower than atmospheric pressure, creating a force that pulls the air from the mouth and pharynx into the esophagus. The higher atmospheric pressure in the mouth and pharynx (+ pressure) compared to the lower esophageal pressure (− pressure) will override the PE segment's sphincteric action allowing the esophagus to insufflate.

Finally, a third technique called the swallow method is mentioned only because it is probably the least efficient method for teaching esophageal speech (Casper & Colton, 1993; Prater, 1984). With this technique the patient is taught to swallow air into the esophagus. By having the patient swallow, it is assumed that the esophagus will open and there will be enough air for vibrating the PE segment and creating vocalization. However, there are many disadvantages with this technique. The main disadvantage is that the amount of time it takes to swallow and produce voice is long compared to the time it takes the two above-mentioned techniques to produce vocalization. Other disadvantages can include extraneous noise following effortful injection of air via the swallow. This noise interferes with the intelligibility of speech and more importantly draws attention to the esophageal speaker.

Tracheoesophageal Fistulization/Puncture

Tracheoesophageal fistulization (TEF) or tracheoesophageal puncture (TEP) currently is the most developed style of ala-

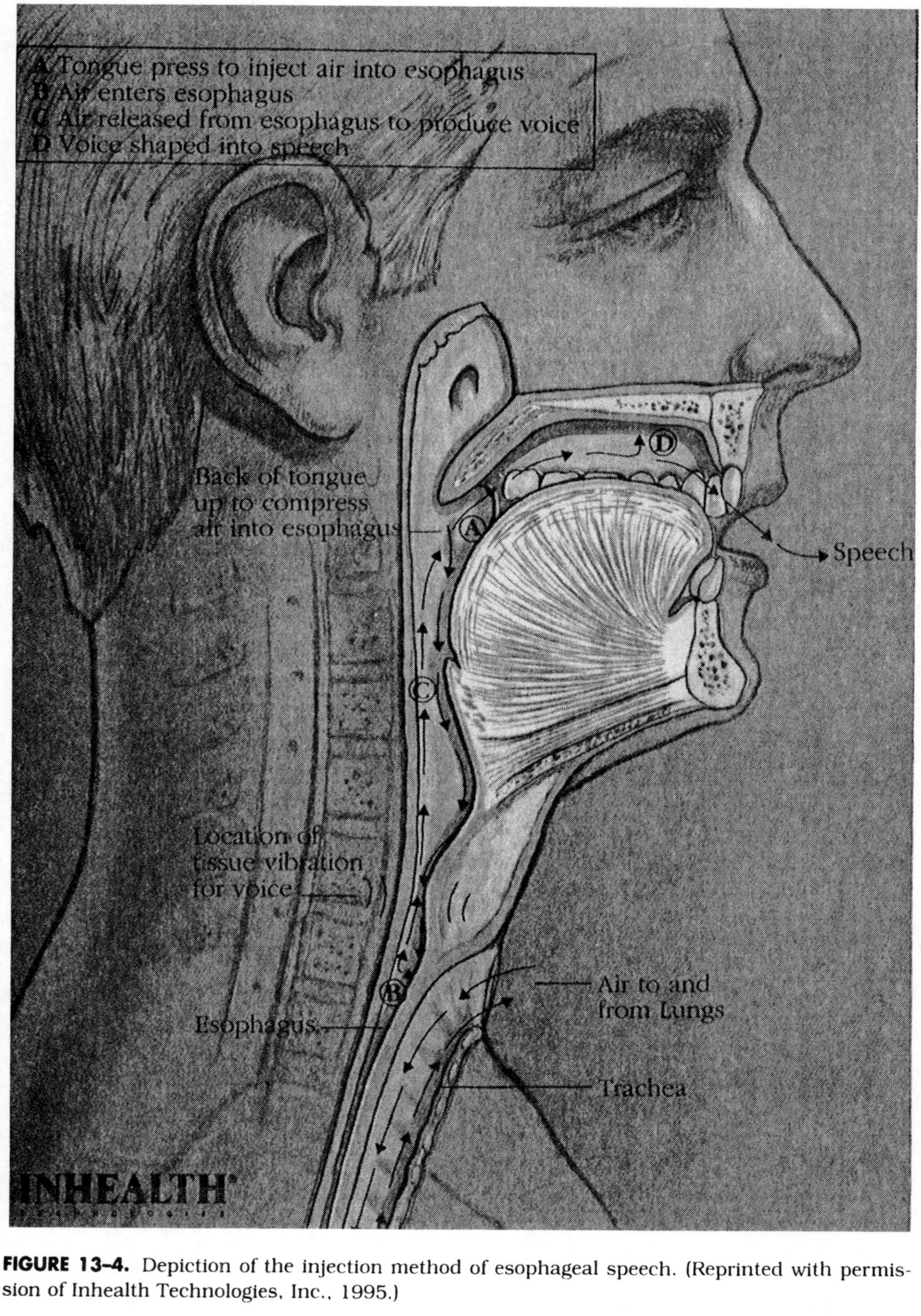
A Tongue press to inject air into esophagus
B Air enters esophagus
C Air released from esophagus to produce voice
D Voice shaped into speech
Back of tongue up to compress air into esophagus
Speech
Location of tissue vibration for voice
Air to and from Lungs
Esophagus
Trachea
INHEALTH

FIGURE 13–4. Depiction of the injection method of esophageal speech. (Reprinted with permission of Inhealth Technologies, Inc., 1995.)

ryngeal speech. Completed through a surgical procedure, it allows air to be directed or shunted from the trachea into the esophagus via a prosthesis (see Figure 13–5). This procedure can be performed at the time of the laryngectomy procedure, referred to as a primary TEP, or later with laryngectomized patients who did not have a puncture at the time of their resection, referred to as a secondary TEP (Garth, McRae, & Rhys-Evans, 1991).

The prosthesis is typically made of silicone and is placed into the surgical opening or fistula of the trachea, providing a pathway for the pulmonary air to be directed into the esophagus (see Figure 13–5). The airflow travels through the PE segment in the same manner as was described for the esophageal speech, and is then modified by the resonating cavities of the upper vocal tract to produce speech sounds.

The voice production associated with tracheoesophageal speech has been previously examined and found to be advantageous over mechanical devices and esophageal speech for a number of reasons (Casper & Colton, 1993). First, because a greater amount of air capacity is available for voice production, the duration of speech can be longer (Baugh, Lewin, & Baker, 1990). Second, loudness and pitch can be varied to a greater extent, and finally, the fluent quality of TEP speech more closely resembles speech associated with laryngeal voice production. For these reasons TEP is considered by some to be advantageous over esophageal speech.

Quer, Burues-Vila, and Garcia-Crespillo, (1992) reported on the cost-efficiency profile of tracheoesophogeal puncture in 23 patients who had received a primary tracheoesophageal procedure. Their findings revealed that 70% (16/23) left

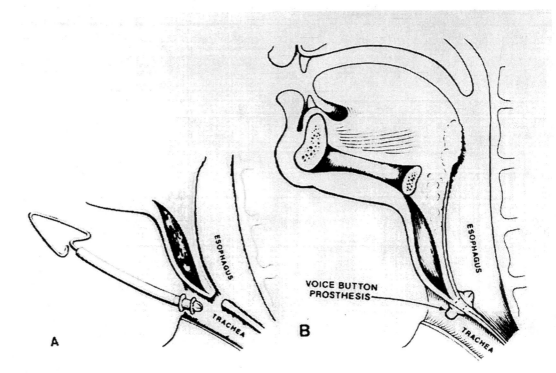

FIGURE 13–5. Schematic of TEP.

the prosthetic voice to use esophageal speech, even though the patients reported the prosthetic voice quality to be superior to the esophageal voice quality.

For those who continue to use tracheo-esophageal speech as the method of voice restoration, the success rate is quite high for most laryngectomees (Baugh et al., 1990). Laryngectomee patients who are good candidates for a TEP are those who are motivated toward their recovery, able to understand how the prosthesis works, and able to insert and clean the prosthesis (Miller, 1990). For TEP speech to be successful, the patient must also be free of postoperative complications such as hypertonicity of the PE segment.

TEP speech is functional only if the PE segment is able to vibrate. If hypertonicity of the PE segment is present, a selective myotomy of the inferior pharyngeal constrictor muscle can be surgically performed to allow the PE segment to be operative for effective sound production (McKenna et al., 1991). Other techniques for relieving hypertonicity of the PE segment are also available (Garth et al.,

1991). Although other pre- or postoperative complications contraindicate success with a TEP (Casper & Colton, 1993; Garth et al., 1991), the most predominant complication for successful TEP use is hypertonicity or scarring of the PE segment.

Adjustable tracheostoma valves are available which allow the prosthesis to shunt the tracheal air to the esophagus without having to occlude the stoma with a finger or thumb (see Figure 13–6). These too have advantages and disadvantages for the laryngectomized patient who chooses to use tracheoesophageal speech. The valve allows the air to be shunted automatically to the esophagus (see Figure 13–7). The tracheoesophageal speaker does not have to occlude the stoma manually, freeing the hands for communicative purpose.

The valve does, however, have to be appropriately fitted to the patient to adjust to the varying degrees of pressure demands during speech and nonspeech tasks. A diaphragm in the valve is sensitive to changes in expiratory air pressure

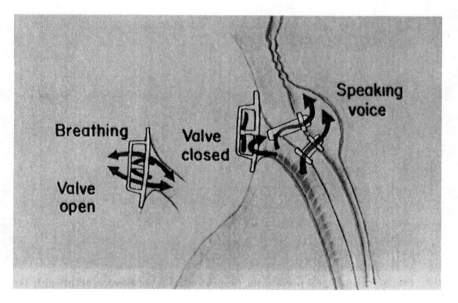

FIGURE 13–6. Schematic of tracheo-esophageal valve.

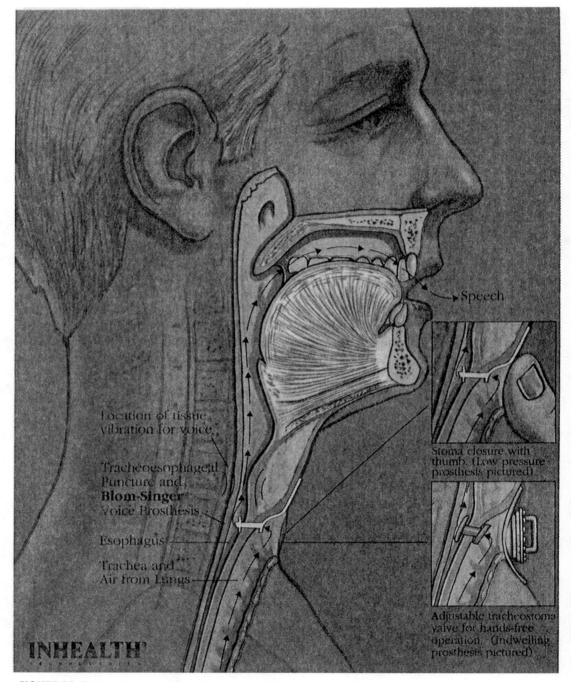

Speech

Location of tissue
vibration for voice.

Tracheoesophageal
Puncture and
Blom-Singer
Voice Prosthesis

Esophagus

Trachea and
Air from Lungs

Stoma closure with
thumb. (Low pressure
prosthesis pictured)

Adjustable tracheostoma
valve for hands-free
operation. (Indwelling
prosthesis pictured)

INHEALTH

FIGURE 13–7. Tracheo-esophageal prosthesis. (Reprinted with permission of Inhealth Technologies, Inc., 1995.)

(McKenna et al., 1991) and must be fitted to respond appropriately to ongoing pressure modifications.

Currently, an indwelling, low pressure voice prosthesis designed by Blom (1995) is available to the laryngectomized person. The indwelling prosthesis is left in place for a longer period of time, approximately 6 months or on an as needed basis. The indwelling prosthesis is replaced by either the physician or clinician. Therefore the routine maintenance is less. This device is ideal for laryngectomized persons who are uncomfortable or unable to change the nondwelling voice prosthesis.

Counseling

Preoperative Counseling

When informing a patient that he or she has cancer, the health-care professional needs to be aware of the impact of the diagnosis on the patient and his or her family and should spend time exploring the social support system available to the patient and his or her family. Blood, Simpson, Raimondi, Kauffman, and Stagaard (1994) found that patients who had intact social support systems were, overall, better adjusted and more equipped to make the necessary adjustments than those without adequate support from their spouses, other family members, and friends. Also, patients who were assertive and communicatively expressive prior to surgery, those who were active, and those who were "information seekers" typically had a more positive rehabilitation outcome (Blood et al., 1992).

In preoperative counseling, the emphasis is on educating the patient and his or her caregiver(s) with regard to the impending surgery, the outcome of the surgery, and alternative methods of communication available to the patient. Adler (1969) listed five goals of preoperative counseling for the patient with laryngeal cancer. The first goal is to explain the operation (laryngectomy) and, secondly, to discuss the postoperative feelings that have been expressed by other patients who have undergone the same operation. It is also critical to prepare the patient for the fact that he or she will lose the ability to use his or her voice to communicate. To accomplish this third goal, Adler relies on a fourth goal of explaining the normal production of speech in terms that can be understood by the patient and his or her family. By explaining the normal process of speech and relating this discussion back to the events that will take place in the surgery, the team member can assist the patient in understanding the impact of the surgery. Finally, Adler stresses the need to reassure the patient that there are several alternative means of communication which can be explored together as a team following the surgery.

The team member designated to provide the preoperative counseling will vary from one setting to the next. However, caution should always be taken to check with the physician to determine exactly what the patient has been told about the impending surgery (Reed, 1988). It may be necessary to review the diagnosis and etiological factors with the patient as well as the actual surgery. The patient may have questions about treatment options and want to review the consequences of all approaches that are available (Kommers et al., 1977). Some treatment teams recommend a visit by a patient who has had a laryngectomy who could more fully explain to the patient the actual impact of the illness and recovery process. The decision to have a recovered patient meet with the patient who is still facing surgery is really a decision to be made by the patient. Many patients would like to meet others who have gone through similar experiences, but the timing of the visit is variable with some patients wanting it to be part of their preoperative education, and others wanting to have the visit following the surgery (Kommers et al., 1977).

It seems a bit ironic that patients with laryngeal cancer, which has one of the best survival rates, would be the patients who require the most counseling. Blood, Luther, and Stemple (1992) point out that, because laryngeal cancer is a very curable cancer, it is critical for the healthcare team to understand the need to assist the patient in achieving his or her desired quality of life. Due to the presence of the stoma and the obvious effect of illness and surgery on speech, laryngeal cancer is a very visible cancer. Psychosocial factors that have been cited by patients and their families are listed in Table 13–2.

Rait and Lederberg (1989) stress that the family and patient who face the diagnosis of cancer typically experience three phases of stress and adaptation. In phase one, the "acute phase," the patient and

Table 13–2. Psychosocial factors related to diagnosis and treatment of laryngeal cancer.

Fear of recurrence of the cancer
Social and emotional isolation
Adjustment to physical changes
Relationship with therapy teams
Critical review of one's priorities
Ability to maintain employment
Insurance concerns
Depression
Anxiety
Nervousness
Denial

Source: Adopted from Coping with Adjustment in Alaryngeal Speakers by G. W. Blood, A. R. Luther, and J. C. Stemple, 1992. *American Journal of Speech Language Pathology, 1*(2), 63–69.

his family are usually shocked and stunned by the diagnosis, and are frightened about the impact of the diagnosis on their family unit. During this phase, they spend a great deal of time trying to figure out how they will cope with the crisis. The "chronic phase" typically begins when the patient comes home from the hospital, and the caregiver(s) assume new responsibilities. These responsibilities relate not only to direct patient care, but also to the assumption of daily chores and responsibilities that previously were shouldered by the patient. During this second phase, the caregiver(s) still tends to function on a day-to-day basis without taking the time to develop and implement long-term solutions to the new set of circumstances they are facing. It is not unusual for feelings of helplessness, anger, and resentment to develop during this phase.

Finally, during the resolution phase, the family unit begins to realize that (a) the immediate threat and concerns about death have resolved and they can now get on with the business of "survivorship" or (b) the patient declines and the family becomes entrenched in the bereavement process.

It is helpful to explain to the patient and his or her family that it is normal for families to go through a myriad of feelings as they approach the beginning of the rehabilitation process. In spite of our own academic recognition and knowledge of the need for preoperative counseling, many studies report that families of laryngectomees, and particularly the spouses, believe that, even when preoperative counseling was provided, either with the patient or separately, it was inadequate (Blood, et al., 1994; Kommers et al., 1977; Kommers & Sullivan, 1979; Mathieson, Stam, & Scott, 1991). A 1983 study conducted in Norway found that approximately 60% of 189 spouses of patients with laryngeal cancer believed that many of the problems faced by their ill family member could have been reduced with better pre-

and postoperative counseling (Natvig, 1983). Similarly, when Salmon (1979) questioned 53 spouses in 15 different states, only 13% of the spouses considered themselves to be well prepared for the surgery and would have liked to have some form of preoperative counseling (Blood et al., 1994). Kommers, Sullivan, and Yonkers (1977) interviewed 45 wives of laryngectomees in Nebraska, Iowa, and Kansas. Over 66% of these spouses reported that their greatest fear during the preoperative period was that the cancer had spread or that their husband would not survive the surgery. Other major concerns expressed by the wives included concern about their husband's ability to cope, uncertainty about the family's future, and fears related to their husband's never speaking again.

In a follow-up study in 1979, Kommers and Sullivan sent questionnaires to 101 wives of laryngeal cancer survivors. Although only 45 questionnaires were returned, the need for more preoperative counseling was strongly expressed. Kommers and Sullivan reported on problems related to laryngectomy in a variety of categories including health and physical care problems, preparation for and reactions to surgery, communication skills, financial situations, and psychosocial factors. Eighty-seven percent of wives of laryngectomees surveyed indicated that the physician was the primary source of information regarding the operation and its consequences. Seventy-eight percent of the wives were with their husbands at the time of diagnosis, but only 31% got preoperative counseling separately from their husbands. However, 62% of the wives did report that they felt fairly well prepared for the surgery. Forty percent of the wives expressed opinions about the content of preoperative counseling and suggested that it should include videotapes of the postsurgical period, more information about the surgery and its consequences,

and a visit from the wife of a husband recovering from laryngeal cancer.

During the preoperative period, the caregiver(s) of laryngeal cancer patients need support in a variety of areas from all members of the health-care team. Care needs to be taken to ensure that they understand the illness, the surgery, and the postoperative experience. They should be introduced to the members of the rehabilitation team who can help to guide them in setting some goals with regard to rehabilitation and maintaining social con-tacts with friends and other family members who are not immediately present (Kommers et al., 1977). Furthermore, because the concerns of the patient may be very different from the concerns of the spouse, it is imperative that counseling be made available to each of them individually as well as together.

Postoperative Counseling

Pre- and postoperative counseling needs vary depending on the age and health status of the patient and spouse prior to the laryngeal cancer. Because elderly caregivers may have health problems of their own, it is especially critical to pay special attention to elderly caregivers (Blood et al., 1994).

The first 6 months of rehabilitation are the months in which caregivers and patients report the most strain and burden with resultant high stress levels. Following the first 6 postoperative months, there is typically a reduction in fear of impending death, and the patient and caregiver typically have worked out a communication system that enables more effective sharing of information. As a result, the level of strain tends to plateau around 6 months postoperatively. Likewise, the sense of extra burden shows evidence of reaching a plateau around 12 months.

Initially, postoperative counseling will focus on reiteration of the preoperative information, particularly with regard to the actual operation and the options available to the patient for alaryngeal speech. Because many patients and caregivers are emotionally labile at the time of diagnosis and presurgical counseling, many will not fully comprehend and remember information provided during the preoperative discussions. Repeating the information from the preoperative counseling session gives the health-care professional a chance to clear up any misunderstandings about the operation and subsequent therapy choices. It also provides the astute clinician clues as to how the patient and caregivers are adapting to the changes that have occurred as a result of the total laryngectomy.

Anxiety, depression, and decreased vigor are documented sequelae of head and neck cancer (Mathieson, Stam, & Scott, 1991). The astute clinician can recognize the development of these detrimental states of mind and address them accordingly. Folkman and Lazarus (Blood et al., 1992) state that there are two ways to deal with stress. The first way is to use a "problem-focused approach" in which the patient and/or caregivers are taught that they can manipulate the external environment. This approach has a more positive effect on postoperative adjustment than does the "emotion-focused approach." In the second approach, the patient views the illness (stressor) as restricting his or her options and requiring changes in the patient's internal affect. Therefore, it is critical that postoperative counseling include coping strategies, discussion of the value of therapy, and establishing realistic goals.

Prognosis

Early Vocal Fold Cancer: T1–T2 and Selected T3 Lesions

Using the philosophy of treating these cancers with radiation therapy for cure and surgical salvage, the ultimate local control site for T1a lesions was 98%, and 93% for T1b lesions. For T2a, the ultimate local control was 97% and for T2b was 88% (Mendenhall, Parsons, Stringer, Cassisi, & Million, 1988). For selected T3 lesions using the same philosophy, the local control after salvage surgery was 73% (Parsons, Mendenhall, Mancuso, Cassisi, Stringer, & Million, 1989). It must be remembered that all of these patients would have received a total laryngectomy.

Supraglottic Laryngeal Cancer

As stated earlier, the results of treatment using either radiation therapy or surgery for early supraglottic cancer are comparable. Bocca, Pignatoro, and Oldini (1983) reported a 5-year survival rate of 80% for T1–T2 supraglottic lesions managed by supraglottic laryngectomy. For T1–T2 supraglottic lesions treated with radiation therapy the local control was 100% for T1 and 81% for T2 lesions, again comparing favorably with the results from supraglottic laryngectomy (Mendenhall et al., 1990).

SUMMARY

Clearly, many advances have been made in the diagnosis and treatment of laryngeal cancers. This has resulted not only in earlier detection, but in a variety of treatment options being available to the patient. In the not-so-distant past, the patient who was diagnosed with laryngeal cancer typically was treated by a total or hemilaryngectomy followed by training in either esophageal speech or the electrolarynx. Many of these advances are the result of interdisciplinary research and clinical interaction, which, again, demonstrates the wisdom of G. Paul Moore in teaching the critical nature of interdisciplinary cooperation.

REFERENCES

Adler, S. (1969). Speech after laryngectomy. *American Journal of Nursing, 69,* 2138–2141.

American Joint Committee on Cancer. (1988). *Manual for staging of cancer* (3rd ed.). Philadelphia: J. B. Lippincott.

Aronson, A. E. (1990). *Clinical voice disorders* (3rd ed.) . New York: Thieme.

Baken, R. J. (1987). *Clinical measurement of speech and voice.* Boston-Toronto-San Diego: College-Hill Press.

Baugh, R. F., Lewin, J. S., & Baker, S. R. (1990). Vocal rehabilitation of tracheoesophogeal speech failures. *Head & Neck, 12,* 69–73.

Blom, E. D. (1995). Tracheoesophageal speech. *Seminars in Speech And Language, 16*(3), 191–204.

Blood, G. W., Luther, A. R., & Stemple, J. C. (1992). Coping and adjustment in alaryngeal speakers. *American Journal of Speech Language Pathology, 1*(2), 63–69.

Blood, G. W., Simpson, K. C., Dineen, M., Kauffman, S. M., & Raimondi, S. C. (1994). Spouses of individuals with laryngeal cancer: Caregiver strain and burden. *Journal of Communication Disorders, 27,* 19–35.

Bocca, E., Pignatoro, O., & Oldini, C. (1983). Supraglottic laryngectomy: 30 years experience. *Annals of Otology, Rhinology, and Laryngology, 92,* 14–18.

Boring, C. C., Squires, T. S., & Tong, T. (1993). Cancer statistics 1993. *Cancer, 43*(1), 7–26.

Case, J. L. (1991). *Clinical management of voice disorders* (2nd ed.). Austin, TX: Pro-Ed.

Casper, J. K., & Colton, R. H. (1993). *Clinical manual for laryngectomy and head and neck cancer rehabilitation.* San Diego, CA: Singular Publishing Group.

Christensen, J. M., & Dwyer, P. E. (1990). Improving alaryngeal speech intelligibility. *Journal of Communicative Disorders, 23,* 445–451.

Devesa, S. S., & Silverman, D. T. (1978). Cancer incidence and mortality trends in the United States: 1935–1974. *JKNCI, 60,* 545–571.

Gardner, W. (1961). Problems of laryngectomees. *Rehabilitation Record, 2,* 15–19.

Garth, R. J. N., McRae, A., & Rhys-Evans, P. H. (1991). Tracheooesophageal puncture: A review of problems and complications. *The Journal of Laryngology and Otology, 105,* 75–754.

Gould, W. J. (1988). The clinical voice laboratory: Clinical application of voice research. *Journal of Voice, 1,* 305–309.

Hammond, E. C., Garfinkel, L., Seidman, H., & Lew, E. A. (1976). "Tar" and nicotine content of cigarette smoke in relation to death rates. *Environmental Research, 12,* 263–270.

Isman, K. A. & O'Brien, C. J. (1992). Videofluoroscopy of the pharyngoesophageal segment during tracheoesophageal and esophageal speech. *Head & Neck, 14*(5), 352–358.

Kommers, M. S., Sullivan, M. D., & Yonkers, A. J. (1977). Counseling the laryngectomized patient. *The Laryngoscope, 87,* 1961–1965.

Kommers, M. S., & Sullivan, M. D. (1979). Wives' evaluation of problems related to laryngectomy. *Journal of Communication Disorders, 12,* 411–430.

Mathieson, C. M., Stam, J. J., & Scott, J. P. (1990). Psychosocial adjustment after laryngectomy: A review of the literature. *The Journal of Otolaryngology, 19*(5), 331–336.

Mathieson, C. M., Stam, J. J., & Scott, J.P. (1991). The impact of a laryngectomy on the spouse: Who is better off? *Psychology and Health, 5,* 153–163.

McKenna, J. P., Fornataro-Clerici, L. M., McMenamin, P. G., & Leonard, R. J. (1991). Laryngeal cancer: diagnosis, treatment and speech rehabilitation. *American Family Physician, 44*(1), 123–129.

Mendenhall, W. M., Parsons, J. T., Stringer, S. P. , Cassisi, N. J., & Million, R. R. (1988). T_1–T_2 vocal cord carcinoma: A basis for comparing the results of radiotherapy and surgery. *Head and Neck Surgery, 10*(6), 373–377.

Mendenhall, W. M., Parsons, J. T., Stringer, S. P. , Cassisi, N. J., & Million, R. R. (1990). Carcinoma of the supraglottic larynx, a basis for comparing the results of radiotherapy and surgery. *Head and Neck Surgery, 12,* 204–209.

Miller, S. (1990). The role of the speech-language pathologist in voice restoration after total laryngectomy. *CA—A Cancer Journal for Clinicians, 40,* 174–182.

Million, R. R., Cassisi, N. J., & Mancuso, A. A. (1994). Larynx. In R. R. Million & N. J. Cassisi (Eds.), *Management of head and neck cancer: A multidisciplinary approach* (2nd ed., Chapter 18, pp. 431–497). Philadelphia, PA: J. B. Lippincott.

Natvig, K. (1983). Laryngectomees in Norway. Study no. 2: Pre-operative counseling and post-operative training evaluated by patients and their spouses. *Journal of Otolaryngology, 12,* 249–254.

Parsons, J. T., Mendenhall, W. M., Mancuso, A. A., Cassisi, N. J., Stringer, S. P., & Million, R. R. (1989). Twice-a-day radiotherapy for T3 squamous cell carcinoma of the glottic larynx. *Head and Neck, 11*(2), 123–128.

Prater, R. J. (1984). *Manual of voice therapy.* Boston, MA: Little, Brown.

Quer, M., Burues-Villa, J., & Garcia–Crespillo. P. (1992). Primary tracheoesophageal puncture versus esophageal speech. *Archives of Otolaryngology, Head–Neck Surgery, 8,* 188–190.

Rait, D., & Lederberg, M. (1989). The family of the cancer patient. In J. C. Holland, & J. H. Rowland, (Eds.), *Handbook of psycho-oncology* (pp. 585–596). New York: Oxford University Press.

Reed, C. G. (1988). Voice disorders in the adult. In N. J. Lass, L. V. McReynolds, J. L. Northern, & D. E. Yoder (Eds.). *Handbook of speech-language pathology and audiology* (pp. 809–834). Toronto: B. C. Decker.

Salmon, S. (1979). Pre- and post-operative conferences with laryngectomized and their spouses. In R. L. Keith (Ed.), *Laryngectomee rehabilitation* (pp. 379–402). Houston: College-Hill Press.

Wagenfield, D. J. H., Harwood, A. R., Bryce, D. P., Van Nostrand, A. W. P. , & DeBoerg, G. (1980). Secondary primary respiratory tract malignancies in glottic carcinoma. *Cancer, 46,* 1883–1886.

Wynder, E. L. (1978). The epidemiology of cancers of the upper alimentary and upper respiratory tracts. *Laryngoscope, 88*(Suppl. 8), 50–51.

VOCAL FOLD
IMMOBILITY

MICHAEL A. CRARY, PH.D.
ANN L. GLOWASKI, M.D.

INTRODUCTION AND DEFINITIONS

Vocal fold mobility may be described in three categories: (a) adduction-abduction, (b) tensing-relaxing, and (c) mucosal wave properties. Each of these categories relies on a distinct physiology and all are interactive. The clinical significance of this categorization lies in a potential framework for understanding abnormalities in vocal fold movement in reference to underlying pathologies.

Adduction and abduction of the vocal folds are accomplished primarily by the lateral cricoarytenoid/interarytenoid and posterior cricoarytenoid muscles, respectively. This antagonistic muscle pair is innervated by the recurrent laryngeal branch of the vagus nerve. The integrity of the cricoarytenoid joint is an important influence on the adduction-abduction movements of the vocal folds. Thus, abnormalities in the neural supply, muscle function, or joint mobility may result in deficits in glottal closure (adduction) or glottal opening (abduction).

Increasing or decreasing tension in the vocal folds is accomplished primarily through action of the cricothyroid mus-cle. This muscle acts to alter the position of the thyroid cartilage in relation to the cricoid cartilage via the cricothyroid joint. Innervation to the cricothyroid muscle comes from the superior laryngeal branch of the vagus. Limitations in the ability to tense or relax the vocal folds may result in pitch range limitations and/or in reduced glottal closure.

Mucosal wave properties refer to the vibratory characteristics of the mucosal covering of the vocal folds during phonation. Any number of abnormalities may interfere with these vibratory characteristics including growths, edema, excessive tension, scar tissue, or other factors that limit mobility of this superficial layer of the vocal fold.

This chapter will focus on the first two areas of vocal fold mobility: adductor-abductor deficits and tensing-relaxing deficits. Both of these contribute to glottal incompetence. Limitations in the vibratory characterists of vocal fold mucosa are discussed in other chapters (see chapters 8, 9, and 10).

PATHOGENESIS

Glottal Incompetence

Any process that interferes with the ability of the larynx to close the glottis during phonation, swallowing, or other activities requiring glottal closure contributes to glottal incompetence. Vocal fold immobility typically results in some degree of glottal incompetence. The characteristics of the immobility often suggest an underlying pathology. Basic observations include whether the deficit is unilateral or bilateral and if functions of the superior laryngeal nerve and the recurrent laryngeal nerve are impaired. Beyond these general observations, position of the immobile vocal fold(s) must be ascertained in addition to the resultant effects of vocal fold immobility including voice characteristics, dysphagia, fatigue, and/or respiratory difficulities. These factors may be interactive in any individual with vocal fold immobility. Certainly, these factors indicate aspects of focus in the clinical examination and hence in considering treatment options. Finally, the common thread running through these factors may be the underlying cause for vocal fold immobility. From this perspective, potential contributors to vocal fold immobility are reviewed, followed by considerations for clinical evaluation and treatment of patients with these laryngeal disorders.

Vagus Nerve Deficits

Cranial nerve X, the vagus nerve, is responsible for laryngeal movements contributing to phonation. Damage to the vagus nerve will contribute to flaccid paralysis and potential atrophy within the innervated musculature. Figure 14–1 is a schematic diagram depicting the various branches of the vagus nerve and the structures and functions subserved by these branches.

Unilateral Deficits of the Vagus Nerve

Processes that impair the vagus nerve above the inferior ganglion (sometimes refered to as high vagal paralysis) will contribute to deficits in pharyngeal-laryngeal musculature. The resulting paresis will be unilateral and ipsilateral to the site of lesion. Typically, the velum is compromised, leading to hypernasality; the pharynx is weakened, leading to dysphagia; and laryngeal adduction (and abduction) is reduced, leading to dysphonia and related symptoms of glottal incompetence. Processes that impair vagal functions below the inferior ganglion (sometimes referred to as low vagal paralysis) are likely to contribute to more selective deficits related to individual branches of the nerve. If the superior and recurrent laryngeal nerves are impaired but the pharyngeal nerve is spared, velar and pharyngeal functions would be intact but the intrinsic laryngeal musculature responsible for adducting-abducting and tensing the vocal folds would be impaired. A selective lesion of the superior laryngeal nerve will impair activity of the cricothyroid muscle on that side limiting the tensing action of the ipsilateral vocal fold. When the internal branch of the nerve also is involved, a sensory deficit in the ipsilateral hemilarynx should be anticipated. Finally, if the recurrent laryngeal nerve is impaired selectively, velar, pharyngeal, and cricothyroid functions will be intact while laryngeal adduction-abduction will be impaired in the ipsilateral hemilarynx.

Bilateral Lesions

Bilateral lesions of the vagus nerve will replicate the above-mentioned deficits to the bilateral larynx, velum, and/or pharynx. The resulting functional deficits often contribute to significant complications for the patient beyond dysphonia. Swallowing is impaired, often with resultant aspiration of swallowed materials. Respiratory complaints are magnified due to poor laryngeal valving for both speech and nonspeech activities. In cases of bilateral recurrent laryngeal nerve damage,

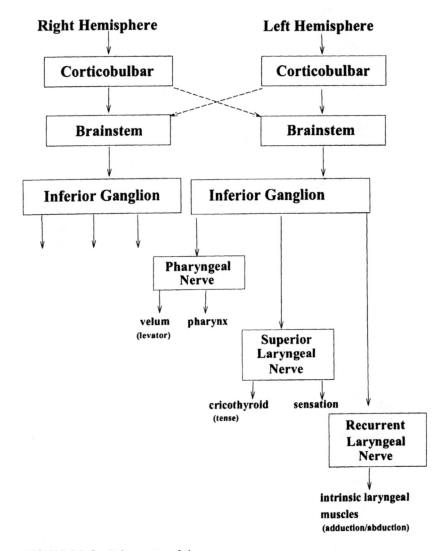

FIGURE 14-1. Schematic of the vagus nerve.

life-threatening airway obstruction may result from midline fixation of the true vocal folds. The voice may be only mildly impaired, but this is of little consequence to the individual who cannot breathe. Table 14–1 summarizes expected clinical deficits associated with various aspects of vagus nerve impairment.

Processes Outside the Vagus Nerve

In addition to lesions of the vagus nerve, numerous pathologic processes have the potential to impair laryngeal functions contributing to phonation. Virtually any process that creates glottal incompetence by limiting adduction or tension of the

Table 14–1. Expected clinical deficits associated with vagus nerve lesions.

Lesion Location	Unilateral	Bilateral

High Vagal (inferior ganglion or above)	Ipsilateral paralysis
	  TVF abducted (intermediate)
	  velum
	  pharyngeal m.
	  cricothyroid m.
	  other intrinsic laryngeal m.
	Hypernasality
	Dysphonia:
	  severe breathiness
	  pitch limitations
	Reduced or absent cough
	Dysphagia
	Aspiration
		Bilateral paralysis
		  Both TVF abducted (intermediate)
		  velum
		  pharyngeal m.
		  cricothyroid m.
		  other intrinsic laryngeal m.
		Severe hypernasality
		Severe dysphonia: near aphonia
		
		Absent cough
		Severe dysphagia
		Severe aspiration

Low Vagal (SLN and RLN)	Same as high vagal without velar or pharyngeal paralysis and related deficits.	

SLN only	TVF may appear normal "tilted" larynx
	Dysphonia:
	  pitch (mild)
	  breathiness
	  hoarseness
		Bilateral bowing of TVF no "tilt"
		Dysphonia:
		  pitch (severe)
		  breathiness
		  hoarseness
		  loudness (reduced)

RLN only	Ipsilateral paralysis TVF abducted (paramedian)
	
	Dysphonia:
	  breathy
	  hoarseness
	  loudness (reduced)
	  possible diplophonia
	  possible high pitch
	
	Possible aspiration
	Reduced cough
		Bilateral paralysis TVF abducted (paramedian)
		Dysphonia:
		  breathy (mild)
		  hoarse (mild)
		  loudness (reduced)
		
		Airway compromise:
		  reduced inspiration
		  inspiratory stridor

TVF = true vocal fold(s), m. = musculature, SLN = superior laryngeal nerve, RLN = recurrent laryngeal nerve.

vocal folds may contribute to dysphonia and related sequelae. The following sections summarize various processes that may contribute to vocal fold immobility through either impairment to branches of the vagus nerve or impairment of nonva-gal laryngeal physiology. Table 14–2 compares results describing the etiology of vocal fold paralysis in two patient series reported by Willatt and Stell (1991) and Woodson and Miller (1981). Although the respective categories were defined slightly

Table 14–2. Frequency of underlying causes of vocal fold paralysis in two patient series reported by Willatt and Stell (1991) and Woodson and Miller (1981).

Etiology	Willatt and Stell (1991)		Woodson and Miller (1981)	
	%	Rank	%	Rank
Malignant disease	31	1	22	3
Surgical trauma	29	2	41	1
Idiopathic	24	3	24	2
Nonsurgical trauma	7	4	8	4
Inflammatory disease	4	5–6	NR	NR
Miscellaneous	4	5–6	5	5
Neurologic disease	1	7	0	–

NR = not reported

differently in the two reports, their results were similar.

Malignant Disease

Tumors originating outside the larynx may impair vocal fold mobility. Carcinoma arising in the lung is a high profile cause of vocal fold deficits and is responsible for nearly half of vocal fold paralyses resulting from malignant disease (Willatt & Stell, 1991). Either by direct compression of the recurrent laryngeal nerve or by nodal extent in the aorto-pulmonary window, these tumors can create vocal fold paralysis.

Esophageal tumors (causing approximately 20% of paralyzed vocal folds from malignant disease) usually impair the recurrent laryngeal nerve in the tracheo-esophageal groove by direct extension. On occasion, esophageal tumors in the cervical esophagus extend directly into the postcricoid area causing fixation of the vocal fold and cricoarytenoid joint.

Malignant thyroid neoplasms contribute to approximately 10% of vocal fold palsies resulting from malignancies via compression of the recurrent laryngeal nerve in the tracheo-esophageal groove.

Less frequently, thyroid enlargement can cause paralysis.

Primary neurogenic tumors of the vagus nerve affect the nerve as tumor growth continues. Deep lobe parotid gland tumors, carotid body tumors, glomus jugulare tumors, glomus vagale tumors, and jugular foramen tumors all can involve the vagus nerve intracranially or in the base of skull.

Mediastinal malignancies may affect the left recurrent laryngeal nerve as it courses through the mediastinum and around the aortic arch. Metastic disease to the cervical lymph nodes is a rare cause of vocal fold paralysis primarily by direct extension to the recurrent laryngeal or vagus nerve.

Surgical Trauma

Surgical trauma often is recognized as another frequent etiology of vocal fold paralysis. Thyroid surgery is the most common surgical procedure resulting in vocal fold paralysis although the frequency is decreasing (Johns & Rood, 1987; Tucker, 1993; Willatt & Stell, 1991). Lung resection, radical neck dissection, and/or carotid artery surgery also may result in damage to various branches of the vagus nerve contributing to vocal fold paralysis. Surgery in the cervical esophagus and cervical approaches to the anterior cervical vertebrae may result in traction injury to the recurrent laryngeal nerve. Less common surgical injuries include transection of the nerve and nerve damage during cardiac surgery.

Intubation Trauma

Arytenoid cartilage dislocation and/or compression of the recurrent laryngeal nerve may result from intubation causing vocal fold immobility, both transient and long-lasting. In cases of long-term intubation, there is increased risk of glottic web, subglottic stenosis, or interarytenoid scarring (Benjamin, 1993). Each has the potential to limit vocal fold mobility.

Nonsurgical Trauma

Nonsurgical trauma is an increasingly common cause of vocal fold paralysis (Tucker, 1993). Gunshot and penetrating wounds to the neck can cause direct or indirect injury to the vagus nerve or to the laryngeal mechanism. Blunt trauma can cause laryngeal fractures (displaced or nondisplaced), laryngeal hematomas, arytenoid dislocations, and even laryngotracheal separation. Chest wounds, either blunt or penetrating, can disrupt the vagus nerve along its thoracic course. Basilar skull fractures through the jugular foramen also may impair the vagus nerve.

Inflammatory Disease

Inflammatory disease is an uncommon cause of vocal fold paralysis. Perhaps the most common contributor in this category is pulmonary tuberculosis that results in mediastinal lymphodenopathy or scarring (Maran, 1979). Other, more remote, causes may include jugular thrombophle-

bitis, syphilis, influenza, and granulomas (Willatt & Stell, 1991).

Peripheral Neurologic Disease

Peripheral neurologic diseases that may impair vocal fold movement result primarily from toxic effects. Causative agents include lead, arsenic, alchohol, and vincristine (Brook & Schreiber, 1971). Systemic diseases such as diabetes, Guillain-Barré, and Charcot-Marie-Tooth syndrome may have peripheral neural consequences that influence vocal fold movement (Willatt & Stell, 1991).

Miscellaneous Causes

A host of other disease processes have the potential to impair vocal fold movement either by damage to the neural supply or alteration of the laryngeal mechanism. Left atrial hypertrophy of the heart with associated mitral stenosis or long-standing congestive heart failure can cause compression of the ipsilateral recurrent laryngeal nerve. An aortic arch aneurysm may exert pressure on the recurrent nerve passing around it. Rheumatoid arthritis can reduce vocal fold mobility through the mechanism of cricoarytenoid joint ankylosis. This condition typically is seen only in long-standing disease. Collagen vascular disorders including systemic lupus erythematosus, dermatomyositis, and relapsing polychondritis may contribute to vocal fold paralysis. Wegener's granulomatosis resulting from vasculitis may impair vocal fold movement, but laryngeal involvement typically is subglottic (Vrabec, 1993).

Idiopathic Causes

Idiopathic or unknown causes of vocal fold immobility are prominent among possible etiologies. A viral process is often presumed, and diagnosis is by exclusion.

In this regard, it is not advisable to offer a diagnosis of idiopathic vocal fold dysfunction in the acute stage because other more problematic pathologies may become evident at a later point in time.

CLINICAL EVALUATION OF PATIENTS WITH VOCAL FOLD IMMOBILITY

The basic principles of voice examination and diagnosis of dysphonia were addressed in Chapter 6. Often, the respective disorders of voice and laryngeal function will have characteristics reflecting the underlying pathology. This section focuses on aspects of the clinical voice/laryngeal examination specific to patients with vocal fold immobility.

Patient Complaints

Individuals with glottal incompetence secondary to limitations in adduction, abduction, or tension in the vocal mechanism may describe both voice and nonvoice complaints. Voice complaints frequently include breathiness, low volume, poor pitch control, and/or hoarseness. Nonvoice complaints may include fatigue when speaking and/or with exercise, reduced ability to cough efficiently, aspiration of liquids, or a more pronounced dysphagia involving various foods. The profile of deficits resulting from vocal fold immobility usually is obvious in the clinical history related by the patient. Subsequent voice and nonvoice laryngeal/pharyngeal evaluation is essential to verify the complaints and grade the relative severity of each.

Clinical History

The clinical history of the patient with vocal fold immobility is an essential aspect of the clinical examination. In cases of unknown etiology, the clinical history often points to potential contributing factors. In all cases, clinicians will want to know the duration of the deficit and how the voice or nonvoice problems have changed since onset. Prior treatment history compared to clinical course will provide indications of potential benefit of various interventions. Clinicians may identify various patient compensatory strategies (both beneficial and nonbeneficial) through a thorough clinical history.

Basic Descriptions of Perceptual Voice Characteristics

Many, if not all, patients with glottal incompetence will demonstrate a breathy voice with reduced loudness, often with low pitch and limited pitch range. These features are the result of air escape between vocal folds that are less than optimally adducted and/or unable to increase tension. Due to the wide array of pathologic processes that may contribute to vocal fold immobility, clinical reality dictates that any number of voice characteristics may be observed. These characteristics may relate directly to the nature of the vocal fold immobility or be a result of compensatory efforts on the part of the patient. For example, the patient with a breathy, low-pitched voice who is unable to raise pitch level may have deficits in both the recurrent and superior branches of the laryngeal nerve. Conversely, the patient who presents with a breathy but high pitched voice who is able to effect pitch changes may have a defict in the recurrent laryngeal nerve, sparing the superior laryngeal nerve. A different example is the patient who demonstrates a breathy but strained voice. This individual may have developed a compensatory strategy of excessive supraglottic compression. In severe cases, false fold phonation may be noted. These examples reflect three clinical variants of patients with an underlying vocal fold immobility. In each case the voice profile and resulting description is different. These differences should be considered in the management of individual cases of vocal fold immobility.

Perceptual Rating Scales for Voice Characterstics

The clinical perception of voice characteristics associated with vocal fold immobility begins at first hearing (or, in some instances, first sighting) of the patient. As mentioned previously, several perceptual attributes are overt to the ear of the examiner including breathiness, pitch deviations, excessive strain, laryngeal-respiratory limitations (i.e., shortness of breath), and other possibilities. Although rating scales may vary in value from one clinician to the next (Bassich & Ludlow, 1986) or from one scale to the next (Krieman, Gerratt, Kempster, Erman, & Berke, 1993), many rating scales are available. Examples may be found in Wilson (1979) and Gelfer (1988). If rating scales are used in cases of glottal incompetence secondary to vocal fold immobility, clinicians should include ratings of nonvoice laryngeal deficits (e.g., fatigue, aspiration, effort involved in speaking, etc.) as well as voice ratings. It also may be valuable to ask the patient to rate his or her voice and nonvoice difficulties before and following intervention if for no other reason than as an index of patient satisfaction.

Maneuvers and Manipulation

Subsequent to documentation of the initial performance profile, voice characteristics should be evaluated under conditions and maneuvers that not only help to characterize the dysphonia, but also might indicate appropriate avenues of intervention. Loudness changes may reveal valuable information regarding performance. Is any voice improvement noted as a result of speaking loudly, from shouting, laughing or other vocal alterations that increase loudness? A related question is whether the vocal folds can adduct in nonvoice functions that increase force of adduction. Coughing and hard glottal attack at the onset of vowel phonation are considered indications of vocal fold adduction with increased effort. Aronson (1990) recommends these forced attempts at adduction as "one of the most useful tests for adductor vocal fold strength" (p. 250). He contends that differences in performance of the cough versus the hard attack at vowel onset can help to grade the severity of vocal fold weakness.

Maximum phonation time (MPT) often is used as a clinical index of laryngeal-respiratory efficiency. Kent, Kent, and Rosenbek (1987) offer a thorough description of this technique and variables that can influence measures of MPT. Inasmuch as glottal incompetence contributes to less efficient use of the expired airstream during phonation, MPT would be expected to be reduced in patients with vocal fold immobility. MPT is dependent on a variety of factors including the effort put forth by the patient and respiratory function independent of laryngeal considerations. Still, this rather simple technique enjoys extensive use in the clinical evaluation of laryngeal-respiratory cooperative function during phonation. Blaugrund, Taira, Dren, Lin, Isshiki, and Gould (1990) demonstrated that MPT increased with manual compression of the thyroid cartilage during evaluation of patients with reduced glottal closure. LaBlance and Maves (1992) and Sasaki, Leder, Petcu, and Friedman (1990) demonstrated that MPT increased following surgical medialization of paralyzed vocal folds resulting in improved glottal closure during phonation. The implication of these reports is that improved glottal closure during phonation contributes to more efficient use of the expired airstream resulting in longer periods of sustained phonation. This position is supported by the findings of Blaugrund et al. (1990) and Ford, Bless, and Prehn (1992). Both of these reports described an inverse relationship between MPT and mean airflow during vowel phonation.

Physical manipulation of the laryngeal structure frequently is employed in the evaluation of patients with glottal incompetence. Turning the head may assist in glottal closure by "stretching" the nonmoving fold into a position closer to the glottal midline where it can be approximated by the mobile vocal fold. In such cases phonation may improve with the head in a turned position (Boone & McFarlane, 1988). Despite the potential logic underlying this technique, Watterson, McFarlane, and Menicucci (1990) reported that head turning had little influence on glottal closure evaluated endoscopically or on vibratory characteristics of the vocal fold(s) evaluated stroboscopically in patients with vocal fold paralysis.

A second physical manipulation, lateral manual compression of the thyroid cartilage, acts to improve glottal closure during phonation by physically approximating the vocal folds via external pressure on the thyroid ala. Isshiki (1989) claims that "in practical terms, this is the most important test in determining the indication for laryngeal framework surgery" (p. 52). He states that voice improvement with this procedure is a good prognostic sign. No voice improvement with manual compression may be explained by at least five possibilities: (a) inadequate manual compression by the examiner; (b) stiff cartilage due to calcification; (c) other problems in the paralyzed vocal fold or in the contraleral fold; (d) inadequate phonation due to pain from the procedure; and (e) excessively wide glottal opening. Any number of these factors may lower the postsurgical expectations for voice improvement.

Watterson et al. (1990) reported that manual pressure to the thyroid improved glottal closure viewed endoscopically. However, they noted little influence on stroboscopic characteristics of vocal fold vibration. Blaugrund and colleagues (1990) described clinical, acoustic, and aerodynamic voice improvement during lateral manual compression in patients with inadequate glottal closure. In four patients who received surgical medialization of paralyzed vocal folds, results of a preoperative lateral manual compression test were a good predictor of postoperative voice improvement. These investigators recommended that this procedure be completed with laryngoscopic monitoring of vocal fold position and with acoustic and aerodynamic documentation of the resultant voice change.

A third physical manipulation of the laryngeal framework, manual cricothyroid approximation, is completed by "thrusting up the lower margin of the cricoid" (Isshiki, 1989, p. 125). During the clinical voice examination this procedure may be attempted by anchoring the thyroid cartilage with gentle downward pressure on the thyroid notch while simultaneously displacing the cricoid cartilage upward with pressure (gently) on the lower margin of the cartilage. The anticipated result of this manipulation is increased tension in the vocal folds contributing to higher pitch. It is conceivable that, in cases of glottal incompetence resulting from bowing in the vocal folds, reduced breathiness and/or increased vocal loudness may result from this manipulation.

In cases where excessive vocal strain suggests increased supraglottic compression, a fourth laryngeal framework manipulation may be used. Gently displacing the thyroid cartilage posteriorly (anteroposterior compression) may assist in reducing some of the perceived strain in the voice by reducing the tension in the laryngeal mechanism (Boone, 1983; Brodnitz, 1958, 1961). The anticipated result is a lowering of pitch secondary to relaxation of the true vocal folds. However, in cases of glottal incompetence in which the patient is compensating with increased supraglottic compression, the result is likely to be perceived as a poorer voice marked by an increase in breathiness. This "decompensation" may be an important clinical observation in patients who demonstrate excessive supraglottic compression as a form of compensation for glottal incompetence. Unfortunately, unlike Watterson's (Watterson et al., 1990) and Blaugrund's (Blaugrund et al., 1990) systematic assessments of the results of the lateral manual compression test, there is little systematic documentation of the results of laryngeal framework manipulation via cricothyroid approximation or posterior displacement of the thyroid. A summary of these laryngeal manipulation techniques is provided in Table 14–3.

Functional Descriptions

Beyond traditional descriptions of vocal performance and change in voice characteristics resulting from various manipulations and maneuvers, clinicians should consider the "functionality" of the voice in patients with glottal incompetence. Functionality, in this context, refers to the degree of impairment in reference to daily activities. Essentially, how well does the voice function in consideration of the daily expectations placed on the patient? Obviously, this concept will change from patient to patient depending on variables such as age, occupation, and personal habits. Unfortunately, no clinical scales exist to describe the degree of functional impairment in the voice for any given patient. This limitation is being amplified in the context of current health care provision changes. Third-party payers, including federal government programs, often request statements on the degree of disability created by the clinical deficit. For example, Social Security Disability Rul-

ings regarding loss of speech (SSR 82-57) request descriptions of "audibility" (the ability to speak at a level sufficient to be heard), "intelligibility" (the ability to articulate . . . with sufficient accuracy to be understood), and "functional efficiency" (the ability to produce and sustain a serviceably fast rate of speech output over a useful period of time). Because many patients with glottal incompetence secondary to vocal fold immobility are members of the workforce, one of the challenges for voice clinicians and researchers is to develop useful methods of rating functional loss of voice that, hopefully, relate to other perceptual and instrumental aspects of the voice evaluation.

Laryngoscopic Examination

Laryngoscopic examination with videotape documentation is necessary to confirm and characterize vocal fold immobility. Flexible nasopharyngoscopy-laryngoscopy provides certain advantages over oral endoscopy in cases of vagus nerve deficits. The primary advantage is a more encompassing view of speech-phonation mechanisms. The transnasal approach with a flexible scope permits examination of the velar mechanism from the superior aspect. This perspective may help to identify paresis in the velum that is missed during oral mechanism examination. The position and movement of the larynx within the pharynx are more easily observed with a flexible scope. Asymmetric paresis in the pharyngeal musculature is observable. Finally, in certain cases of bilateral vocal fold paralysis, an inferior view of the vocal folds via a tracheostomal site may be desirable or required to obtain an adequate evaluation of the larynx. A related consideration is the nature of the performance tasks that patients can attempt. Flexible scope imaging permits a wider variety of attempted speech-phonation tasks than rigid oral endoscopy. In

Table 14–3. Manipulation of the laryngeal framework during clinical examination and expected voice changes.

Manipulation	Technique	Influence on Larynx	Expected Voice Change	Documentation
Head turn	Turn head toward each shoulder	Improved glottal closure	Reduced breathiness Reduced hoarseness Louder voice	No consistent benefit (Watterson et al., 1990)
Lateral thyroid compression	Use fingers to compress thyroid ala	Improved glottal closure	Reduced breathiness Reduced hoarseness Louder voice	Consistent benefit (Blaugrund et al., 1990; Watterson et al., 1990)
Cricothyroid approximation	Anchor notch with finger and elevate cricoid inferior border with another finger	Increased tension on vocal folds	Increased pitch Reduced breathiness Increased loudness	None
Thyroid displacement posteriorly (anteroposterior compression)	Gentle pressure posteriorly on the thyroid angle	Decrease tension on vocal folds Decrease supraglottic compression	Decrease pitch Decrease loudness Increase breathiness	None

cases of reported dysphagia or suspected aspiration, swallowing functions also may be evaluated during flexible endoscopy (Langmore, Schatz, & Olson, 1988).

Vocal Fold Position

Regardless of the imaging technique employed, certain observations are indicated in cases of vocal fold immobility. Initially, the position of the vocal folds at rest should be described. A simple technique to describe asymmetry in paired structures is to draw a mental line through the midline of the structure and compare the right and left halves. In the case of laryngeal paralysis, envision a line along the glottal midline from the posterior commissure to the anterior commissure. The position of the vocal folds may be described using general terms such as midline, paramedian, or intermediate describing the position of the vocal folds in refrence to the glottal midline (Brewer, Woo, Casper, & Colton, 1991). Rontal and Rontal (1986) claim that "an examination of the vocal cords will help determine the exact location of the initiating neurologic disturbance" (p. 2061). To a certain extent this may be a valid assertion. If the superior laryngeal nerve is spared, the nonmoving vocal fold may still be able to tense. Tensing the vocal fold contributes to adduction. Therefore, the paralyzed vocal fold may lie in a more paramedian position if the superior laryngeal nerve is spared. Conversely, if the superior laryngeal nerve is damaged, the vocal fold may lie in a more intermediate position. Despite the conventional wisdom of this logic, Ballenger (1985) described several factors that may influence the position of a paralyzed vocal fold. These include: (a) function of the cricothyroid muscle; (b) degree of atrophy and fibrosis in the deinnervated muscle(s); (c) residual tone associated with autonomic nerve supply; (d) function of the cricoarytenoid joint; (e) function of the interarytenoid muscle; and (f) tension of the conus elasticus.

Other Observations

In addition to vocal fold position, movement characteristics and degree of glottal opening at maximum adduction should be described. Specific observations should include any residual movement in the impaired fold, degree of compensation by the intact fold, position and movement of the arytenoid cartilages, level of the vocal folds in reference to each other, and the presence of any compensatory activities during phonation (i.e., false fold adduction, pharyngeal squeezing, etc.). Examine tensing activity during attempted pitch changes as an evaluation of superior laryngeal nerve integrity. Superior laryngeal nerve deficits also may contribute to a tilted laryngeal position within the pharynx (Tucker, 1987). Describe relative sizes of the vocal folds in an attempt to identify potential atrophy in the musculature of the impaired fold. Finally, describe the vocal fold edge(s). Especially in cases of laryngeal trauma or prolonged intubation, irregular vocal edges may result from scarring or other abnormal processes.

Stroboscopic Evaluation

Stroboscopic evaluation is not essential to identify immobility in the vocal folds. However, stroboscopic assessment is useful in evaluating the mucosal vibratory characteristics of the impaired vocal fold(s) and the intact fold. This aspect of vocal fold evaluation may be particularly important in cases in which trauma, intubation, prior surgery, or other factors that contribute to irregularities in vocal fold mucosa are present. Stroboscopic findings reported in cases of unilateral vocal fold paralysis include increased amplitude of vibration (mucosal wave) and aperiodocity of vibration (Kitzing, 1985; Watterson, et al., 1990). However, caution should be extended against overinterpretation of these observations. Differing degrees of paresis/paralysis, influence of the underlying pathology, and presence of other mucosal irregulatories will have a direct effect on stroboscopic results.

Acoustic Characteristics

Acoustic descriptions of dysphonia resulting from vocal fold immobility present both benefits and challenges to clinical practitioners. A potential benefit of acoustic description is a degree of objectivity in measures that describe specific aspects of vocal performance. Potential challenges range from the choice of equipment (Titze & Winholtz, 1993) and procedures (Read, Buder, & Kent, 1992) used to acquire the voice signal to the method of acoustic analysis (Titze & Liang, 1993). Assuming the practitioner is aware of the potential problems associated with acoustic analysis and has prepared accordingly, the next step is to select acoustic measures that reflect one or more dimensions of dysphonia in cases of vocal fold immobility and will reflect change in the voice resulting from treatment.

Signal-to-Noise Ratio

One measure used to describe characteristics of dysphonia secondary to vocal fold immobility is the signal-to-noise (S/N) ratio (also referred to as the harmonic-to-noise ratio). As the name implies this acoustic measure is a ratio of the harmonics (signal) to the breathy component (noise) in the voice (Yumoto, Sasaki, & Okamura, 1984). A voice with little noise will have a high signal-to-noise ratio (S/N). As the amount of noise (in this context, breathiness) increases, the S/N decreases. Noise (breathiness) resulting from glottal incompetence should be lessened as a result of successful intervention (i.e., the S/N should be lower following successful treatment). Blaugrund and colleagues (1990) demonstrated a lower "breathiness index" (similar, but not identical, to S/N) during the lateral manual compression test in patients with incomplete glottal closure. Conversely, Ford, et al. (1992) reported little change in signal-to-noise ratios obtained from 16 patients with glottic insufficiency tested pre- and postsurgical medialization of a single vocal fold. (*Note:* Their patient group was not limited to cases of vocal fold paralysis.) Despite offering a degree of logic as a measure of voice in cases of vocal fold immobility, the S/N has yet to be established firmly as a sensitive index of change.

Spectrographic Patterns

Air escape during phonation from an underadducted glottis is expected to contribute to increased high-frequency noise in the vocal spectrum. Isshiki (1989) refers to spectrographic changes to demonstrate reduced breathiness following surgical medialization of paralyzed vocal folds. Yanagihara (1967) has described four types of spectrograms that reflect the degree of noise relative to harmonics. Clinicians with access to spectrographic analysis may opt for this form of documentation.

Percent Voicing

An indirect method of documenting breathiness is to assess the percent of voicing in a sustained vowel. This acoustic attribute may be obtained from the Visipitch™ (Kay Elemetrics, Pine Brook, NJ). A voice produced by an underadducted glottis might be expected to result in a lower percent voicing value. Likewise, following successful treatment, percent voicing would be expected to increase. Caution is advised in using this application however, because many laryngeal-phonatory irregularities may contribute to interruptions in voicing during vowel prolongation.

Pitch-Frequency Measures

Pitch-frequency measures might include fundamental frequency, variation in fundamental frequency, pitch range (typically in semitones), and perturbation measures. Sasaki et al. (1990) described increases in fundamental frequency as an index of voice improvement following surgical medialization of paralyzed vocal folds. LaBlance and Maues (1992) reported both increases and decreases in fundamental frequency (F_0) following the same surgical procedure in individual patients. Crary, Moore, and Cassisi (1991) reported that 9 of 14 patients demonstrated F_0 increases and 5 of 14 demonstrated fundmental frequency decreases following surgical medialization. Their conclusion was that appropriateness of presurgical F_0 in consideration of age and gender of the patient was perhaps the most important factor in determining change in the fundamental frequency postoperatively.

Perturbation measures reflect the degree of irregularity of vocal fold vibration. Abnormal voices are expected to have higher degrees of variability and therefore higher perturbation values. Postmedialization decreases in perturbation measures were reported by LaBlance and Maues (1992) and by Ford et al. (1992). Caution should be exercised in interpreting these measures because excessive aperiodicity may render perturbation values meaningless.

Loudness-Amplitude

Reduced loudness typically is associated with vocal fold immobility. Amplitude (acoustic correlate of loudness) may be measured rather simply using a sound-level meter. Loudness variations also may be estimated by asking the patient to produce the softest and the loudest speaking voice possible. Sasaki et al. (1990) used the relative intensity measure from the Visipitch™ obtained during a reading task to evaluate loudness changes in their group of thyroplasty patients. Similar to frequency perturbations, variations in the amplitude of the vibratory cycle may be expressed as amplitude perturbation or shimmer. LaBlance and Maues (1992) and Ford et al. (1992) both demonstrated reduction in shimmer values following surgical correction of glottal incompetence.

A Caution

Although a great deal of attention and effort is being given to developing acoustic models and databases to describe various dysphonias, it would be premature to suggest that any measure, or group of measures, is diagnostic of a specific dysphonia at this juncture. Perhaps the best application of acoustic measures at this time lies in the documentation of voice change resulting from maneuvers and manipulations during the evaluation and from treatment.

Aerodynamic Characteristics

Aerodynamic measures are applied less frequently than acoustic measures in the description of voice pathology. However, these measures may have particular application in cases of vocal fold immobility and resulting glottal incompetence. Simply stated, if glottal incompetence creates less resistance to the expired phonatory air stream, airflow should increase and air pressure below the vocal folds should decrease. Aerodynamic measures seem well suited to the description of glottal incompetence secondary to vocal fold immobility and changes in laryngeal-phonatory function resulting from treatment. Mean airflow measured during vowel production in normal speaking adults ranges roughly from 80–200 ml/s (Colton & Casper, 1990; Isshiki, 1989). Higher flow rates may be indicative of glottal incompetence. In this respect improved glottal closure should result in lower rates of mean airflow. Blaugrund and colleagues (1990) demonstrated lower mean airflow rates during lateral manual compression of the thyroid ala in 10 out of 10 patients with reduced glottal closure. Ford and colleagues (1992) reported lower mean airflow rates in 11 of 15 patients post surgical medialization of a single vocal fold. Few, if any, studies have detailed air pressure or laryngeal airway resistance characteristics in cases of vocal fold immobility pre- or posttreatment. Clinicians using these measures to document change in individual patients are reminded that aerodynamic measures are influenced by a variety of laryngeal and human performance factors.

Electromyography

One of the more prominent causes of vocal fold immobility is vocal fold paralysis secondary to peripheral neurological deficit. Intramuscular electromyographic (IEMG) evaluation may be a useful technique to document the nature and extent of vocal fold paralysis (Hiroto, Hirano, & Tomita, 1968). IEMG evaluation may help to identify deinnervation in the thyroarytenoid and/or the cricothyroid muscles helping to confirm recurrent and/or superior laryngeal nerve deficits. Prognostic information also may be obtained from IEMG investigations of laryngeal musculature (Parnes & Satya-Murti, 1985); however, IEMG information should be supplemented with other diagnostic and evaluative findings.

Laryngeal IEMG does not enjoy widespread clinical application at this time. Among the primary reasons are the invasive nature of the technique and the high degree of expertise required in head and neck anatomy and the application and interpretation of IEMG.

Respiratory Functions

Respiratory complaints may be prominent among patients with vocal fold immobility. Mean airflow measures provide some indication of respiratory support for phonation, but a more thorough evaluation of inspiratory and expiratory airflow is obtained from the flow-volume loop spirogram (FVLS). Kashima (1984, 1991) reported that characteristic FVLS patterns are obtained in cases of either bilateral or unilateral vocal fold paralysis. Although many clinicians will not have the instrumentation available for this procedure, a preliminary examination of respiratory functions may be completed via spirometry techniques available in many speech clinics. This cursory examination may be especially useful in older patients with suspected limitations in respiratory function or in patients with known respiratory disease. When respiratory limitations beyond those resulting from laryngeal valving deficiencies are suspected, appropriate medical referral should be pursued. Beyond medical concerns, the role of lung volume measures as part of the voice evaluation is unclear. Colton and Casper (1990) suggested that information regarding the control of respiration during speech may be more valuable to the voice evaluation process than information on lung volumes.

Fluorography

Videofluorographic evaluation of the upper aerodigestive tract may be beneficial, if not mandatory, in certain cases of vocal fold immobility. Lateral views of the head and neck area obtained during speech under fluorographic examination provide information on lingual, velar, pharyngeal, and laryngeal movements. Anterior views are helpful in evaluating pharyngeal and laryngeal movement patterns. In cases where aspiration is suspected, a videofluorographic swallowing examination is indicated to determine the nature and extent of aspiration (Groher, 1984; Logemann, 1983, 1986).

TREATMENT: OPTIONS AND OUTCOMES

Pharmacologic Treatment

Pharmacologic treatments for vocal fold immobility are limited. In most cases of vocal fold paralysis or fixation, irreversible damage has occurred prior to the voice examination. Steroidal treatments may be beneficial in certain inflammatory disease processes; however, these treatments are probably more effective prior to vocal fold fixation.

Laryngeal irritation also may play a role in vocal performance and/or postoperative recovery of voice in cases of vocal fold immobility. Either symptomatically or prophylactically, treatments focused on reducing laryngeal irritation should be considered when surgical intervention is planned.

Surgical Treatment

General Considerations

In most cases of vocal fold immobility, surgical intervention is a primary treatment consideration. The decision to perform surgery and the type of surgery performed depends on the etiology of immobility, the time history of the disease process, and the patient's symptoms. Arytenoid dislocation, for example, is treated by relocation with laryngeal spatula usually within 48 hours of the injury. Reported results have been variable (Tucker, 1993). Once the joint is ankylosed it is difficult to relocate. A different situation is seen following laryngeal trauma. Laryngeal fractures and mucosal injuries may be repaired either endoscopically or via thyrotomy. The primary goal, however, is airway maintenance; good voice production is a secondary concern. Similar considerations are faced in bilateral vocal fold paralysis in which the vocal folds rest in the adducted or paramedian position. These patients often require a tracheostomy for variable time periods. Voice production is a secondary concern to airway maintenance.

Unilateral Vocal Fold Immobility

Surgical interventions for a single nonmoving vocal fold have expanded in recent years. These avenues of intervention may be considered in three categories: injectables, medializations, and reinnervations. The common goal of these procedures is to improve glottal closure and efficiency for voice production and airway protection.

Injection Procedures

Many materials have been injected into the vocal folds to improve glottal closure. Detailed reviews of these procedures may be found in Miller and Duplechain (1993) and Tucker (1993). Gelfoam is intended as a temporary medium for patients expected to recover vocal fold mobility. Typically, it is reserved only for patients experiencing significant functional deficits resulting from glottal incompetence. Col-

lagen may be injected to effect small adjustments in medialization of a nonmoving vocal fold. Patients should be tested for allergic reaction prior to injection. Autologous fat (Mikaelian, Lowry, & Sataloff, 1991) injection shows promise as a medialization technique. Initial overinjection may be indicated with the expectation of resorption or expression of the fat. Rejection is unlikely because the fat is harvested from the patient. Teflon injection was once the primary injection method to improve glottal incompetence. Usually the injection is done endoscopically with placement of the material in the lateral area of the vocal fold causing a medialization of the soft tissues. Inappropriate placement, overinjection, migration, potential for formation of granulomas, and difficulty removing implanted Teflon have lessened its desirability in recent years.

Medialization Procedures

Perhaps the most popular surgical technique used presently to medialize a nonmoving vocal fold is the Type I Thyroplasty. The basic procedure described by Isshiki (1989) involves creating a small window in the thyroid ala, medializing the vocal fold, and placing a small silastic implant to keep the nonmoving vocal fold in a medialized position. Reports of this procedure almost uniformly claim a high success rate for voice restoration with minimal complications (Ford et al., 1992; LaBlance & Maues, 1992; Netterville, Stone, Civantos, Luken, & Ossoff, 1993). This procedure also has been described in combination with other surgical attempts to improve glottal closure including arytenoid adduction (Slavit & Maragos, 1994) and vocal fold lengthening (Type IV thyroplasty: Isshiki, 1989).

Reinnervation Procedures

Attempts to reinnervate paralyzed vocal folds have included nerve-muscle pedicle procedures (Tucker, 1990) and nerve transfer procedures (Crumley, 1990). Generally, these have not enjoyed widespread use.

Voice Therapy

Voice therapy techniques may be appropriate in certain cases of vocal fold immobility resulting from unilateral paralysis. Unfortunately, a paucity of information is available to guide clinical decisions in the application of voice therapy in these cases. Furthermore, there is a distinct possibility that certain voice therapy techniques may contribute to other laryngeal difficulties in patients with unilateral paralysis. Three published observations should serve to portray the complicated nature of the decision to pursue voice therapy in these cases. McFarlane, Holt-Romeo, Lavorato, and Warner (1991) suggested that "voice therapy be considered as a primary treatment choice to restore voice in cases of unilateral vocal fold paralysis when aspiration is not a problem" (p. 48). Their study evaluated 16 patients with unilateral vocal fold paralysis who had been treated with voice therapy, Teflon injection, or muscle-nerve reinnervation techniques. Listener ratings of six vocal parameters served as the basis of comparison for outcome of the respective techniques. Voice samples from patients receiving Teflon injection were rated lower (less desirable) on all vocal parameters than either the voice therapy or surgery groups. The only feature distinguishing treatment outcome between the voice therapy and muscle-nerve reinnervation groups was the rating for breathiness. Patients in the surgery group were felt to have greater improvement in this vocal parameter than patients in the voice therapy group. This report contains many intriguing features. First, the duration of therapy averaged 9 hours with a range from 3 to 24 hours. This observation speaks to the efficiency of the applied techniques (basically techniques to enhance or force adduction of the vocal folds). Second, no complications were reported as a result of voice therapy. This is not always the case as will be noted momentarily. From the converse perspective, however, the findings of this study must be approached cautiously. Each treatment group contained a small number of patients (four or six). Although etiology of paralysis was noted, there was no discussion of the laryngeal condition prior to treatment or the rationale for the choice of treatment among the patients. The authors seem to gloss over the observation that the voice therapy group improved less than the muscle-nerve reinnervation group on the vocal attribute of breathiness—one of the major clinical features of vocal fold paralysis. Finally, as discussed by the authors, surgical medialization by thyroplasty has become a popular choice of treatment in these cases and should be considered in future studies of treatment efficacy.

The second observation is that offered by Yamaguchi, Yotsukura, Hirosaky, Watanabe, Hirose, Kobayashi, and Bless (1993). These investigators completed a systematic evaluation of pushing exercises as a treatment approach in cases of glottal incompetence secondary to paralysis or sulcus vocalis. Three patients were described as exemplars of the treatment technique. The first case (unilateral vocal fold paralysis) required 3 months (weekly sessions of 20–30 minutes) to reach a criterion point for loudness during vowel production but failed to utilize the louder voice in connected speech. The second case (bilateral sulcus vocalis) was treated for 10 months with pushing exercises following which she had improved but not normal voice. The third case (congenital recurrent laryngeal paralysis noted in an adult patient) required a combination of surgical medialization and pushing exercises (7 months) to reach criterion for termination of treatment. Clearly, the cases reported by these investigations demonstrated some improvement in voice abilities following treatment with pushing exercises; however, the degree of improvement and the effectiveness of the treatment should be questioned by their results. The authors include an insightful discussion of indications and contraindications for this treatment approach, including limitations on the duration of therapy prior to surgical intervention. They also advocate that voice therapy be completed in the acute phase (3 to 6 months) of unilateral vocal fold paralysis "to recover the compensatory capacity of the healthy side of the vocal fold" (Yamaguchi et al., 1993, p. 255). Finally, they discuss the potential for laryngeal complications including inflammation secondary to the therapy in some cases. Despite the specifics of improved voice described in their three patients, their overall results do not support a clear choice of voice therapy via pushing exercises in cases of glottal incompetence secondary to unilateral paralysis or sulcus vocalis.

The third observation point is offered by Colton and Casper (1990), "In our own experience, we have not been impressed by the results obtained in voice therapy using effort closure techniques" (p. 265). As a result of their experiences, they do not recommend the routine use of these excerises in cases of unilateral vocal fold paralysis. They do note that high pitch or falsetto techniques may produce clearer and less breathy voice in such cases, but question the generalization of improved voice to an acceptable pitch level. This point is emphasized in a patient described by Case (1991). This patient demonstrated unilateral vocal fold paralysis secondary to thyroid surgery. His voice was of "essentially normal quality"

but of high pitch with breaks into falsetto range. Voice therapy techniques focused on lowering pitch were successful over a 3-week duration. However, the resultant voice was breathy and lacked adequate loudness. Subsequent surgical intervention (Teflon injection) resulted in significant voice improvement. This case demonstrates the principle of decompensation voice therapy. The high pitch noted in this patient presumably reflected compensation for inadequate closure via the cricothyroid muscles (superior laryngeal nerve was intact). The result was improved glottal closure at the expense of an acceptable pitch range. Voice therapy techniques were effective in removing this nonfunctional compensation following which surgical intervention was successful in restoring a more normal voice.

These observations present a range of opinions regarding the role of voice therapy in cases of vocal fold immobility secondary to unilateral paralysis. Simply stated, the available evidence is insufficient to advocate voice therapy as an efficient and cost-effective intervention avenue in *all* cases of vocal immobility. Our approach has been to use vocal hygiene techniques to facilitate a "healthy, nonirritated larynx" prior to surgical medialization via thyroplasty. In certain cases, decompensation therapy is pursued to remove nonfunctional compensations either prior or subsequent to phonosurgery. Cases in which the vocal folds approximate (i.e., the nonmoving fold is in the midline or paramedian position) may benefit from voice therapy.

SUMMARY

Vocal fold immobility may result from numerous pathologic processes to the neural innervation and/or laryngeal structures involved in glottal closure. Comprehensive assessment involves both voice and nonvoice functions of the larynx. Assessment is typically multidimensional, but minimally includes documentation of voice characteristics and laryngeal deviations. Vocal rehabilitation focuses on establishing improved glottal efficiency which translates simply to improved approximation of the vocal folds. Primary treatments incorporate surgical medialization of the nonmoving vocal fold. Voice therapy may be indicated as either an adjunctive therapy prior to or following surgery or a primary treatment for voice improvement.

REFERENCES

Aronson, A. E. (1990). *Clinical voice disorders* (3rd ed.). New York: Thieme.

Ballenger, J. J. (1985). *Diseases of the nose, throat, ear, head and neck* (13th ed.). Philadelphia: Lea & Febiger.

Bassich, C. J., & Ludlow, C. (1986). The use of perceptual methods by new clinicians for assessing voice quality. *Journal of Speech and Hearing Disorders, 51,* 125–133.

Benjamin, B. (1993). Prolonged intubation injuries of the larynx: Endoscopic diagnosis, classification, and treatment. *Annals Otolology, Rhinology, and Laryngology, 102* (Suppl. 160), 1–15.

Blaugrund, S. M., Taira, T., Dren, A. E., Lin, P., Isshiki, N., & Gould, W. J. (1990). Effects of lateral manual compression upon glottic incompetence: Objective evaluations. *Annals of Otology, Rhinology and Laryngology, 99,* 248–255.

Boone, D. R. (1983). *The voice and voice therapy* (2nd ed.). Englewood Cliffs, NJ: Prentice-Hall.

Boone, D. R., & McFarlane, S. C. (1988). *The voice and voice therapy* (3rd ed.). Englewood Cliffs, NJ: Prentice-Hall.

Brewer, D. W., Woo, P., Casper, J. K., & Colton, R. H. (1991). Unilateral recurrent laryngeal nerve paralysis: A re-examination. *Journal of Voice, 5,* 178-185.

Brodnitz, F. S. (1958). The pressure test in mutational voice disturbance. *Annals of Otology, Rhinology, and Laryngology, 67,* 235–240.

Brodnitz, F. S. (1961). *Vocal rehabilitation* (2nd ed.). Washington, DC: American Academy of Ophthalmology and Otolaryngology.

Brook, J. W., & Schreiber, W. (1971). Vocal cord paralysis: A toxic reaction to vinblastine therapy. *Cancer Chemotherapy and Pharmacology, 55,* 591–593.

Case, J. L. (1991). *Clinical management of voice disorders* (2nd ed.). Austin, TX: Pro-Ed.

Colton, R. H., & Casper, J. K. (1990). *Understanding voice problems: A physiologic perspective for diagnosis and treatment.* Baltimore, MD: Williams & Wilkins.

Crary, M. A., Moore, G. P., & Cassisi, N. J. (1991, November). *Surgical voice restoration via Type 1 thyroplasty.* Seminar presented at the Annual Convention of the American Speech-Language and Hearing Association, Atlanta, GA.

Crumley, R. L. (1990). Teflon versus thyroplasty versus nerve transfer: A comparison. *Annals of Otology, Rhinology, and Laryngology, 99,* 759–763.

Ford, C. N., Bless, D. M., & Prehn, R. B. (1992). Thyroplasty as primary and adjunctive treatment of glottic insufficiency. *Journal of Voice, 6,* 277–285.

Gelfer, M. P. (1988). Perceptual attributes of voice: Development and use of rating scales. *Journal of Voice, 2,* 320–326.

Groher, M. E. (1984). *Dysphagia diagnosis and management.* Stoneham, MA: Butterworth Publishers.

Hiroto, I., Hirano, M., & Tomita, H. (1968). Electromyographic investigation of human vocal cord paralysis. *Annals of Otology, Rhinology, and Laryngology, 77,* 296–304.

Isshiki, N. (1989). *Phonosurgery theory and practice.* New York: Springer-Verlag.

Johns, M. E., & Rood, S. R. (1987). *Vocal cord paralysis: Diagnosis and management.* Washington, DC: American Academy of Otolaryngology—Head and Neck Surgery Foundation, Inc.

Kashima, H. K. (1984). Documentation of upper airway obstruction in unilateral vocal cord paralysis: Flow-volume loop studies in 43 subjects. *Laryngoscope, 94*, 923–937.

Kashima, H. K. (1991). Bilateral vocal fold motion impairment: Pathophysiology and management by transverse cordotomy. *Annals of Otology, Rhinology, and Laryngology, 100*, 717–721.

Kent R. D., Kent, J., & Rosenbek, J. (1987). Maximum performance tests of speech production. *Journal of Speech and Hearing Disorders, 52*, 367–387.

Kitzing, P. (1985). Stroboscopy: A pertinent laryngological examination. *Journal of Otolaryngology, 14*, 151–157.

Krieman, J., Gerrat, B. R., Kempster, G. B., Erman, A., & Berke, G. S. (1993). Perceptual evaluation of voice quality: Review, tutorial, and a framework for future research. *Journal of Speech and Hearing Research, 36*, 21-40.

LaBlance, G. R., & Maves, M. D. (1992). Acoustic characteristics of post-thyroplasty patients. *Otolaryngology—Head and Neck Surgery, 107*, 558–563.

Langmore, S. E., Schatz, K., & Olson, N. (1988). Fiberoptic endoscopic examination of swallowing safety. *Dysphagia, 2*, 216–219.

Logemann, J. A. (1983). *Evaluation and treatment of swallowing disorders*. San Diego, CA: College-Hill Press.

Logemann, J. A. (1986) *Manual for the videofluorographic study of swallowing*. Boston, MA: College-Hill Press.

Maran, A. G. (1979). Vocal cord paralysis. In A. G. Maran & P. M. Stell (Eds.), *Clinical otolaryngology*, (pp. 405–411). Oxford: Blackford Scientific Publications.

McFarlane, S. C., Holt-Romeo, T. L., Lavorato, A. S., & Warner, L. (1991). Unilateral vocal fold paralysis: Perceived vocal quality following three methods of treatment. *American Journal of Speech-Language Pathology: A Journal of Clinical Practice, 1*, 45–48.

Mikaelian, D. O., Lowry, L. D., & Sataloff, R. T. (1991). Lipoinjection for unilateral vocal cord paralysis. *Laryngoscope, 101*, 465–468.

Miller, R. H., & Duplechain, J. K. (1993). Hoarseness and vocal cord paralysis. In B. Bailey (Ed.), *Head and neck surgery—oto-laryngology* (pp. 620–629). Philadephia: J. B. Lippincott.

Netterville, J. L., Stone, R. E., Civantos, F. J., Luken, E. S., & Ossoff, R. H. (1993). Silastic medialization and arytenoid adduction: The Vanderbilt experience. *Annals of Otology, Rhinology, and Laryngology, 102*, 413–424.

Parnes, S. M. & Satya-Murti, S. (1985). Predictive value of laryngeal electromyography in patients with vocal cord paralysis of neurogenic origin. *Laryngoscope, 95*, 1323–1326.

Read, C., Buder, E. H., & Kent, R. D. (1992). Speech analysis systems: An evaluation. *Journal of Speech and Hearing Research, 35*, 314–332.

Rontal, E., & Rontal, M. (1986). The immobile cord. In C. W. Cummings, J. M. Frederickson, L. A. Harker, C. J. Krause, & D. E. Schuler (Eds.), *Head and neck surgery* (pp. 2055–2071). St. Louis: C. V. Mosby.

Sasaki, C. T., Leder, S. B., Petcu, L., & Friedman, C. D. (1990). Longitudinal voice quality changes following Isshiki thyroplasty type I: The Yale experience. *Laryngoscope, 100*, 849–852.

Slavit, D. H., & Maragos, N. E. (1994). Arytenoid adduction and type I thyroplasty in the treatment of aphonia. *Journal of Voice, 8*, 84–91.

Titze, I. R., & Liang, H. (1993). Comparison of fo extraction methods for high-precision voice perturbation measurements. *Journal of Speech and Hearing Research, 36*, 1120–1133.

Titze, I. R., & Winholtz, W. S. (1993). Effect of microphone type and placement on voice perturbation measurements. *Journal of Speech and Hearing Research, 36*, 1177–1190.

Tucker, H. M. (1987). *The larynx*. New York: Thieme Medical.

Tucker, H. M. (1990). Combined laryngeal framework medialization and reinnervation for unilateral vocal fold paralysis. *Annals of Otology, Rhinology, and Laryngology, 99*, 778–781.

Tucker, H. M. (1993). *The larynx* (2nd ed.). New York: Thieme Medical.

Vrabec, D. P. (1993). Inflammatory diseases of the larynx. In G. M. English (Ed.), *Otolaryngology* (pp. 1–30). Philadelphia: J. B. Lippincott.

Watterson, T., McFarlane, S. C., & Menicucci, A. l. (1990). Vibratory characteristics of Teflon-injected and noninjected paralyzed vocal folds. *Journal of Speech and Hearing Disorders, 55 , 61–66.

Willatt, D. J., & Stell, P. M. (1991). Vocal cord paralysis. In M. M. Paparella (Ed.), *Otolaryngology* (pp. 2289–2306). Philadelphia: W. B. Saunders.

Wilson, D. K. (1979). *Voice problems in children* (2nd ed.). Baltimore, MD: Williams & Wilkins.

Woodson, G. E., & Miller, R. H. (1981). The timing of surgical intervention in vocal cord paralysis. *Otolaryngology—Head and Neck Surgery, 89,* 264–267.

Yamaguchi, H., Yotsukura, Y., Hirosaky, S., Watanabe, Y., Hirose, H., Kobayashi, N., & Bless, D. M. (1993). Pushing exercise program to correct glottal incompetence. *Journal of Voice, 7,* 250–256.

Yanagihara, N. (1967). Hoarseness: Investigation of the physiological mechanisms. *Annals of Otology, Rhinolology, and Laryngology, 76,* 472–488.

Yumoto, E., Sasaki, Y., & Okamura, H. (1984). Harmonics-to-noise ratio and psychophysical measurement of the degree of hoarseness. *Journal of Speech and Hearing Research, 27,* 2–6.

CHAPTER 15

NEUROLOGICAL DISORDERS OF THE VOICE

LORRAINE OLSON RAMIG, PH.D.

INTRODUCTION AND DEFINITIONS

Voice disorders accompanying damage or disease to the nervous system are called neurological voice disorders. Because these disorders reflect a wide range of characteristics and etiologies, a number of classification systems have been proposed to assist in their description, diagnosis, and treatment planning.

Historically, neurological voice disorders were viewed in the context of dysarthria or motor speech disorders. Aronson (1980) labeled them "dysarthrophonias" and referred to them in relation to the classic dysarthria classification system of flaccid, spastic, ataxic, hypokinetic, hyperkinetic, and mixed dysarthrias (Darley, Aronson, & Brown, 1969a, 1969b). Ward, Hanson, and Berci (1981) proposed a similar framework to consider neurological voice disorders which included the efferent motor subcategories of upper motor neuron (cortex and pyramidal tracts), extrapyramidal (reticular substance), cerebellar, and nuclear (lower motor neuron).

Aronson (1980) proposed an additional classification system which was based on the constancy or variability of the acoustic symptoms accompanying the neurological voice disorders. He proposed the following categories: relatively constant (flaccid, spastic, pseudobulbar), mixed flaccid-spastic and hypokinetic, arhythmically fluctuating (ataxic, choreic, dystonic), rhythmically fluctuating (palatopharyngolaryngeal myoclonus and organic essential tremor), paroxysmal (Gilles de la Tourette's syndrome), and loss of volitional phonation (apraxia, akinetic mutism, and dysprosody of pseudo-foreign dialect). These approaches are based on an association between the voice disorder and the corresponding site of neurological damage and have made important contributions to the description and diagnosis of neurological voice disorders.

Ramig and Scherer (1992) proposed a system for considering neurological voice disorders with specific application to *treatment*. Rather than relating the neurological disorder to the site of neural damage, this classification system focuses on the existing laryngeal physical pathology and resulting voice characteristics. They proposed the following categories of neural laryngeal physical pathologies: adduction problems (hypoadduction and hyperadduction), stability problems (short-term, e.g., hoarseness, and long-term, e.g., tremor), and coordination problems (phonatory incoordination, e.g., dysprosody). Ramig and Scherer (1992) used these categories to organize approaches to treatment of neurological voice disorders which focused on modification of laryngeal physical condition with corresponding changes in perceptual characteristics of voice. This approach, which has been further developed by Smith and Ramig (1995) and Ramig (1995b), is discussed in detail in the section on speech pathology treatment later in this chapter.

PATHOGENESIS

The etiologies of neurological voice disorders are varied. Any damage or disease of the components of the peripheral or central nervous system that control laryngeal function can affect voice production. The most common etiologies of neurological voice disorders include trauma, cerebral vascular accidents, tumors, and diseases of the nervous system.

Flaccid neural laryngeal disorders involve damage or disease to one or more components of the motor unit (nucleus, ambiguus, vagus nerve, myoneural junctions, or laryngeal muscles). Viral infections, tumors, strokes, trauma, or degeneration of the cell bodies in the nucleus ambiguus or a wound to the recurrent laryngeal nerve branch of the vagus nerve (cranial nerve X) could result in laryngeal muscle paralysis. Myasthenia gravis is caused by autoimmune mechanisms that reduce available acetylcholine receptors at the neuromuscular junction and reduce laryngeal neuromuscular transmis-

sion. Muscular dysphonias or myopathies such as myotonic dystrophy, an autosomal dominant disorder with variable expression, may cause atrophy of laryngeal muscle fibers. The flaccid neural laryngeal disorders resulting from laryngeal nerve involvement are discussed in Chapter 14. This chapter will focus on the flaccid disorders associated with myasthenia gravis and myotonic muscular dystrophy.

Spastic (pseudobulbar) neural laryngeal disorders are associated with bilateral upper motor neuron damage. Such damage may occur with multiple, bilateral cerebral vascular accidents, any lesion of the corticobulbar tracts bilaterally, and vascular and degenerative diseases involving motor cortical areas bilaterally. In addition, vascular diseases and tumors of the internal capsule or brainstem, degenerative diseases involving the entire corticobulbar tract system, infectious diseases, and the congenital disorder of spastic cerebral palsy may be etiologies for spastic neural laryngeal disorders. Consequent release of inhibition of excitatory nerve impulses to vagal nuclei (Aronson, 1985) may result in hyperadduction of the true and false vocal folds observed in these disorders. It is important to distinguish spastic neural laryngeal voice disorders resulting from bilateral upper motor neuron damage from adductor spasmodic dysphonia (see Chapter 16).

Ataxic neural laryngeal disorders may occur following cerebellar damage resulting from strokes, traumas, toxins, tumors, or diseases such as Friedreich's ataxia.

Hypokinetic neural laryngeal disorders have been most commonly related to the degenerative neurological disorder idiopathic Parkinson disease. The etiology of this disease of the extrapyramidal system is unknown; however, it has been associated with both genetic and environmental factors. In Parkinson disease, degenerative changes in the substantia nigra result in depletion of the neurotransmitter dopamine. Parkinsonism is an umbrella term for other disorders that have some of the characteristics of idiopathic Parkinson disease but are the result of a virus, head trauma, carbon monoxide poisoning, toxic build-up, or the historic influenza epidemic (Darley, 1975). Disorders included under the term of Parkinsonism include postencephalitic Parkinsonism, progressive supranuclear palsy, and Shy-Drager syndrome.

Hyperkinetic neural laryngeal disorders are generally associated with diseases of the extrapyramidal system and include a range of diseases such as Huntington's disease, organic essential tremor, orofacial dyskinesia, dystonia, athetosis, palatopharyngolaryngeal myoclonus, and Gilles de la Tourette's syndrome. This chapter will focus on the hyperkinetic disorders associated with Huntington's disease and essential tremor. The abnormal "choreiform" movements accompanying the autosomal dominant disease of Huntington's disease are associated with the loss of neurons in the caudate nucleus. Vocal tremor accompanies a number of neurological diseases including organic essential tremor and has been associated with both a central and peripheral mechanism. Oscillations occurring in the olivocerebellorubral loop system have been suggested as the cause of essential tremor.

Mixed neural laryngeal disorders occur from damage or disease to multiple neural subsystems. For example, both lower motor neurons and bilateral upper motor neurons may be affected in amyotrophic lateral sclerosis (ALS) which is considered a flaccid and spastic dysarthria. The etiology of ALS is unknown; theories include viral infection and environmental factors. Demyelinization of both upper motor and cerebellar neurons occurs in multiple sclerosis (MS) which is considered a spastic and ataxic dysarthria. Etiologies of MS include an environmental agent (e.g., unspecified viral infection) in a genetically susceptible population.

DEMOGRAPHIC INFORMATION

The incidence of neurological voice disorders varies according to the incidence of the disorder or disease it accompanies. Not every patient with a neurological disorder will have a voice disorder; however, in some cases, voice disorders may be the first sign of a neurological disease.

For example, myasthenia gravis has a prevalence of 2–10 per 100,000 persons (Newsom-Davis, 1992) and at least 15% of affected individuals have a speech or voice disorder (Grob, 1958). Twice as many females as males have myasthenia gravis. Myotonic muscular dystrophy has a prevalence of 3–5 cases per 100,000 persons (Barchi & Furman, 1992) and speech and voice disorders are reported to occur commonly.

There are 500,000 new stroke cases per year; the frequency of co-occurring voice disorders has not been reported. At least 400,000 school-aged children have cerebral palsy with the incidence of dysarthria ranging from 31–59% (Wolfe, 1950) to 88% (Achilles, 1955).

Ataxic involvement can result from neoplasms, trauma, infarct, and neural degeneration. It has been reported that the prevalence of Friedreich's ataxia is 1 or 2 per 100,000 (Harding, 1983, 1984) with 63–93% of patients having dysarthria (Heck, 1964; Joanette & Dudley, 1980).

The prevalence of Parkinson disease is 1,000 per 100,000 in persons over age 60 and 100 in 100,000 under age 60. It has been reported that 1.5 million Americans have idiopathic Parkinson disease with 89% of these patients having a voice disorder (Logemann, Fisher, Boshes, & Blonsky, 1978).

The autosomal dominant disorder of Huntington's disease affects 4 to 8 per

100,000 individuals, with voice and speech disorders reported to occur frequently. The neurologic symptom of tremor occurs in a number of neurological disorders such as Parkinson disease, cerebellar disorders, and essential tremor. The neurological disorder of essential tremor is the most prevalent, occurring in 414.6 per 100,000 individuals and affecting 5 million people (Haerer, Anderson, & Schoenberg, 1982; Hubble, Busenbark, & Koller, 1989). Vocal tremor occurs in 4–20% of essential tremor patients (Elble & Koller, 1990) and may be the first or only sign of the disorder.

The mixed dysarthria of amyotrophic lateral sclerosis has an incidence of between 0.4 and 1.8 per 100,000 population. Its peak incidence is at the fifth to seventh decade of life. The male to female ratio is 1.5 to 1.0. Brainstem or bulbar involvement occurs in 30% of cases (Carpenter, McDonald, & Howard, 1979) and progresses more rapidly than spinal involvement.

In the northern part of the United States, the prevalence of the mixed dysarthria of multiple sclerosis (MS) is 100 per 100,000. Below the 37th parallel the prevalence is 35.5 per 100,000, and above the 37th parallel, the prevalence is 68.8 per 100,000. Approximately 40% of patients with MS have disordered speech and/or voice. The ratio of females to males is 1.5 to 1. Darley, Brown, and Goldstein (1972) reported that 59% of patients with MS had normal speech.

ONSET AND COURSE OF THE DISORDER

The onset and course of neurological voice disorders vary according to the etiology of the related neurological disorder. In the case of a voice disorder resulting from one discrete trauma, the disorder would be static with no expected deterio-

ration. In contrast, the voice disorder resulting from a degenerative neurological disease may deteriorate as the disease progresses. The relationship between the rates of progression of the neurological disease and the voice disorder is variable. In some cases, the deterioration appears parallel; in other cases, the rates of progression appear unrelated.

In females, the onset of myasthenia gravis is typically in the third decade of life, whereas in males onset most frequently occurs during the sixth decade. Myasthenia gravis patients reach a maximum level of weakness in 3 years (Grob, 1981); however, the disease has an unpredictable course. The mortality rate is 3.3%. Although the onset of the progressive disorder of myotonic dystrophy can be in childhood, typically it is in early adulthood, between ages 20–30 years. Death usually occurs in the fifth or sixth decade of life.

Friedreich's ataxia, one example of an autosomal recessive cerebellar disorder, usually has onset of symptoms between 8–15 years (Harding, 1981).

Although Parkinson disease is generally considered a disease of the elderly, with the diagnosis typically occurring in the sixth decade, the onset can occur as early as 35 years of age. Patients with Parkinson disease can live 10–20 years after diagnosis. In contrast, the parkinsonism disorder of Shy-Drager has a progressive course of about 5 years.

The average age of onset for Huntington's disease is 30–50 years of age, but cases have been reported as early as 5 and as late as 70 years of age. The mean age of onset of Essential Tremor (ET) is 48 or 57 years (Aronson & Hartman, 1981). Larsson and Sjogren (1960) report that essential tremor occurs more often in males.

The average age of onset of amyotrophic lateral sclerosis is 58 years with the average life expectancy of 17 months postdiagnosis. Death occurs in 50% of cases 3 years after diagnosis (Mulder, 1980; Tandan & Bradley, 1985); however, there are reports of patients stabilizing or progressing gradually over 15 years (Rosen, 1978; Rowland, 1980). Patients with bulbar signs deteriorate faster, with death usually resulting from aspiration pneumonia and respiratory paralysis. Ten percent of ALS patients survive 10 years.

The onset and course of multiple sclerosis varies. The exacerbating remitting type is most common under age 40. The acute progressive and chronic progressive types are most common after age 40. Ninety-five percent of the cases begin between 10 and 50 years of age, with the median age of onset being 27 years with a life expectancy of 35 years after onset.

MEDICAL CONSIDERATIONS

Certain classic medical symptoms contribute to the diagnosis of the neurological disorder and, subsequently, the accompanying voice disorder. For example, in myasthenia gravis, the common initial symptom is in the extraocular muscles. Other classic symptoms of myasthenia gravis include fatiguability and fluctuation and restoration of function after rest. In myotonic muscular dystrophy, the classic symptom of clinical myotonia is seen as the delayed relaxation of skeletal muscle after voluntary contraction.

In Friedreich's ataxia, the most frequent first symptom is ataxia of gait. Diagnostic criteria include progressive gait and limb ataxia. Hypotonia and incoordination of muscles may also be observed in ataxia.

In Parkinson disease, the physical pathologies of rigidity, tremor, reduced range of movement, and slowness of movement are observed together with the classic symptoms of mask-like face and micrographia. Diagnosis is made when three of these primary symptoms are observed plus a positive response to L-dopa.

In Huntington's disease, the choreiform movements (abrupt, jerky, purposeless) and progressive mental deterioration (loss of memory and intellectual capacity) are classic symptoms. Tremor has been observed in varied neurological disorders as well as in normal individuals under stress. The tremor accompanying the disease may appear at rest and is finer and less rhythmic than Parkinson tremor. It may occur first in the hand and progress to the face, arms, and neck. It can be accentuated by voluntary movement of the extremities or by emotional or physical stress.

The initial manifestations of ALS include muscle weakness, cramps, and fasciculations (Carpenter, McDonald, & Howard, 1978). It has been reported that 28% of patients with ALS presented with symptoms in the head, neck, larynx, or voice (Bonduelle, 1975; Carpenter et al., 1978; Dworkin & Hartman, 1979; Mulder, 1980; Tandan & Bradley, 1985). Classic signs of multiple sclerosis are varied: optic neuritis and sensory or motor disturbance of the limbs may be common presentations. Approximately two thirds of the patients have exacerbation and remission of symptoms; in the other third, the symptoms are progressive.

THE VOICE EVALUATION

Unlike many other voice disorders, neurological voice disorders may exist in the company of disorders of the speech subsystems of respiration, articulation, and resonance. In addition, swallowing problems are common in these neurological disorders. These co-occurring speech mechanism disorders must be considered in the assessment of the voice. Furthermore, patients may compensate laryngeally for disorders in another part of the speech mechanism and cognitive or emotional changes may accompany the neu-

rological dis
sider these va⌐.
to the disordered ⌐
voice disorders have b⌐
earliest symptom of a neu⌐
der, and this should be consid⌐
sessment as well.

Voice Characteristics

The primary perceptual descriptions of neurological voice disorders come from the work of Darley, Aronson, and Brown (1969a, 1969b, 1975); Aronson, Brown, Litin, and Pearson (1968); and Aronson (1980, 1985, 1990).

Myasthenia gravis has been characterized perceptually by inhalatory stridor, breathy voice, hoarseness, flutter, and tremor. Loudness is reduced, and there is a restriction of pitch range. There is progressively increased dysphonia including breathiness and reduced loudness while speaking (Walton, 1977). Mild breathy dysphonia and hypernasality have been reported (Aronson, 1971; Neiman, Mountjoy, & Allen, 1975; Wolski, 1967). Myotonic muscular dystrophy is characterized by weak, hoarse, and nasal voices (Ramig, Scherer, Titze, & Ringel, 1988).

Spastic (pseudobulbar palsy) voice is characterized by harshness (97%), strained-strangled quality (67%), abnormally low pitch (87%), monopitch (97%), pitch breaks and voice tremor (30%) (Aronson, et al., 1968). Nasality, monotone, and reduced intensity have also been reported (Aring, 1965). These characteristics typically occur in the presence of accompanying dysarthria.

The voice of the patient with an ataxic disorder is frequently within normal limits. When it is disordered, it may be characterized by a hoarse-harsh voice quality, sudden bursts of loudness, irregular increases in pitch and loudness, or coarse voice tremor. The voice may also be monopitch, too low, have a strain-strangled

⌐ality, and have pitch breaks (Aronson, ⌐). In addition, the voice disorder typ-⌐urs in the presence of accompa-⌐thria (Aronson, 1990). The ⌐accompanying Friedreich's ⌐een reported to be harsh ⌐ pitch breaks, prosodic ex-⌐phonatory-prosodic insufficien-⌐tte & Dudley, 1980).

⌐ voice of the patient with Parkinson disease has been described as reduced in loudness, monopitch, breathy, rough, hoarse, and, in some cases, tremorous. Reduced volume and monotone pitch may be the first signs of Parkinson disease (Aronson, 1990). Logemann et al. (1978) found that 89% of 200 patients with Parkinson disease demonstrated laryngeal dysfunction, and 45% had laryngeal dysfunction as the only symptom. They reported the following voice characteristics: breathiness (15%), roughness (29%), hoarseness (45%), and tremulousness (13.5%). These observations are consistent with those of Pawlas and Ramig (in review) who reported the following voice characteristics in addition to reduced loudness in a group of 45 patients with Parkinson disease: hoarseness (71%), monotone (49%), reduced stress (49%), unnatural prosody (40%), vocal fry (36%), mucous crackle (24%), and tremor (20%).

The voice of the individual with Huntington's disease is characterized by irregular pitch fluctuations and voice arrests (Ramig, 1986). Darley et al. (1969a) reported sudden forced inspiration or expiration, harsh voice quality, excess loudness variations, strained/strangled phonation, monopitch, monoloudness, reduced stress, transient breathiness, and voice arrests (Aronson, et al., 1968; Aronson, 1985) in the voices of patients with Huntington's disease. The tremorous voice accompanying essential tremor is characterized by "quavering intonation" (Aronson, 1990; Brown & Simonson, 1963; Colton & Casper, 1990). The pitch, loudness, and regularity of vocal tremor have been reported to vary, and there may be arrests of phonation.

The voices of individuals with ALS have been described in a number of studies. Carrow, Rivera, Mauldin, and Shamblin (1974) studied 79 patients with ALS and reported that 80% had harsh voice quality, 65% were breathy, 63% had tremor, 60% were strain-strangled, 41% had audible inhalation, 38% had excessively high pitch, and 8% had excessively low pitch. Darley et al. (1975) reported voices in ALS patients that were harsh (79.75%), strained-strangled (59.5%) with some breathiness (64.5%), reduced loudness, audible inhalation, "wet hoarseness," and hypernasality (74.7%). Rapid tremor or flutter on vowel prolongation was reported in 63.3% of the patients with ALS studied by Aronson, Ramig, Winholtz, and Silber (1992). It was suggested that the specific profile of voice characteristics in ALS (e.g., more flaccid or spastic) depended on the site of lesion. Darley et al. (1972) studied 168 patients with MS and reported that the 59% who were vocally disordered had voices characterized by the following: impaired loudness control (77%), harsh voice (72%), impaired intonation, inappropriate pitch, and breathiness. Farmakides and Boone (1960) reported impaired loudness, harshness, and hypernasality in patients with multiple sclerosis.

Endoscopy

Comprehensive endoscopic descriptive data sets do not exist on the majority of neurological voice disorders.

Myasthenia gravis or myotonic muscular dystrophy may reveal bilateral weakness of intrinsic laryngeal muscles. The vocal folds may adduct incompletely, and there may be bowing. Sluggish vocal fold adduction and increasing weakness of arytenoid and vocal fold motion has

been suggested in myasthenia gravis (Colton & Casper, 1990). Velopharyngeal inadequacy has been observed frequently in both myasthenia gravis and myotonic dystrophy.

Aronson (1990) suggests that the voice disorder accompanying spastic (pseudobulbar) dysarthria is caused by hyperadduction of the true and false vocal folds (i.e., glottic constriction and resistance to the exhalatory airflow). Aronson (1990) reports that the folds appear normal in structure. Kitzing (1985) suggested that, when hyperadduction occurs, there would be reduced vocal fold amplitudes, diminished mucosal waves, and excessive glottal closure.

Hanson, Gerratt, and Ward (1984) reported bowing and greater amplitude of vibration and laryngeal asymmetry in patients with Parkinson disease. Smith, Ramig, Dromey, Perez, and Samandari (1995) reported one of the first stroboscopic descriptions of these patients. They noted that 12 of 21 patients with Parkinson disease had a form of glottal incompetence (bowing, or anterior or posterior chink) on nasal fiberoptic views. Perez, Ramig, Smith, and Dromey (in press) recently reported visually rated laryngeal tremor in 55% percent of the 29 patients with idiopathic Parkinson disease they studied; the primary site of tremor was vertical laryngeal motion. The most striking stroboscopic findings for these individuals with idiopathic Parkinson disease were abnormal phase closure and phase asymmetry. Amplitude and mucosal waveform were essentially within normal limits in the majority of these patients.

Endoscopic descriptions of one individual with Huntington's disease revealed adductory movements at rest and termination of phonation seemingly by adductory laryngospasm (Ramig & Wood, 1983). Endoscopic descriptions of vocal tremor have revealed multiple sites of tremor including the posterior tongue and/or the posterior pharyngeal wall as well as laryngeal structures (Ardran, Kinsbourne, & Rushworth, 1966; Koda & Ludlow, 1992; Ludlow, Bassich, Connor, & Coulter, 1986; Smith & Ramig, 1995).

Endoscopic reports of ALS reveal that, if there is spastic involvement, patients may adduct normally or may hyperadduct with the false folds. If there is flaccid involvement, there is less abductory, adductory excursion (Aronson, 1990). Garfinkel and Kimmelman (1982) reported pooling of saliva in the pyriform sinuses and related that finding to the ALS "gurgle." Although endoscopic reports on MS are limited, the voice characteristics of "breathy" or "pressed" suggested that hypo- or hyperadduction may be observed (Smith & Ramig, 1995). Hypoadduction was observed in one patient with MS (Ramig, Countryman, Pawlas, & Fox, 1995).

Acoustic Analysis

Acoustic analysis of voice characteristics accompanying neurological disease has focused primarily on descriptions of frequency and intensity during sustained vowel phonation and reading. Application of acoustic analysis to the neurologically disordered voice may be challenging because of the variability and severity of many neurologically disordered voices.

Acoustic characteristics of voice in myasthenia gravis have included evidence of aperiodicity and high-frequency noise with improved periodicity of vocal fold function after edrophonium chloride injection (Rontal, Rontal, & Leuchter, 1978). Acoustic characteristics of voice in myotonic muscular dystrophy revealed elevated aperiodicity (Ramig et al., 1988).

Acoustic reports of voice in spastic pseudobulbar palsy are limited. Kammermeier (1969) reported fundamental frequency in male patients to be equal or

slightly higher than aged-matched control subjects. He also suggested that frequency and intensity ranges were reduced in these patients (Kammermeier, 1969).

Acoustic reports of voice characteristics of ataxic speakers have included the "aberration in control of F_0 (Kent, Netsell, & Abbs, 1979) and "monotone F_0 contours" (Kent & Netsell, 1975).

Acoustic studies of voice in Parkinson disease have included reports of intensity and frequency and their variability, as well as duration of sustained vowel phonation. Although perceptual reports consistently document patients with Parkinson disease as having reduced loudness, acoustic data are not always consistent with these perceptual observations. Canter (1963) reported that intensity was not reduced in a reading passage when individuals with Parkinson disease were compared to age-matched control subjects. However, Canter (1963) reported that, when "shouting," the vocal intensity of individuals with Parkinson disease was lower than normal. Ludlow and Bassich (1983) reported that intensity is reduced in Parkinson disease. Recently, Fox, Ramig, and Countryman (1995) reported that females with Parkinson disease were lower in intensity across speech tasks (average 1–3 dB less at 30 cm) when compared with an age- and gender-matched control group. Acoustic studies have reported higher speaking fundamental frequency in Parkinson disease (Canter, 1963, 1965a, 1965b; Kammermeier, 1969; Schley, Fenton & Niimi, 1982). It has been reported that patients with Parkinson disease read at an average of 129 Hz as compared to the mean frequency of 102 Hz of a control group. In contrast, Aronson et al. (1968) reported a very low speaking pitch level for individuals with Parkinson disease. It has been reported that frequency variability (Grewel, 1957) and pitch range (Schilling, 1925) were much less for individuals with Parkinson disease compared to control subjects. Canter (1965a, 1965b) also reported that individuals with Parkinson disease had much shorter maximum duration of sustained vowel phonation times (9.5 sec) compared to control subjects (20.6 sec). Recent findings following intensive voice treatment administered to individuals with idiopathic Parkinson disease (Lee Silverman Voice Treatment), document post-treatment increases in maximum duration of sustained vowel phonation, maximum fundamental frequency range, fundamental frequency variation (Ramig, Bonitati, Lemke, & Horii, 1994), and sound pressure level (Ramig, Countryman, Thompson, & Horii, 1995).

In an acoustic study of females with Huntington's disease, Jarema, Kennedy, and Shoulson (1985) reported statistically significantly shorter maximum phonation times for individuals with Huntington's disease when compared to controls. Ramig (1986) studied sustained vowel phonation and measured low-frequency segments (abrupt drops in frequency and return to original frequency; subharmonics), voice arrests, and reduced vowel duration in the phonation of individuals with Huntington's disease. Most of the acoustic data on vocal tremor have been obtained from visual displays of waveform data or graphic level recorded displays of amplitude contours of sustained vowel phonation. Tremor of essential tremor has been reported to be a rhythmic oscillatory movement of 4 to 12 Hz with variable amplitude.

Acoustic analysis of voice in ALS has documented increased cycle-to-cycle phonatory stability (Ramig, Scherer, Klasner, Titze, & Ringel, 1990; Strand, Yorkston, Buter, & Ramig, 1994) as well as 9–13 Hz frequency and amplitude variation associated with the perception of "flutter" (Aronson et al., 1992).

Aerodynamics

There are few data sets on aerodynamic characteristics of voice disorders accompanying neurological disease. The majority of papers describing aerodynamic data do so for flaccid involvement resulting in vocal fold paralysis. For example, von Leden (1968) reported mean airflow rate of 845 cc and 346 cc per second compared to 130 cc for normal male subjects and 94 cc for females (Koike, Hirano, & von Leden 1968) with recurrent laryngeal nerve paralysis. Hirano, Koike, and von Leden (1968) reported shorter maximum phonation time (excess expenditure of air) in 10 of 13 patients; mean flow rates in 8 of the 13 were greater than normal; and in 7 of 11, phonation quotients were greater. Given the likelihood that individuals with myasthenia gravis and myotonic muscular dystrophy have characteristics of hypoadduction, aerodynamic data may not be dissimilar to these data observed in vocal fold paralysis cases. Unfortunately, aerodynamic data for myasthenia gravis or muscular dystrophy are not available at this time.

For spastic dysphonia (pseudobulbar palsy), aerodynamic studies also are limited. It has been reported that mean airflow rate is decreased in individuals who phonate with hyperadduction of the vocal folds (von Leden, 1968). Measures of laryngeal resistance were 85% higher than average in a case of multiple bilateral strokes and marked strain-strangled voice quality (Smitheran & Hixon, 1981). Colton and Casper (1990) predict higher than normal subglottal air pressure in these patients because of hyperadduction.

Only recently have there been reports of aerodynamic data on patients with Parkinson disease. Recent findings support increases in subglottal air pressure from 6.6 (2.5) to 8.6 (2.9) cm H_2O accompanying increases of sound pressure level of 68.5 (4.2) to 75.0 (5.8) dB at 50 cm following intensive voice treatment administered to a group of 10 individuals with Parkinson disease (Dromey, Ramig & Johnson; 1995; Ramig, & Dromey, in press).

Aerodynamic data from patients with Huntington's disease (Jarema et al., 1985) report higher airflow rates than for normal controls.

Aerodynamic data from patients with ataxia, essential tremor, amyotrophic lateral sclerosis, and multiple sclerosis are not available at this time.

EMG

Although electromyographic studies are frequently reported for limb musculature and at times for lip musculature, there are limited electromyographic studies of laryngeal muscles in individuals with neurological voice disorders.

The primary data on laryngeal electromyographic activity have been reported on Parkinson disease. Hirose and Joshita (1987) reported data from the thyroarytenoid (TA) muscle in a patient with idiopathic Parkinson disease who had limited vocal fold movement. They reported no reduction in the number of motor unit discharges and no pathological discharge patterns (such as polyphasic or high amplitude voltages). They reported loss of reciprocal suppression of the TA during inspiration and interpreted this as evidence of deterioration in the reciprocal adjustment of the antagonist muscles associated with Parkinson rigidity. Guidi, Bannister, Gibson, and Payne (1981) reported higher resting activity and background activity in the interarytenoids (IA) and posterior cricoarytenoids (PCA) in a patient with Parkinsonism. Electromyographic study of eight patients with essential tremor found predominant involvement of the TA muscles as well as other extrinsic laryngeal muscles (Koda & Ludlow, 1992).

Social Implications

Patients with neurological voice disorders frequently present with a variety of social and emotional issues that may affect the diagnosis and treatment of their voice disorder.

Emotional

In addition to each patient's emotional response to disordered voice and impaired communication, emotional responses to neurological damage or progressive neurological disease have been well documented. For example, depression is frequently reported in patients with neurological diseases such as Parkinson disease (Mayeux, Williams, Stern, & Cote, 1986). Emotional lability is a frequently reported characteristic of pseudobulbar palsy (Darley, Aronson, & Brown, 1969a, 1969b).

Psychosocial

Various neurological disorders and diseases are characterized by neuropsychological problems such as memory, learning, language problems, and dementia. For example, it has been reported that it is not uncommon for individuals with Parkinson disease (Mayeaux et al., 1986; Mayeaux, Chen, & Mirabello, 1990), Huntington's disease (Bamford, et al., 1989), and multiple sclerosis (Rao, 1990) to have neuropsychological problems.

Educational and Vocational

Only limited data are available on the effects of neurolaryngeal disorders on education and vocational aspects of daily functioning. However, recently, Countryman, Ramig, King, and Pawlas (1995) reported positive effects of intensive voice treatment (Lee Silverman Voice Treatment; Ramig, Pawlas, & Countryman, 1995) on maintaining employment and quality of life in three employed individuals with Parkinson disease.

TREATMENT: OPTIONS AND OUTCOMES

Treatment of neurological voice disorders must be considered in the context of treatment for the overriding neurological disorder. Frequently, patients with neurological voice disorders are receiving neuropharmacological treatment or may have had neurosurgical treatment. Either or both of these treatments may influence their voices.

Surgical

Treatment for a neurological voice disorder may include neurosurgical treatment to treat the overriding neurological disorder or laryngeal surgical treatment to treat the disordered larynx. For example, patients with myasthenia gravis may receive a thymectomy to treat this disorder. This is especially useful for adolescents and young adults (Seybold, 1983).

Various neurosurgical procedures have been used to treat Parkinson disease: adrenal cell transplant, fetal cell transplant (Freed et al., 1992), and pallidotomy (Iacono & Lonser, 1994). Data on corresponding speech and voice changes following these procedures are accumulating. For example, Larson, Ramig, Freed, and Johnson (1994) reported that, although measures of limb movement improved following fetal cell transplant, measures of speech and voice did not show systematic changes. Thalamectomy has been used for a number of years to successfully reduce limb tremor (Manen, van Speelman, & Tans, 1984). However, reduced vocal volume has been associated with bilateral thalamectomy (Allan, Turner, & Gadea-Ciria, 1966; Selby, 1967).

In 1993, Countryman and Ramig reported pre- and post-treatment and follow-up data following an intensive voice treatment program (Lee Silverman Voice Treatment [LSVT]) administered to a patient with idiopathic Parkinson disease who had had bilateral thalamotomies. Although the patient demonstrated statistically significant improvements following treatment on various measures of phonatory stability, intensity, and fundamental frequency variation, she was unable to maintain these changes at 6- and 12-month follow-up. Data are variable in terms of the effect of surgical treatment on speech and voice production in Parkinson disease, but it appears that the magnitude and consistency of these effects are not adequate to consistently impact functional communication.

Pharmacological

Neuropharmacological treatments can be very useful in treating general motor symptoms of the neurological condition. For example, in myasthenia gravis, positive effects of tensilon/pyridostigmine (Mestinon) have been documented on symptoms of myasthenia gravis including the voice (Rontal et al., 1978). Neuropharmacological treatment for Parkinson disease supports amelioration of general motor symptoms with dopamine precursors (levodopa) or agonists (bromocriptine, pergolide mesylate). It has been suggested that Deprenyl may slow progression of disability (Shoulson & Fahn, 1989). However, the impact of these drugs on speech or voice production has not been established. Although there are papers to support positive effects of medication on voices of individuals with Parkinson disease (Audelman, Hoel, & Lassman, 1970; Mawdsley & Gamsu, 1971; Wolfe, Garvin, Bacon, & Waldrop, 1975), the findings do not support consistent and significant effects of neuropharmacological treatment on functional voice production. For example, in a study of on-off effects of medication on acoustic and electroglottographic measures of vocal function in two patients with Parkinson disease, Larson, Ramig, and Scherer (1994) reported no systematic or consistent relationship between drug cycle fluctuations and these measures. Medical treatment of Huntington's disease has involved pharmacological attempts to control the choreic movements with antidopaminergic agents, phenothiazines, benzodiazepines, or antiseizure medications (Brin et al., 1992). The effects of these drugs on voice in Huntington's disease have not been documented. Smith and Ramig (1995) report improved voice quality and ease of phonation in an individual with hyperadductory voice arrests associated with Huntington's disease following botulinum toxin injections into the thyroarytenoid muscle. The neuropharmacological treatment of essential tremor has involved various drugs (e.g., propranolol, primidone, acetazolamide, alprazolam, phenobarbital) with mixed results (Elble & Koller, 1990). Recently, Stager and Ludlow (1994) reported positive findings on use of BOTOX® for treatment of vocal tremor.

Speech Pathology

Behavioral treatment for neurological voice disorders has only recently been addressed systematically (Ramig, 1995b; Ramig & Scherer, 1992; Smith & Ramig, 1995). In contrast to previous approaches to speech treatment that have been directed to the etiological classification of disorders, the approach suggested by Ramig and colleagues presents a treatment framework in relation to the physical pathology in the laryngeal mechanism (see Table 15–1). Neurolaryngeal disorders have been classified as disorders of adduction (hypoadduction and hyperadduction) and instability (short- and long-term).

Treatment for Disorders Associated with Hypoadduction

Certain neurological disorders are accompanied by inadequate vocal fold adduction or hypoadduction. The particular type and extent of hypoadduction may be associated with the site and extent of the related neurological damage. Hypoadduction may accompany a variety of neurological disorders, but is often associated with lower motor neuron (flaccid) involvement, which is characterized by paresis (weakness) or paralysis (immobility), atrophy, and fatigue. Recently the hypoadduction accompanying Parkinson disease has received attention (Ramig, Paulas, & Countryman, 1995; Smith et al., 1995).

Recently, Lee Silverman Voice Treatment (LSVT) has been developed and studied for administration to patients with Parkinson disease (Ramig et al., 1994; Ramig, Countryman, & Pawlas, 1995). It is an intensive treatment program consisting of 16 sessions in 1 month. The focus of the LSVT is increasing vocal loudness by increasing respiratory or phonatory effort to maximize phonatory efficiency and functional speech productions. In addition to vocal loudness, the LSVT trains patients' self-monitoring of effort and loudness levels. Recent data (Ramig et al., in press) support maintenance of treatment effects for at least 1 year.

In general, in treatment approaches for patients with neurological disorders characterized by reduced adduction, the primary treatment goal is to increase loudness and reduce breathy, hoarse voice quality by increasing vocal fold adduction. Procedures used to accomplish this include pushing, pulling, and lifting while phonating (Froeschels, Kastein, & Weiss, 1955). The goal is to maximize adduction by "reinforcing the sphincter action of the laryngeal muscles engaged in phonation" (Froeschels et al., 1955). Other techniques used to increase adduction in-

Table 15–1. Therapeutic goals in treating perceptual characteristics of laryngeal disorders.

Laryngeal Disorders	Examples of Associated Neurologic Disorder	Perceptual Characteristics	Therapy Goals and Techniques
Hypoadduction	Laryngeal nerve paralysis Parkinson disease	Reduced loudness, breathy, hoarse voice quality	Increase loudness Increase adduction and respiratory support
Hyperadduction	Spasticity Extrapyramidal disorders	Pressed, harsh, strain-strangled voice quality	Reduce strained quality Relax laryngeal and respiratory musculature
Phonatory	Most neurologic disorders of the larynx	Tremorous, rough hoarse voice quality; pitch breaks; fry	Increase steady, clear phonation Maximize respiratory and laryngeal coordination

Source: Adapted from "Voice Therapy for Neurologic Disease" by L. O. Ramig, 1995. *Otolaryngology and Head and Neck Surgery, 3,* 174–182.

clude hard glottal attack, digital manipulation of the thyroid cartilage, and turning the head to one side or the other (to increase tension on the paralyzed fold) (Aronson, 1990). It is never the goal of these treatments to cause patients to hyperfunction, but rather to generate a maximally efficient voice source.

To facilitate the goal of increased loudness and improved quality, the respiratory system also is often a focus of treatment. The goal of respiratory treatment is to achieve a consistent subglottal pressure during speech that is produced with minimal fatigue and appropriate breath group lengths (Netsell & Daniel, 1979). Stabilization of posture may be considered first (Collins, Rosenbek, & Donahue, 1982; Murphy, 1965; Putnam & Hixon, 1985; Rosenbek & LaPointe, 1985). This may be followed by training to increase subglottal air pressure to "5 cm of water pressure for 5 sec" (Netsell & Hixon, 1978). Other techniques include exercises against a resistive load and controlled exhalation (Putnam, 1988). To train improved coordination of respiration and phonation, various techniques such as maximum duration vowel phonation (Ramig et al., 1994, 1995; Stemple, Lee, D'Amico, & Pickup, 1994) and phonation with simultaneous respiratory and vocal feedback have been suggested (Yorkston, Beukelman, & Bell, 1988). The patient with hypoadduction also may be encouraged to maximize oral resonance to increase loudness and quality. Details of these approaches have been reported by Ramig and Scherer (1992), Smith and Ramig, (1995), Ramig (1995b), and Ramig, Pawlas, and Countryman (1995).

Treatment for Disorders Associated with Hyperadduction

Certain neurological diseases result in excess vocal fold adduction, or hyperadduction. In some cases, the ventricular (false) vocal folds may hyperadduct as well (Aronson, 1990). The particular type and extent of hyperadduction may be associated with the site and extent of the related neurological damage. Hyperadduction most frequently occurs in cases of upper motor neuron system disorders characterized by spasticity and hypertonicity and extrapyramidal system diseases accompanied by abnormal involuntary movements (e.g., tics, chorea, dystonia) that may be focal or generalized. In addition, hyperadduction may be compensatory. For example, a patient may have weak respiratory support or velopharyngeal closure and hyperadduct to manage the air stream for adequate loudness (Putnam, 1988).

The primary focus of voice therapy for patients with hyperadduction is to decrease the pressed strained voice by reducing vocal fold hyperadduction. Procedures used to accomplish this are designed to relax laryngeal musculature and facilitate easy voice onset. These techniques may begin with whole body relaxation (Jacobson, 1976; McClosky, 1977) and then focus on laryngeal musculature. Other approaches include laryngeal massage, the chewing approach, the yawn-sigh, chanting, and delayed auditory feedback (Boone, 1983; Froeschels, 1952; Pershall & Boone, 1986). These techniques are based on the hypothesis that, when phonation is produced in the context of these reflex-like (Aronson, 1990) or continuous phonation responses, it will be more relaxed and less hyperadducted.

To facilitate the goal of improved voice quality, the respiratory system is often a focus of treatment in patients with hyperadduction. The goal of respiratory treatment is to achieve consistent, steady airflow with relaxed respiratory musculature (Aten, 1983). Once the patient's posture is stabilized, relaxed abdominal breathing may be trained to provide the greatest respiratory support with minimum muscle tension (Prater & Swift, 1984). These activities may be combined with progressive relaxation exercises. To encourage reduced hyperadduction and remove the laryngeal focus, some clinicians (Cooper & Cooper, 1977) encourage

"placement" of the vocal resonance in the front nasal area.

Instability

Certain neurological disorders are accompanied by increased phonatory instability. The particular type, extent, and regularity of the instability may be associated with the site and extent of the related neurological damage. Long-term fluctuations and short-term changes can occur as well as random or continuous use of alternative modes of voicing such as ventricular phonation, glottal fry, or diplophonia (Aronson, 1990; Ramig et al., 1988). These forms of instability may occur singly or in combination and may be related to the problems of adduction discussed previously.

The main focus of therapy for patients with phonatory instability is to reduce the unsteady, hoarse, rough voice quality by targeting steady, clear phonation. Patients are encouraged to maximize respiratory and laryngeal coordination, as discussed previously, to sustain steady voicing with consistent good quality. Treatments discussed earlier to promote more efficient vocal fold adduction have been reported to have positive effects on phonatory stability as well. For example, improved phonatory stability has been measured in patients with Parkinson disease after therapy designed to promote increased vocal fold adduction (Dromey et al., 1995).

Use of Augmentative/Alternative Communication Devices

In some cases, severity of the neurolaryngeal disorder in combination with breakdowns in other parts of the speech mechanism makes a form of augmentative or alternative communication the best choice to facilitate communication. These devices can range from a simple manual board up to devices which cost in the range of $3–8,000. The more advanced devices offer synthesized or digitized speech output which can be customized to the patient's needs. Some also include environmental control systems which enable the patient to maintain a higher level of independence. Regardless of the level of sophistication of the augmentative/alternative communication system, the patient, the patient's family, and the speech-language pathologist should work cooperatively in determining the vocabulary to be included and deciding which system to use.

Prognosis

Recently, data have been presented on the efficacy of voice treatment for patients with neurolaryngeal disorders. These data have been generated primarily around an intensive voice treatment program designed for patients with Parkinson disease called the Lee Silverman Voice Treatment (LSVT). Data from administration of this treatment (Ramig, Pawlas, & Countryman, 1995) support improved sound pressure level, fundamental frequency variation, vocal fold adduction, and subglottal air pressure as well as maintenance of these changes for 6 to 12 months without additional treatment when compared with a group of patients with Parkinson disease who received placebo treatment (Ramig, Countryman, O'Brien, Hoehn, & Thompson, in press). The rationale and techniques for the treatment have been summarized elsewhere (Ramig, Pawlas, & Countryman, 1995). These findings are consistent with data reported by others on the usefulness of intensive voice treatment for patients with idiopathic Parkinson disease (Scott & Caird, 1983; Robertson & Thompson, 1984). Application of these treatment concepts to selected patients with multiple sclerosis, stroke, ataxic dysarthria, and closed head injury has generated positive findings as well (Countryman, Ramig, & Pawlas, 1994; Ramig, Countryman, Pawlas, & Fox, 1995).

SUMMARY

The past few years have seen a great increase in academic and clinical interest in neurological voice disorders. Knowledge of the neural bases and physiology underlying these disorders continues to grow. Surgical, pharmacological, and behavioral treatments offer the potential to enhance speech production in individuals with these disorders. The combined efforts of the speech-language pathologist, neurologist, and otolaryngologist can provide optimal speech intelligibility for individuals with neurological disorders of the larynx.

REFERENCES

Achilles, R. (1955). Communication anomalies of individuals with cerebral palsy: I. Analysis of communication processes in 151 cases of cerebral palsy. *Cerebral Palsy Review, 16*, 15–24.

Allan, C. M., Turner, J. W., & Gadea-Ciria, M. (1966). Investigations into speech disturbances following stereotaxic surgery for Parkinsonism. *British Journal of Speech Communication Disorders, 1*, 55–59.

Ardran, G., Kinsbourne, M., & Rushworth, G. (1966). Dysphonia due to tremor. *Journal of Neurology, Neurosurgery, and Psychiatry, 29*, 219–223.

Aring, C. (1965). Supranuclear (pseudobulbar) palsy. *Archives of International Medicine, 115*, 198–199.

Aronson, A. E. (1971). Early motor unit disease masquerading as psychogenic breathy dysphonia: A clinical case presentation. *Journal of Speech and Hearing Disorders, 36*, 116–124.

Aronson, A. E. (1980). *Clinical voice disorders: An interdisciplinary approach.* New York: B. C. Decker.

Aronson, A. E. (1985). *Clinical voice disorders* (2nd ed.). New York: Thieme-Stratton.

Aronson, A. E. (1990). *Clinical voice disorders* (3rd ed.). New York: Thieme-Stratton.

Aronson, A. E., Brown, J. R., Litin, E., & Pearson, J. S. (1968). Spastic dysphonia II: Comparison with essential (voice) tremor and other neurologic and psychogenic dysphonias. *Journal of Speech and Hearing Disorders, 33,* 220–231.

Aronson, A. E., & Hartman, D. E. (1981). Adductor spastic dysphonia as a sign of essential (voice) tremor. *Journal of Speech and Hearing Disorders, 46,* 52–58.

Aronson, A. E., Ramig, L., Winholtz, W., & Silber, S. (1992). Rapid voice tremor or "flutter" in amyotrophic lateral sclerosis. *Annals of Otology, Rhinology, and Laryngology, 101,* 511–518.

Aten, J. (1983). Treatment of spastic dysarthria. In W. H. Perkins (Ed.), *Current therapy of communication disorders: Dysarthria and apraxia* (pp. 69–78). New York: Thieme.

Audelman, J. U., Hoel, R. L., & Lassman, F. M. (1970). The effect of L-dopa treatment on the speech of subjects with Parkinson's disease. *Neurology, 20*(4), 410–411.

Bamford, K. A., Caine, E. D., Kiddo, D. K., et al. (1989). Clinical pathological correlation in Huntington's disease: A neuropsychological and computed tomography study. *Neurology, 39,* 796–801.

Barchi, R. L., & Furman, R. E. (1992). Pathophysiology of myotonia and periodic paralysis. In A. K. Ashbury, G. M. McKhan, & W. I. McDonald (Eds.), Diseases of the nervous system. *Clinical neurobiology* (2nd ed., pp. 146–163). Philadelphia, PA: W. B. Saunders.

Bonduelle, M. (1975). Amyotrophic lateral sclerosis. In P. J. Vinten, & G. W. Gruyn (Eds.), *Handbook of clinical neurology* (pp. 281–338). Amsterdam: North Holland.

Boone, D. (1983). *The voice and voice therapy* (3rd ed.). Englewood Cliffs, NJ: Prentice-Hall.

Brin, M. F., Fahn, S., Blitzer, A., Ramig, L., & Stewart, C. (1992). Movement disorders of the larynx. In A. Blitzer, M. F. Brin, C. T. Sasaki, & K. Harris (Eds.), *Neurologic disorders of the larynx* (pp. 248–278). New York: Thieme Medical.

Brown, J. R., & Simonson, I. (1963). Organic voice tremor. *Neurology, 13,* 520–525.

Canter, G. J. (1963). Speech characteristics of patients with Parkinson disease: I. Intensity, pitch, and duration. *Journal of Speech and Hearing Disorders, 28,* 221–229.

Canter, G. J. (1965a). Speech characteristics of patients with Parkinson's disease: III. Articulation, diadochokinesis, and overall speech adequacy. *Journal of Speech and Hearing Disorders, 30,* 217–224.

Canter, G. J. (1965b). Speech characteristics of patients with Parkinson's disease: II. Physiological support for speech. *Journal of Speech and Hearing Disorders, 30,* 44–49.

Carpenter, R. J., III, McDonald, T. J., & Howard, F. M., Jr. (1978). The otolaryngologic presentation of amyotropic lateral sclerosis. *Otolaryngology, 86*(1), 479–484.

Carpenter, R. J., III, McDonald, T. J., & Howard, F. M., Jr. (1979). The otolaryngologic presentation of mysathenia gravis. *Laryngoscope, 89*(6, Pt 1), 922–928.

Carrow, E., Rivera, V., Mauldin, M., & Shamblin, L. (1974). Deviant speech characteristics in motor neuron disease. *Archives of Otolaryngology, 100,* 212–218.

Collins, M., Rosenbek, J., & Donahue, E. (1982). The effects of posture on speech in ataxic dysarthria. *Journal of the American Speech and Hearing Association, 24,* 767.

Colton, R., & Casper, J. (1990). *Understanding voice problems.* Baltimore: Williams & Wilkins.

Cooper, M., & Cooper, M. H. (Eds.). (1977). *Modern techniques of vocal rehabilitation.* Springfield, IL: Charles C Thomas.

Countryman, S., & Ramig, L. (1993). Effects of intensive voice therapy on speech deficits associated with bilateral thalamotomy in Parkinson disease: A case study. *Journal of Medical Speech-Language Pathology, 1,* 233–250.

Countryman, S., Ramig, L., King, J., & Pawlas, A. (1995, December). *The effect of intensive voice treatment on employability of patients with Parkinson disease.* Paper presented at the annual convention of the American Speech-Language-Hearing Association, Orlando, FL.

Countryman, S., Ramig, L., & Pawlas, A. (1994). Speech and voice deficits in Parkinson plus syndromes: Can they be treated?

Journal of Medical Speech-Language Pathology, 1, 233–250.

Darley, F. L. (1975). Treatment of acquired aphasia. *Advances in Neurology, 7,* 111–145.

Darley, F. L., Aronson, A. E., & Brown, J. R. (1969a). Differential diagnostic patterns of dysarthria. *Journal of Speech and Hearing Research, 12,* 246–269.

Darley, F. L., Aronson, A. E., & Brown, J. R. (1969b). Clusters of deviant speech dimensions in the dysarthrias. *Journal of Speech and Hearing Research, 12,* 462–496.

Darley, F. L., Aronson, A. E., & Brown, J. R. (1975). *Motor speech disorders.* Philadelphia: W. B. Saunders.

Darley, F. L., Brown, J. R., & Goldstein, N. (1972) Dysarthria in multiple sclerosis. *Journal of Speech and Hearing Research, 15,* 229–245.

Dromey, C., Ramig, L. O., & Johnson, A. B. (1995). Phonatory and articulatory changes associated with increased vocal intensity in Parkinson disease: A case study. *Journal of Speech and Hearing Research, 38,* 751–764.

Dworkin, J., & Hartman, D. (1979). Progressive speech deterioration and dysphagia in patients with amyotrophic lateral sclerosis: A case report. *Archives of Physical Medicine & Rehabilitation, 60,* 423–425.

Elble, R. J., & Koller, W. C. (1990). *Tremor.* Baltimore: John Hopkins University Press.

Farmakides, M. N., & Boone, D. K. (1960). Speech problems of patients with multiple sclerosis. *Journal of Speech and Hearing Disorders, 25,* 385–390.

Fox, C., Ramig, L., & Countryman, S. (1995, December). *Acoustic and perceptual characteristics of voice in females with idiopathic Parkinson disease and an age-matched control group.* Paper presented at the annual convention of the American SpeechLanguage-Hearing Association, Orlando, FL.

Freed, C., Breeze, R., Rosenberg, M., Schneck, S. A., Kriek, E., Qi, J., Lane, T., et al. (1992). Survival of implanted fetal dopamine cells and neurologic improvement 12 to 46 months after transplantation for Parkinson's disease. *New England Journal of Medicine, 327*(22), 1549–1555.

Froeschels, E. (1952). Chewing method as therapy. *Archives of Otolaryngology, 56,* 427–434.

Froeschels, E., Kastein, S., & Weiss, D. A. (1955). A method of therapy for paralytic conditions of the mechanisms of phonation, respiration, and glutination. *Journal of Speech and Hearing Disorders, 20,* pp. 365–370.

Garfinkle, T. J., & Kimmelman, C. P. (1982). Neurologic disorders: Amyotrophic lateral sclerosis, myasthenia gravis, multiple sclerosis, poliomyelitis. *American Journal of Otolaryngology, 3,* 204–212.

Grewel, F. (1957). Dysarthria in post-encephalitic Parkinsonism. *Acta Psychiatrica Neurologica Scandinavica, 32,* 440–449.

Grob, D. (1958). Myasthenia gravis: Current status of pathogenesis, clinical manifestations and management. *Journal of Chronic Disorders, 8,* 536–566.

Grob, D. (1981). Myasthenia gravis—retrospect and prospect. *Annals of the New York Academy of Sciences, 377,* xiii–xvi.

Guidi, G. M., Bannister, R., Gibson, W. P. R., & Payne, J. K. (1981). Laryngeal electromyography in multiple system atrophy with autonomic failure. *Journal of Neurology, Neurosurgery, and Psychiatry, 44,* 49–53.

Haerer, A. F., Anderson, D. W., & Schoenberg, B. S. (1982). Prevalence of essential tremor. Results from the Copiah County Study. *Archives of Neurology, 39*(12), 750–751.

Hanson, D. G., Gerratt, B. R., & Ward, P. H. (1984). Cinegraphic observations of laryngeal function in Parkinson's disease. *Laryngoscope, 94,* 348–353.

Harding, A. E. (1981). Friedreich's ataxia: A clinical and genetic study of 90 families with an analysis of early diagnostic criteria and intrafamilial clustering of clinical features. *Brain, 104,* 589–620.

Harding, A. E. (1983). Classification of the hereditary ataxias and paraplegias. *Lancet, 1,* 1151–1155.

Harding, A. E. (1984). *The hereditary ataxias and related disorders.* Edinburgh: Churchill Livingstone.

Heck, A. F. (1964). A study of neural and extraneural findings in a large family with Friedreich's ataxia. *Journal of the Neurological Sciences, 1,* 226–255.

Hirano, M., Koike, Y., & von Leden, H. (1968). Maximum phonation time and air usage during phonation. Clinical study. *Folia Phoniatrica, 20,* 185–201.

Hirose, H., & Joshita, Y. (1987). Laryngeal behavior in patients with disorders of the central nervous sytem. In M. Hirano, J. A. Kirchner, & D. M. Bless (Eds.), *Neurolaryngology: Recent advances* (pp. 258–266). Boston: Little, Brown.

Hubble, J. P., Busenbark, K. L., & Koller, W. C. (1989). Essential tremor. *Clinical Neuropharmacology, 12*(6), pp. 453–482.

Iacono, R. P., & Lonser, R. R. (1994). Posteroventral pallidotomy in Parkinson's disease. *Journal of Clinical Neuroscience, 2*(2), 140–145.

Jacobson, E. (1976). *You must relax* (5th ed.) New York: McGraw-Hill.

Jarema, A. D., Kennedy, J. L., & Shoulson, I. (1985, November). *Acoustic and aerodynamic measurements of hyperkinetic dysarthria in Huntington's disease.* Paper presented at the convention of the American Speech-Language-Hearing Association, Washington, DC.

Joanette, Y., & Dudley, J. G. (1980). Dysarthric symptomatology of Friedreich's ataxia. *Brain and Language, 10*(10), 39–50.

Kammermeier, M. A. (1969). *A comparison of phonatory phenomena among groups of neurologically impaired speakers.* Dissertation, University of Minnesota, Minneapolis.

Kent, R. D., & Netsell, R. (1975). A case study of an ataxic dysarthric: Cineradiographic and spectrographic observations. *Journal of Speech and Hearing Disorders, 40*(1), 115–134.

Kent, R. D., Netsell, R., & Abbs, J. H. (1979). Acoustic characteristics of dysarthria associated with cerebellar disease. *Journal of Speech and Hearing Research, 22*(3), 627–648.

Kitzing, P. (1985). Stroboscopy-a pertinent laryngological examination. *Journal of Otolaryngology, 14*(3), 151–157.

Koda, J., & Ludlow, C. (1992). An evaluation of laryngeal muscle activation in patients with voice tremor. *Otolaryngology, Head and Neck Surgery, 107*(5), 684–696.

Koike, Y., Hirano, M., & von Leden, H. (1968). Vocal initiation: Acoustic and aerodynamic investigations of normal subjects. *Folia Phoniatrica, 19*, 173–182.

Larson, K., Ramig, L., Freed, C., & Johnson, A. (1994, March). *Fetal cell transplant: Effects on acoustic characteristics of voice and speech.* Paper presented at the Motor Speech Conference, Sedona, AZ.

Larson, K., Ramig, L., & Scherer, R. (1994). Acoustic and glottographic voice analysis during drug-related fluctuation in Parkinson disease. *Journal of Medical Speech-Language Pathology, 2*, 227–239.

Larsson, T., & Sjogren, T. (1960). Essential tremor: A clinical and genetic population study. *Acta Physiologic Scandinavia, 36* (Suppl. 144), 1–176.

Logemann, J. A., Fisher, H. B., Boshes, B., & Blonsky, E. R. (1978). Frequency and occurrence of vocal tract dysfunctions in the speech of a large sample of Parkinson's patients. *Journal of Speech and Hearing Disorders, 42*, 47–57.

Ludlow, C. L., & Bassich, C. J. (1983). Relationships between perceptual ratings and acoustic measures of hypokinetic speech. In M. R. McNeil, J. C. Rosenbek, & A. E. Aronson (Eds.), *Dysarthria of speech: Physiology-acoustics-linguistics-management.* San Diego: College-Hill Press.

Ludlow, C., Bassich, C. J., Connor, N. P., & Coulter, D. C. (1986). Phonatory characteristics of vocal fold tremor. *Journal of Phonetics, 14*, 509–515.

Manen, J., van Speelman, J. D., & Tans, R. J. (1984). Indications for surgical treatment of Parkinson's disease after levodopa therapy. *Clinical Neurology and Neurosurgery, 86*, 207–212.

Mawdsley, C., & Gamsu, C. V. (1971). Periodicity of speech in parkinsonism. *Nature, 231*, 315–316.

Mayeaux, R., Chen, J., & Mirabello, E. (1990). An estimate of the incidence of dementia in idopathic Parkinson's disease. *Neurology, 40*, 1513–1517.

Mayeux, R., Williams, J., Stern, Y., & Cote, L. (1986). Depression and Parkinson's disease. In M. D. Yahr, & K. J. Bergmann (Eds.), *Advances in neurology* (pp. 241–250). New York: Raven Press.

McClosky, D. G. (1977). General techniques and specific procedures for certain voice problems. In M. Cooper, & M. H. Cooper, (Eds.), *Approaches to vocal rehabilitation* (pp. 138–152). Springfield, IL: Charles C Thomas.

Mulder, D. S. (1980). *The diagnosis and treatment of amyotrophic lateral sclerosis.* Boston: Houghton-Mifflin.

Murphy, A. T. (1965). *Functional voice disorders* (2nd ed.). Englewood Cliffs, NJ: Prentice-Hall.

Neiman, R. F., Mountjoy, J. R., & Allen, E. L. (1975). Myasthenia gravis focal to the larynx. *Archives of Otolaryngology, 101*, 56–570.

Netsell, R., & Daniel, B. (1979). Dysarthria in adults: Physiologic approach to rehabilitation. *Archives of Physical Medicine and Rehabilitation, 60*, 502–508.

Netsell, R., & Hixon, T. (1978). A noninvasive method for clinically estimating subglottal air pressure. *Journal of Speech and Hearing Disorders, 43*, 326–330.

Newsom-Davis, J. (1992). Diseases of the neuromuscular junction. In A. K. Ashbury, G. M. McKhann, & W. I. McDonald, W. I. (Eds.), *Disease of the nervous system, clinical neurobiology* (2nd ed., pp. 197–212). Philadelphia: W. B. Saunders.

Pawlas, A., & Ramig, L. (in review). Perceptual characteristics of speech and voice in idiopathic Parkinson disease. *Neurology.*

Perez, K., Ramig., L. O., Smith, M. E., & Dromey, C. (in press). The Parkinson larynx: Tremor and videolaryngostroboscopic findings. *Journal of Voice.*

Pershall, K. E., & Boone, D. R. (1986). A videoendoscopic and computerized tomographic study of hypopharyngeal and supraglottic activity during assorted vocal tasks. *Transcripts of the Fourteenth Symposium: Care of the Professional Voice* (pp. 276–282). New York: The Voice Foundation.

Prater, R. J., & Swift, R. W. (1984). *Manual of voice therapy.* Boston: Little, Brown.

Putnam, A. H. B. (1988). Respiratory dysfunction management. In D. E. Yoder, & R. D. Kent (Eds.), *Decision making in speech-language pathology* (pp. 121–131). Philadelphia: B. C. Decker.

Putnam, A. H. B., & Hixon, T. (1985). Respiratory kinematics in speakers with motor neuron disease. In M. McNeil, J., Rosenbek, & A. Aronson (Eds.), *The dysarthrias.* San Diego: College-Hill Press.

Ramig, L. A. (1986). Acoustic analysis of phonation in patients with Huntington's disease: Preliminary report. *Annals of Otology, Rhinology, and Laryngology, 95*, 288–293.

Ramig, L. O. (1995a). Speech therapy for patients with Parkinson's disease. In W. Koller, & G. Paulson (Eds.), *Therapy of parkinson's disease* (pp. 539–548). New York: Marcel Dekker.

Ramig, L. O. (1995b). Voice therapy for neurologic disease. *Current Opinion in Otolaryngology, Head and Neck Surgery, 3*, 174–182.

Ramig, L., Bonitati, C., Lemke, J., & Horii, Y. (1994). Voice treatment for patients with Parkinson disease: Development of an approach and preliminary efficacy data. *Journal of Medical Speech-Language Pathology, 2*, 191–209.

Ramig, L., Countryman, S., O'Brien, C., Hoehn, M., & Thompson, L. (in press). Intensive speech treatment for patients with Parkinson disease: Short- and long-term comparison of two techniques. *Neurology.*

Ramig, L., Countryman, S., Thompson, L., & Horii, Y. (1995). A comparison of two forms of intensive speech treatment for Parkinson disease. *Journal of Speech and Hearing Research, 38, 6*, 1232–1251.

Ramig, L., Countryman, S., Pawlas, A., & Fox, C. (1995, December). *Voice treatment for Parkinson disease and other neurological disorders.* An Institute presented at the annual convention of the American Speech-Language-Hearing Association, Orlando, FL.

Ramig, L., & Dromey, C. (in press). Aerodynamic mechanisms underlying treatment-related changes in vocal intensity in patients with Parkinson disease. *Journal of Speech and Hearing Research.*

Ramig, L., Pawlas, A., & Countryman, S. (1995). *The Lee Silverman Voice Treatment: A practical guide for treating the voice and speech disorders in Parkinson disease.* Iowa City: National Center for Voice and Speech, University of Iowa.

Ramig, L. O., & Scherer, R. C. (1992). Speech therapy for neurologic disorders of the larynx. In A. Blitzer, M. F. Bri, C. T. Sasaki, S. Fahn, & K. S. Harris (Eds.), *Neurologic disorders of the larynx* (pp. 163–181). New York: Thieme Medical.

Ramig, L., Scherer, R., Klasner, E., Titze, I., & Ringel, S. (1990). Acoustic analysis of voice in amyotrophic lateral sclerosis: A longitudinal case study. *Journal of Speech and Hearing Disorders, 55,* 2–14.

Ramig, L. A., Scherer, R. C., Titze, I. R., & Ringel, S. P. (1988). Acoustic analysis of voices of patients with neurologic diseases: Rationale and preliminary data. *Annals of Otology, Rhinology, and Laryngology, 97,* 164–172.

Ramig, L. O., & Wood, R. (1983). Personal notes.

Rao, S. M. (1990). *Neurobehavioral aspects of multiple sclerosis.* New York: Oxford University Press.

Robertson, S., & Thompson, F. (1984). Speech therapy in Parkinson's disease: A study of the efficacy and long-term effect of intensive treatment. *British Journal of Disorders of Communication, 19,* 213–224.

Rontal, M., Rontal, E., & Leuchter, W. (1978). Voice spectrography in the evaluation of myasthenia gravis of the larynx. *Annals of Otology, Rhinology, and Laryngology, 87,* 722–728.

Rosen, A. D. (1978). Amyotrophic lateral sclerosis: Clinical features and prognosis. *Archives of Neurology, 35,* 638–642.

Rosenbek, J., & LaPointe, L. L. (1985). The dysarthrias: Description, diagnosis, and treatment. In D. F. Johns (Ed.), *Clinical management of neurogenic communicative disorders* (2nd ed., pp. 97–152). Boston: Little, Brown.

Rowland, L. P. (1980). Motor neuron diseases: The clinical syndromes. In D. W. Mulder (Ed.), *The diagnosis and treatment of amyotrophic lateral sclerosis* (p. 7–33). Boston: Houghton-Mifflin.

Schilling, R. (1925). Experimentell-phonetische untersuchunger bei Erkrankunger des extrapyramidalen systems. *Arch. Psychiatr. Neuenkr., 75,* 419–471.

Scott, S., & Caird, F. L. (1983). Speech therapy for Parkinson's disease. *Journal of Neurology, Neurosurgery, and Psychiatry, 46,* 140–144.

Selby, G. (1967). Stereotactic surgery for the relief of Parkinson disease: 2. An analysis of the results in a series of 303 patients (413 operations). *Journal of Neurological Science, 5,* 342–375.

Seybold, M. E. (1983). Myasthenia gravis. A clinical and basic science review. *Journal of the American Medical Association, 250*(18), 2516–2521.

Shoulson, I., & Fahn, S. (1989). Parkinson study group. Effect of deprenyl on the progression of disability in early Parkinson's disease. *New England Journal of Medicine, 321,* 1364–1371.

Smith, M.E., & Ramig, L. O. (1995). Neurological disorders and the voice. In J. S. Rubin, R. T. Sataloff, G. S. Korovin, & W. J. Gould (Eds.), *Diagnosis and treatment of voice disorders* (pp. 203–224). New York: Igaku-Shoin.

Smith, M. E., Ramig, L. O., Dromey, C., Perez, K. S., & Samandari, R. (1995). Intensive voice treatment in Parkinson's disease: Laryngostroboscopic findings. *Journal of Voice, 9*(4), 453–459.

Smitheran, J., & Hixon, T. (1981). A clinical method for estimating laryngeal airway resistance during vowel production. *Journal of Speech and Hearing Research, 46,* 138–146.

Stager, S., & Ludlow, C. (1994). Responses of stutterers and vocal tremor patients to treatment with botulinum toxin. In J. Jankovic, M. Hallet, (Eds.). *Therapy with botulinum toxin* (pp. 481–490). New York: Marcel Dekker.

Stemple, J., Lee, L., D'Amico, B., & Pickup, B. (1994). Efficacy of vocal function exercises as a method of improving voice production. *Journal of Voice, 8*(3), 271–278.

Strand, E., Yorkston, K., Buter, E., & Ramig, L. (1994). Differential phonatory characteristics of four women with amyotrophic lateral sclerosis. *Journal of Voice, 8*(4), 327–339.

Tandan, R., & Bradley, W. G. (1985). Amyotrophic lateral sclerosis: Part 1. Clinical features, pathology, and ethical issues in management. *Annals of Neurology, 18,* 271–280.

von Leden, H. (1968). Objective measures of laryngeal function and phonation. *Annals of the New York Academy of Science, 155,* 56–67.

Ward, P. H., Hanson, D., & Berci, G. (1981). Photographic studies of the larynx in central laryngeal paresis and paralysis. *Acta Otolaryngologica* (Stockholm), *91,* 353–367.

Walton, J. (1977). Muscular dystrophy: Some recent developments in research. *Israel Journal of Medical Sciences, 13*(2), 152–158.

Wolfe V. I., Garvin, J. S., Bacon, M., & Waldrop, W. (1975). Speech changes in Parkinson's disease during treatment with L-dopa. *Journal of Communication Disorders,* 8, 271–279.

Wolfe, W. G. (1950). Comprehensive evaluation of 50 cases of cerebral palsy. *Journal of Speech and Hearing Disorders, 15,* 234–251.

Wolski, W. (1967). Hypernasality as the pre-senting system of myasthenia gravis. *Journal of Speech and Hearing Disorders, 32*(1), 36–38.

Yorkston, K., Beukelman, D., & Bell, K. (1988). *Clinical management of dysarthria of speech.* Boston: College-Hill Press.

CHAPTER 16

SPASMODIC DYSPHONIA

THOMAS MURRY, PH.D.
GAYLE E. WOODSON, M.D., F.R.C.S.

INTRODUCTION AND DEFINITIONS

Spasmodic dysphonia is a chronic voice disorder of unknown origin, characterized by excessive or inappropriate contraction of laryngeal muscles during speech. It was first described by Traube (1871) who believed it to be a form of nervous hoarseness. For many years the disorder was referred to as "spastic dysphonia," but more recently the term "spasmodic dysphonia" has gained wide acceptance. The terms "spastic" and "spasticity" refer to muscle rigidity, such as that associated with corticospinal tract lesions (Basmajian & DeLuca, 1985). In contrast, the excessive muscle contraction in spasmodic dysphonia is intermittent and occurs during phonation (Miller & Woodson, 1991); hence, the term "spasmodic dysphonia."

Spasmodic dysphonia (SD) may be manifested by excessive glottic closure (adductor spasmodic dysphonia), incomplete, irregular vocal fold approximation (abductor dysphonia), or a combination of the two. Adductor dysphonia, the form originally described and most commonly

observed clinically, is characterized by strained-strangled phonation and irregular voice stoppages. Abductor spasmodic dysphonia presents with a breathy voice or brief absences of voicing, associated with abrupt widening of the glottis. This second form was first described by Aronson (1977). Since then, it has been recognized that some patients have a combination of both types of vocal symptoms (Aronson, 1980; Cannito & Johnson, 1981).

PATHOGENESIS

Neither the cause nor the pathophysiologic mechanism of spasmodic dysphonia is known. Originally, it was thought to be a psychological problem, because of the disparity between the vocal handicap and the apparently normal anatomy of the larynx, and because variations in symptom severity usually correlate with stress. Numerous reports in the literature describe a psychogenic basis for the disorder (Arnold, 1959; Boone, 1971; Brodnitz, 1976; Critchley, 1939; Heaver, 1959). However, an increasing body of evidence supports an organic cause and suggests that, in most cases, the disorder is a focal dystonia of the larynx (Blitzer, Brin, Fahn, & Lovelace, 1988a).

In a landmark study, Robe, Brumlik, and Moore (1960) identified a specific neurologic disease in 4 of 10 patients studied. Moreover, eight had a positive history of neurologic disturbance prior to the onset of their disorder. Eight years later, Aronson, Brown, Litin, and Pearson (1968) described neurologic signs in 20 of 27 patients. These included voice tremor, facial and tongue twitches, increased sucking reflexes and torticollis. Additional early support of a neurological basis for spasmodic dysphonia was provided by several investigators using acoustic, perceptual, and familial history data (Aminoff, Dedo, & Izdebski, 1978; Aronson & Hartman, 1981; Dordain & Dordain, 1972; Rabuzzi & McCall, 1972).

The case for an organic basis was strengthened when Dedo (1976) produced a dramatic improvement in the speech of SD patients by transecting the recurrent laryngeal nerve. Although the voice did not return to normal in all cases, the success of a surgical procedure in treating a problem so resistant to psychiatric and speech therapy strongly suggested an organic rather than a psychologic cause.

Additional support for a neurological basis of the disorder was provided by Schaffer (1983) who performed three independent evaluations of brainstem function on patients with spasmodic dysphonia and on a normal control group matched by age and sex. Schaffer found statistically significant differences between the two groups. In addition, he found a significant correlation between severity of CNS impairment and vocal tremor, number of associated neurologic signs, and duration of illness. Vital or traumatic factors did not correlate with severity of brainstem impairment. Schaffer concluded that SD appeared to be a spasmodic brainstem disorder.

The prevailing opinion today is that the vast majority of patients with spasmodic dysphonia have a medical disease: a focal dystonia of the larynx. The term dystonia refers to a syndrome of sustained muscle contractions. Dystonic movements are aggravated or become manifest during voluntary movement, and get worse with fatigue or physical or emotional stress. Dystonia may be generalized (as in postural torsion dystonia involving the limbs or trunk), regional, or focal (involving an isolated, typically task-related muscle group). SD is most often a focal dystonia, but may present as a regional dystonia such as Meige's Syndrome, blepharospasm, and/or torticollis. Primary generalized dystonia is clearly a genetic disorder, and has been attributed to a defect on chromosome 9q32-34 (Ozelius, Kramer, & Moskowitz, 1989). It is not known whether patients with primary focal dystonias, such as SD, have a genetic defect.

Isolated SD, like other organic neuromotor disorders, is frequently associated with tremor. Essential tremor, a common neurologic disorder of middle to late adulthood, causes 6–8 Hz shaking, primarily of the hands, head, and voice. In SD, the tremor may be isolated to the larynx, or may involve the pharynx, head, or even the hands. In a recent video endoscopic study of 38 patients with spasmodic dysphonia, Woodson et al. noted tremor of the larynx or pharynx in 29 of the patients (Woodson, Zwirner, Murry, & Swenson, 1991). Rosenfield et al. found essential tremor in 71 of 100 subjects with SD, involving the larynx and/or pharynx (Rosenfield et al., 1991). Other authors also have noted a high incidence of tremor in association with SD (Aronson & Hartman, 1981; Freeman, Cannito, & Finitzo-Hieber, 1984; Parnes, Lavarato, & Meyers, 1978).

The results of EMG studies by Ludlow et al. (Ludlow, Hallet, Sedory, Fujita, &

Naughton, 1990; Ludlow, Naughton, Sedory, Schulz, & Hallett, 1988) suggest that the voluntary movement abnormalities seen in SD are characteristic of a focal dystonia. SD patients have abnormally high resting EMG activity levels in both the thyroarytenoid (TA) and cricothyroid (CT) muscles and an imbalance between TA and CT muscles which results in increased adduction and tension in anterior-posterior dimension during speech, swallow, and quiet breathing. It has been suggested that SD may involve increased sensitivity of motoneuron pools in the brainstem. Alternatively, there may be some other defect in the feedback control of motor function in speech.

The pathophysiology of dystonia is not known. Although primary dystonia is not associated with any particular brain lesion, secondary generalized dystonia is often associated with lesions in the basal ganglia (Burton, Farrell, Li, & Calne, 1984; Jankovic & Patel, 1983). Electrophysiologic studies implicate dysfunction in the pyramidal tract or basal ganglia. A few biochemical studies of autopsied brains have demonstrated altered levels of neurotransmitters in various regions of the midbrain (Hornykiewicz, Kish, Becker, Farley, & Shannon, 1986; Jankovic, Svendson, & Bird, 1988). A neurotransmitter defect is also suggested by the finding that some dystonia patients improve significantly on L-dopa therapy (Nygaard, 1989). The preponderance of evidence, therefore, suggests that idiopathic dystonias are due to an abnormality of neurotransmitters in the basal ganglia.

Some patients have spasmodic dysphonia symptoms which have been clearly attributed to psychiatric causes. Other patients develop spasmodic dysphonia after head trauma or toxic exposure. It is likely that pathophysiology is variable and that SD is not a homogeneous entity.

DEMOGRAPHIC INFORMATION

Early textbooks reported that SD was a relatively rare voice disorder; however, recent reports in the literature would suggest that it is not a rare disorder, but rather one that is not frequently diagnosed and reported. In most studies, the disorder affects more females than males. Reported male to female ratios range from 1:1 (Miller & Woodson, 1991) to 1:8 (Aronson, 1985). In our population of 155 subjects (Woodson & Murry, 1993), one male SD patient presented for every 4.2 females over a 3.5-year period.

The onset of SD is generally in the age range of 40–60 years (Aronson, 1977); however, it may occur as early as the teens in rare exceptions and as late as 80. Reports of the mean age of SD patients are typically in the 48–50 year range. Woodson et al. (1991) described 38 SD patients with a mean age of 51 years; however, symptoms had been present for a mean of 7.5 years. This indicates onset at a younger age than previously reported. Although a genetic basis has not been established for SD, some patients report relatives with similar voice problems or other dystonias. Blitzer and his colleagues (Blitzer, Lovelace, Brin, Fahn, & Fink, 1985) found that 23% of 110 patients reported a family history of dystonia.

ONSET AND COURSE OF DISORDER

Most SD patients relate some potential precipitating factor which was temporally related to the onset of the voice disorder. Tables 16–1 and 16–2 summarize these factors in two categories: physical symptoms reported to be present at or near the time of diagnosis and emotional factors occurring near the time of onset or felt to be related to the onset by the patient, respectively.

Table 16–1. Physical symptoms commonly associated with onset of spasmodic dysphonia.

Physical Symptoms	Reference
"Sore throat"	Rosenfield (1991)
Familial tremor	Freeman and Cannito (1972) Dordain and Dordain (1972)
Traumatic head/neck injury (whiplash) Viral infection Arthritis Following laryngeal surgery	Freeman, Cannito, and Finitzo-Hieber (1985)
Nonspecific hoarseness	Aronson (1980)
Disease of CNS	Aronson and DeSanto (1983)
Focal dystonias	Blitzer et al. (1985)
Tremor	Aronson, Brown, Litin, and Pearson (1968)
Central brainstem abnormality	Feldman, Nixon, Finitzo-Hieber, and Freeman (1984)
Brainstem abnormality	Finitzo-Hieber and Freeman (1989) Sharbrough, Stockard, and Aronson (1978)
Familial neurologic disease CNS disease Multiple sclerosis	Robe, Brumlik, and Moore (1960)

Table 16–2. Emotional symptoms commonly associated with onset of spasmodic dysphonia.

Emotional Symptoms	Reference
Job stress Family death Marital discord Emotionally traumatic events	Freeman, Cannito, and Finitzo-Hieber (1985)
Interpersonal conflicts	Aronson (1979)
Suppression of aggression	Brodnitz (1976) Heaver (1959)

It should be pointed out that Tables 16–1 and 16–2 do not necessarily reflect cause and effect. Probably no single cause of this disease exists. Nonetheless, numerous physical findings and emotional events have been frequently detected in the course of evaluating these patients. Associated factors may be implicated as causing SD or merely as unmasking the disorder by hindering compensatory function. Finitzo and Freeman (1989) reported that 84% of the SD subjects they studied had multifocal structural, metabolic and/or electrophysiologic abnormalities of the central nervous system. This heterogeneity of factors associated with onset of the disease is congruent with the multiple descriptive voice and speech characteristics associated with SD.

MEDICAL CONSIDERATIONS

It is apparent that a neurological disorder is present in the majority of SD patients (Cannito & Johnson, 1981; Finitzo & Freeman, 1989; Schaffer, 1983). Dystonias may be primary or result from some other disease process. It is also true that some patients with symptoms similar to SD actually suffer from some other neurologic problem, such as parkinsonism, pseudobulbar palsy, or cerebellar disorders. The history and physical examination should therefore particularly focus on searching for evidence of an underlying cause and ruling out disorders with similar vocal symptoms (Swenson, Zwirner, Murry, & Woodson, 1992).

A careful drug history should include specific questioning regarding previous psychotropic medication. Some antihypertensive medications can cause similar dyskinesias. Transient ischemic attacks (TIAs), strokes, head trauma, previous brain surgery, or infections may also be factors. A family history of dystonia, tremor, or similar voice problems would be consistent with, but not diagnostic of, a primary dystonia.

The physical examination in SD usually is remarkable only for the dystonic movements or associated tremor. Indeed for many years the sine qua non of spasmodic dysphonia was the finding of a severely impaired and strangled sounding voice in the absence of any apparent physical deficit. More recently, the use of fiberoptic laryngeal examination during connected speech reveals that, although the larynx is structurally normal, its movements are not. In adductor dysphonia, the vocal folds are rigid or tightly adducted, either continuously or episodically. In abductor dysphonia, the vocal folds abruptly open, most commonly during the transition from a plosive consonant to a vowel, as in "Pay Paul a penny." As noted above, a high percentage of patients also have endoscopically observable laryngeal and/or pharyngeal tremor, and spasmodic movements are sometimes noted during quiet breathing. The presence of supralaryngeal hyperfunction (false vocal fold closure or anterior-posterior laryngeal compression) and movement in associated structures (epiglottis, tongue) during speech and quiet respiration have been observed (Woodson, Zwirner, Murry, & Swenson, 1991).

An important part of the medical evaluation is a careful neurologic examination. The occurrence of other neurologic signs, aside from other dystonias or tremor, suggests that SD is secondary to another disease process. A thorough investigation for the cause is then warranted. The neurologic examination also may detect signs of other neurologic disorders that may be misconstrued as spasmodic dysphonia.

In routine clinical management, a careful history and physical examination will establish the disorder as a primary focal or segmental dystonia. Thyroid function tests, erythrocyte sedimentation rate, CBC, and chemistry panel are useful to rule out other systemic disorders. However, brain imaging should be reserved for patients with focal findings on neurologic examination beyond the distribution of the dystonia. There is no current indication for the routine clinical use of electrophysiologic testing.

THE VOICE EVALUATION

The voice evaluation for spasmodic dysphonia is necessary to: (a) rule out other disease that may present with similar vocal characteristics as spasmodic dysphonia; (b) determine the severity and variability of the disease over various speaking conditions; and (c) plan a course of treatment that will maximize communication.

Voice Characteristics

Some vocal characteristics of SD are present in other generalized neurological disorders. Thus, evaluation of the voice should discriminate signs of focal laryngeal dystonia from those of other neurological disorders. The classic perceptual sign of SD is strained voice quality, heard in contextual speech but not necessarily in singing, laughing, falsetto voice, or crying. Although easily recognized, objective description and assessment of SD is quite difficult due to symptom variability over time and speaking conditions. It is important to separate other neurological disorders from spasmodic dysphonia. These disorders (e.g., Parkinson disease, pseudobulbar palsy, cerebellar disorders, multiple sclerosis and essential tremor) all share variants of the strained, strong, or harsh voice qualities of SD. However, careful evaluation of speech and voice will show that, while SD is focal to the larynx, the other disorders present with characteristics such as slow labored speech, dysarthria and possibly altered resonance (Parkinson, pseudobulbar palsy) or explosive speech and dysmetria (cerebellar disorders). Frequent accompaniments to SD are voice tremor, oromandibular dystonia (Meige's syndrome), and blepharospasm (Blitzer et al., 1988a). At present, there are no clinically conclusive tests to confirm SD and no uniform guidelines to follow in evaluating patients for SD. Recent studies have provided clinicians with acoustic and perceptual characteristics (Zwirner, Murry, & Woodson, 1993a) of the disorder as well as the general movement characteristics of the vocal folds seen through endoscopic analysis. Further, it has been reported that, as a group, SD patients tend to have elevated scores on depression and anxiety scales (Murry, Cannito, & Woodson, 1994). Nonetheless, as Woodson et al. (1991) point out, it is not possible to objectively measure the physical and emotional difficulty the patient experiences when trying to communicate. Acoustic, physiologic, and endoscopic data provide only an index of severity. SD reflects a problem much more aberrant than physical measures alone depict.

Endoscopy

Several investigators have described movements of the larynx and related structures in patients with spasmodic dysphonia (Ludlow, et al., 1988; McCall, Skolnick, & Brewer, 1971; Schaffer, 1983). In the study by Woodson et al. (1991), the presence of extrinsic muscle hyperfunction was noted along with intrinsic laryngeal muscle hyperfunction tremor and spasms at rest. Thirty-five of the 38 subjects studied exhibited intrinsic hyperfunction, specifically, excessive arytenoid adduction. Twenty-nine of the 38 patients had laryngeal or pharyngeal tremor; in 19, tremor was also observed at rest. Extrinsic muscle hyperfunction, including false vocal fold adduction and anterior-posterior compression of the glottis, was present in 33 of 38 patients. Thus, visual observation demonstrates that, along with the abrupt vocal fold closures, a constellation of intrinsic and extrinsic muscle hyperfunction behaviors exists during phonation and at rest.

Acoustic Analysis

Acoustic analysis of spasmodic dysphonia must take into account both sustained phonation and contextual speech. The fundamental frequency (F_0) characteristics of patients with SD are similar to those of non-SD patients (Miller & Woodson, 1991) with the possible exception of a reduced F_0 range in the SD group. However, other acoustic measures such as the standard deviation of the fundamental frequency and jitter (measured in milliseconds) and shimmer are significantly higher in patients with SD. The measure of signal-to-noise ratio is generally lower in patients with SD than in normal controls.

Ludlow and Conner (1987) reported acoustic evidence of a movement disorder in spasmodic dysphonia. They found that patients with SD were slow to achieve phonation onset, although they had no difficulty with the onset of a nonvocal laryngeal movement using a reaction time paradigm. Others have found that patients with SD speak slower (Ludlow et al., 1988) and have slower reaction times (Reich & Till, 1983).

Zwirner, Murry, Swenson, and Woodson (1991) have used the term "voice break factor" to describe the breaks in phonation of patients with SD. This measure, which is defined as the number of voice breaks divided by the maximum phonation time, reflects the stability of phonation without the confounding factors of contextual speech or length of speech sample. Although spasmodic dysphonia differs significantly from normal phonation and other neurological disorders, it should be kept in mind that acoustic measures alone should not be regarded as diagnostic tests for SD but rather as an indication of vocal function (Zwirner et al., 1991).

Aerodynamics

The characteristic description of spasmodic dysphonia as being a strained-strangled type of phonation would suggest that airflow is reduced and/or disrupted. In adductor SD, mean airflow rates have been shown to range from normal to extremely low (Zwirner, Murry, Swenson, & Woodson, 1992).

When patients with adductor spasmodic dysphonia are injected with botulinum toxin, airflow rates increase to normal or above normal values. Moreover, the sudden drops in airflow associated with spasms are virtually eliminated. In abductor spasmodic dysphonia mean phonatory airflow rate is generally above normal (i.e.,

greater that 220 cc/sec) with bursts of airflow occurring with the abductor spasm. Data for airflow patterns in abductor SD generally indicate that flow rates decrease after botulinum toxin injection.

Subglottal pressure measures were estimated from esophageal pressure recordings in two patients with adductor spasmodic dysphonia (Miller, Woodson, & Jancovic, 1989) and found to be in the range 40–50 cm H_2O. After BOTOX® injections these values dropped to a normal range of 3.5–5.0 cm H_2O.

It is apparent that it is necessary to examine aerodynamic parameters associated with SD before and after treatment. Phonatory airflow rate may be a useful clinical parameter for monitoring the treatment of SD because changes in airflow rate would reflect changes in glottal resistance. Moreover, reduced variability in the airflow rate pattern may be useful in describing the stability of voice production after treatment. The changes in subglottal air pressure and airflow rate ultimately may provide objective, noninvasive indications of vocal function.

Electromyographic Analysis

Electromyographic data have been reported for patients with adductor spasmodic dysphonia (Blitzer et al., 1985; Ludlow, Baker, Naughton, & Hallett, 1987; Schaffer, 1983; Shipp, Izdebski, Reed, & Morrissey, 1985) and for abductor SD (Finitzo & Freeman, 1989; Watson et al., 1991). In adductor SD, there are generally increased peak and activation levels of the intrinsic muscles (thyroarytenoid and cricothyroid). Ludlow and Connor (1987) found this during quiet respiration as well as phonation. However, when comparing the increase in activity between the minimum and maximum activation during the respiratory cycles, Ludlow et al. (1987) found that the SD group had the same proportional increase as the normal control group.

Little data are available for large numbers of subjects with abductor spasmodic dysphonia. From the data of Finitzo and Freeman (1989) and Watson, MacIntire, Roark, and Schaffer, (1992), it appears that high levels of activity are present in both the posterior cricoarytenoid and the thyroarytenoid muscles. As yet, qualitative and quantitative analysis of the EMG signals from patients with abductor SD do not differentiate this group from the adductor patients with SD. It may be that subjects with SD, regardless of the perceived symptoms (i.e., abductor or adductor), show abnormalities in the adductor musculature. EMG findings may be interpreted to indicate that SD represents a common neuropathophysiology which is unrelated to the acoustic/perceptual signs and symptoms or that there may be neurological subtypes that are not related to perceived signs. It is important to keep in mind that abnormal muscle activity varies with different tasks as well as within tasks. As the complex neurophysiology of this disorder becomes further understood, the use of EMG for diagnostic purposes in SD may prove highly valuable in directing treatment. With the use of EMG, treatment may be directed toward altering neuromotor performance rather than attempting to effect a change in the acoustic, perceptual, or aerodynamic output.

SOCIAL IMPLICATIONS

Emotional

Spasmodic dysphonia is debilitating from a socioeconomic as well as from a communication standpoint. When one considers the psychosocial aspects of trying to speak with intermittent voice breaks, reduced loudness, and increased effort, one can imagine the number of limitations that SD produces, from cheering at a sporting event to talking in a restaurant, department store, or in a car where background noise is present. It is not un-

common to review case histories that outline an individual's withdrawal from social settings due to the inability to be heard above the ambient noise or due to continuous questions about his or her health or simply being asked, "What's wrong with your voice?" Patients report the need to change jobs due to the inability to meet the communication demands whether they are answering a telephone, conducting staff meetings, or teaching in a classroom. In clinics where a significant number of patients with SD have been treated, reports of job changes or even retirement by athletic coaches, ministers, teachers, and dispatchers are far too common. Of further significance is the social aspect of speech and voice. Patients report less social interaction over the telephone, at work, or church and even at home with their spouses. The uncertainty of the voice, the anticipation of the voice breaks, and the need to explain to the listener that one does not have a cold nor does it "hurt to talk" tends to lead to a life of increasing silence and iconoclasm.

Psychosocial

Early descriptions of spasmodic (spastic) dysphonia often characterized the patient as nervous, withdrawn, and/or tense. More recent examinations of patients suggest that, although anxiety and depression levels may be elevated in as many as 50% of those with spasmodic dysphonia, the emotional changes are the result of, rather than the basis for, the disorder. Murry, Cannito, and Woodson (1994) report that, following successful treatment of spasmodic dysphonia with botulinum toxin, patients who were clinically anxious or depressed showed a significant reduction in both measures. Figure 16–1 shows that patients exhibiting mild depression had a reduction in state anxiety (the anxiety associated with a particular state such as talking) and trait anxiety (the anxiety associated with basic person-

Anxiety

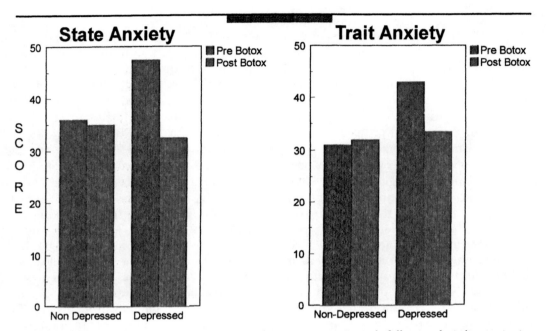

FIGURE 16-1. Changes in state anxiety and trait anxiety 1 week following botulinum toxin injection. (Data from *Spasmodic Dysphonia's Emotional Status and Botulinum Toxin Treatment* by T. Murry, M. Cannito, and G. E. Woodson, 1994, *Journal of Voice, 9*, 310–316.).

ality traits) 1 week following botulinum injection and subsequent reduction of the strained, strangled voice quality.

Despite the fact that the patients did not have completely normal voices, they reported increased voice use, reconsideration of returning to work, and a reduction in communication avoidance, especially on the telephone. Through patient interviews, the authors found that the persistence of breathiness or softness did not carry the same interference with speaking as did the voice breaks and the perceptually strained quality associated with adductor spasmodic dysphonia. Although continued study of the emotional effects of SD is warranted, it is clear that reduction of symptoms in a vast majority of patients influences the patient's psychological condition.

TREATMENT: OPTIONS AND OUTCOMES

Prior to the use of botulinum toxin, treatment of spasmodic dysphonia was attempted through speech therapy or surgical lysis of one recurrent laryngeal nerve. Although neither speech therapy nor recurrent laryngeal nerve resection offered a completely normal voice, both offered some relief from the strained-strangled voice associated with adductor spasmodic dysphonia.

Surgical Treatment

Dedo (1976) introduced a surgical transection of the recurrent laryngeal nerve as treatment for adductor spasmodic dysphonia. This procedure results in a paralysis of one vocal fold which reduces the laryngeal tightness and increases flow of air through the glottis. Early results were quite encouraging to many despite the lack of a completely normal voice. However, Levine, Wood, Batza, Rusnov, and Tucker (1979) and Aronson and Hartman (1981) reported less success with this procedure when the patients were reassessed over a longer term. They reported excess breathiness as well as return of tightness and adductor spasms, sometimes more severe than the original problem. The return of spasms has been explained by regeneration of the nerve over time as seen in canine studies (Crumley, 1990). Dedo and Izdebski (1984) described vocal fold "thinning" with a laser to treat recurrent spasm and Teflon® injection for the persistent breathiness problem. Although recurrent laryngeal nerve resection offers an improvement for many with adductor spasmodic dysphonia, there are no acceptable selection criteria to predict long-term results. General enthusiasm for the procedure has waned in recent years.

Pharmacologic Treatment

The use of botulinum toxin A (oculinum) for treatment of spasmodic dysphonia evolved out of the success of treating other muscle movement disorders. The principle behind this approach was that injection of botulinum toxin (BOTOX®) into a muscle produces a temporary paralysis or paresis. When injected into the thyroarytenoid muscle for the treatment of adductor spasmodic dysphonia, there is a resultant reduction or elimination of the adductor spasms and an increase in the average breath flow rate during speech. The result of the injection is a 3- to 8-month reduction of spasms and improved phonation. For abductor spasms, BOTOX® is injected into the posterior cricoarytenoid muscle to reduce the abductor spasms.

The intracellular molecular mechanism of action of the botulinum toxin is not fully understood. It acts presynaptically at the motor end plate to block the release of acetylcholine, thereby preventing muscle activation and contraction. Depending on the number of end plates involved, the result is either paresis or paralysis. In treating both SD and blepharospasm, it has been noted that botulinum toxin reduces spasm on both the injected (paretic) and the noninjected (grossly unweakened) side. This is likely a central effect on the feedback control of muscle activity (Sanders, Massey, & Buckley, 1985).

Injection of BOTOX® for SD is usually performed percutaneously, using EMG guidance, but may also be accomplished per orally, via mirror or flexible laryngoscope (Ford, Bless, & Lowery, 1989). The EMG technique utilizes a small gauge hypodermic needle, insulated except at the hub and tip, to serve as the both the electrode and the port of injection. Lidocaine may be used sparingly and superficially to anesthetize the skin, taking care to avoid diffusion to underlying muscles or motor nerves.

For adductor spasms, the needle is passed through the skin overlying the superior edge of the cricoid, and advanced through the cricothyroid membrane into the right or left vocal fold to reach the thyroarytenoid muscle. By entering slightly off the midline, the injection usually can be accomplished totally submucosally, without entering the airway. This minimizes discomfort and complicating reflexes, such as cough or spasm. The oscilloscope and auditory output of the EMG apparatus are monitored to detect muscle activity. When crisp action potentials are obtained with phonation and not with neck flexion or breathing, needle position in a laryngeal adductor muscle is confirmed. Once the position is assured, the toxin is slowly injected. Although the dosage of toxin ranges widely, from as little as 0.625 to as high as 50 units, the dilution should be adjusted to keep the volume of the injection to between 0.1 to 0.3 cc.

To reach the posterior cricoarytenoid muscle for treatment of abductor spasmodic dysphonia, the larynx is rotated manually to move the anterior larynx away from the side of interest. The posterior cricoid cartilage is located by palpation, and the EMG needle is passed through the lateral neck skin and advanced just superficial to the cricoid cartilage. Care is taken to avoid the vascular sheath, including the carotid artery, jugular vein, and vagus nerve. As for adductor injection, the EMG output is monitored to detect activation. PCA placement is confirmed by activation during inhalation. Clinical experience with PCA injection is far more limited than that for thyroarytenoid injection.

The results of botulinum toxin may be best described by their effects on the vocal output after injection. Adductor spasmodic dysphonia is far more common than abductor and the reports of improvement in spasmodic dysphonia are generally reported for larger numbers of adductor patients. Ludlow et al. (1988) reported significant reductions in pitch and voice breaks in addition to phonatory periodicity and sentence duration in 16 patients with adductor spasmodic dysphonia 2 weeks after botulinum toxin injection. These authors also reported a reduction in speech volume.

Zwirner et al. (1992) examined acoustic parameters, airflow rate, and videoendoscopic changes 1 week and 1 month after BOTOX® injection in 11 patients. They found that four acoustic measures, standard deviation of the fundamental frequency, jitter, shimmer, and signal-to-noise ratio all improved at 1 week after injection with further improvement 1 month after injection. The most significant improvements were in the fundamental frequency standard deviation, shimmer, and signal-to-noise ratio. In addition, they obtained a measure of irregular stoppages which they called the "voice break factor." This is defined as the number of voice breaks (signal stoppage with a length longer than two cycles divided by the fundamental frequency) divided by

the maximum phonation time (MPT). The voice break factor was significantly reduced 1 week after injection and was very near to zero at 1 month post-injection.

Figure 16–2 shows the results of mean airflow rate prior to and following BOTOX® injection. Prior to injection, the 11 Patients with SD had significantly lower mean airflow rates during phonation than a matched group of control subjects. One week following BOTOX® injection, mean airflow rates increased to a level generally associated with the flow rates found in vocal fold paralysis. One month after injection, however, the flow rates of the SD group were only slightly higher than those of the normal controls.

Zwirner et al. (1992) also obtained ratings for intrinsic and extrinsic laryngeal muscle hyperfunction and indications of underlying movement disorders from endoscopic recordings made prior to injection and 1 week and 1 month after injection. A four-point scale described by Woodson et al. (1991) with 0 equal to normal and 3 equal to highly abnormal was used to obtain the ratings. Table 16–3 summarizes the ratings. Intrinsic muscle parameters and signs of neurologic involvement were significantly reduced after injection. However, the extrinsic parameters did not change. It should be noted from Table 16–3 that the primary response was one week after injection.

Murry, Zwirner, and Woodson (1991) and Zwirner, Murry, and Woodson (1993b) also reported on the effects of unilateral and bilateral BOTOX® injections in adductor spasmodic dysphonia. When injected unilaterally, a dosage of approximately 5–10 units produced significantly improved phonation in the majority of patients. A bilateral injection of 1.25 units on each side was found to be sufficient for improved phonation. The major differences in the unilateral versus bilateral injections are the patterns of change in the jitter, standard deviation of the fundamental frequency and the mean airflow rate. The differences obtained from 24 pa-

MEAN AIRFLOW RATE

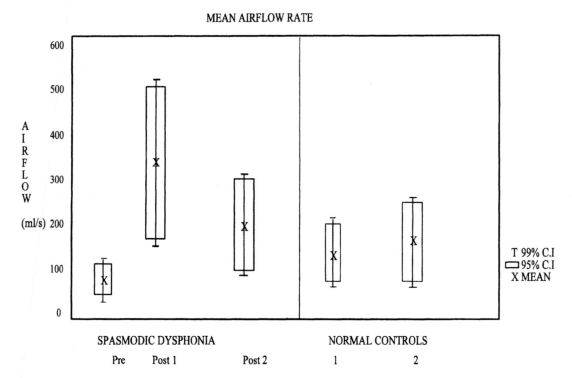

FIGURE 16–2. Effect of BOTOX® injection on the mean airflow rate. Confidence intervals (CI) of 99% and 95% and mean values for the mean airflow ratio (in ml/sec) for the spasmodic dysphonia group before (pre) and 1 week (post 1) and 1 month (post 2) after unilateral BOTOX® injection and the two trials (1, 2) within a 2-week interval for the normal control group. (Data from Effects of Botulinum Toxin in Patients with Adductor Spasmodic Dysphonia: Acoustic, Aerodynamic, and Videoendoscopic Findings by P. Zwirner, T. Murry, and M. Swenson, 1992. *Laryngoscope, 102*(4), 400–406.)

tients with adductor spasmodic dysphonia are presented in Figure 16–3.

In the unilateral injection, there is a significant drop in jitter and F_0 standard deviation 1 week after injection, whereas in the bilateral injection, jitter increases somewhat and the F_0 standard deviation has a statistically nonsignificant drop. For mean airflow rate, the rise in mean airflow rate 1 week after injection is approximately 10 times that of the preinjection levels in the bilateral group whereas it is four times greater than the preinjection levels in the unilateral group. One month following injection, flow rates are nearly the same for both groups.

It should also be pointed out that there is an increase in reported tempo-rary aspiration in the bilateral group compared to the unilateral group. Although there are no definite criteria for selecting a unilateral versus bilateral injection, it appears that patients with more severe symptoms are best managed by bilateral injections because a greater effect (i.e., increased airflow rate and reduced voice break factor) is produced with less toxin injected bilaterally compared to a unilateral injection. When the patient presents with a mild or moderate condition of spasmodic dysphonia, a unilateral dose achieves reduced spasms with an acceptable level of breathiness.

To understand more about the mechanisms of persisting vocal dysfunction ollowing BOTOX® injection, Woodson et

Table 16-3. Means *(M)* and Standard Deviations *(SDs)* of videolaryngoscopic rating scores of nine parameters assessing three categories of dysfunction: Intrinsic hyperfunction (intrinsic), extrinsic hyperfunction (extrinsic), and indicators of underlying movement disorders (neurologic), and total score for each category of dysfunction.

Parameters	Pre-BOTOX®	Postinjection 1 Week M (SD)	Postinjection 1 Month M (SD)
Intrinsic			
Hyperadduction	1.7 (0.7)	0.5 (0.7)*	0.6 (0.4)*
Rigidity	1.3 (0.4)	0.3 (0.8)*	0.3 (0.4)*
Abduction	0.1 (0.3)	0	0
Total Score	3.1 (1.1)	0.8 (1.4)*	0.9 (0.8)*
Extrinsic			
False closure	1.3 (0.9)	1.0 (0.6)	1.1 (0.8)
AP compression	1.3 (0.9)	1.2 (0.9)	1.3 (0.6)
Epiglottis spasms	0.5 (0.9)	0.6 (1.0)	0.1 (0.1)
Total Score	3.1 (2.0)	2.8 (1.4)	2.5 (1.3)
Neurologic			
Tremor with phonation	1.3 (0.8)	0.3 (0.4)*	0.4 (0.7)*
Tremor with respiration	0.5 (0.5)	0.2 (0.5)	0.1 (0.3)
Spasms with respiration	0.4 (0.5)	0.2 (0.5)	0.1 (0.3)
Total Score	2.2 (1.1)	0.7 (1.4)*	0.6 (1.0)*

*Significantly lower than pre-BOTOX® injection ($p < .05$).

Source: Data from Effects of Botulinum Toxin in Patients with Adductor Spasmodic Dysphonia: Acoustic, Aerodynamic, and Videoendoscopic Findings by P. Zwirner, T. Murry, M. Swenson, and G. E. Woodson, 1992. *Laryngoscope, 102*(4), 401–406.

al. (1991) performed detailed analyses of videolaryngoscopy of 17 patients before and after injection. Video segments were randomized on a cassette and then evaluated by three independent observers without knowledge of the recording condition. Excessive glottic closure and vocal fold rigidity were evaluated as indicators of intrinsic laryngeal muscle spasm. Extrinsic laryngeal activity was also assessed. Tremor was detected and scored. After BOTOX® injection, intrinsic laryngeal muscle hyperfunction was abolished or diminished in all cases. Mean tremor score was reduced, but not all patients improved. Extrinsic muscle hyperfunction was not significantly improved: it was judged to be worse in three patients. This suggests that the results of BOTOX® may improve if tremor was controlled and extrinsic muscle hyperfunction was treated with voice therapy.

Other factors may limit the success of BOTOX® injection. The weakening of the muscle by the toxin reduces or eliminates the spasms at the expense of volume. Some patients are uncomfortable with the reduced vocal volume or with the amount of breathiness present. It is important that the patient understand the tradeoff so as not to be disappointed with a soft voice despite the elimination of the spasms. Along with reduced volume, patients may experience reduced inflection or other limitations of vocal output that do not allow them to have a completely normal voice.

Results of BOTOX® injection to treat abductor spasmodic dysphonia are less encouraging than for adductor dyspho-

Jitter

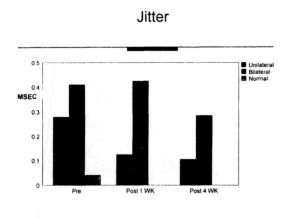

SDFO

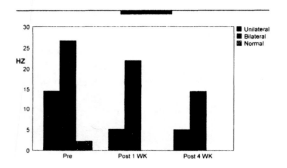

Mean Air Flow Rate

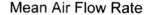

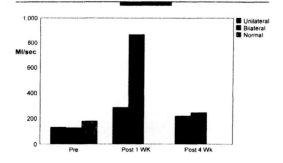

FIGURE 16–3. Mean jitter (msec), standard deviation of the fundamental frequency (Hz), and mean airflow rate (ml/sec) ratio (dB) for two groups of patients with adductor spasmodic dysphonia (unilateral, *n* = 11; bilateral, *n* = 11) and a group of normal controls (*n* = 10). The SD patients were seen prior to injection and 1 week and 1 month after BOTOX® injection.

nia. The abductor muscle, the posterior cricoarytenoid, is located between the larynx and pharynx and is more difficult to inject. The treatment also has a greater potential for complications related to aspiration because of the proximity of the pharyngeal constrictors. If the toxin is subject to migration, as suggested earlier, the swallowing mechanisms as well as the airway may be at risk. Injection of the cricothyroid muscle, located in the anterior larynx is less risky and may be beneficial to control abductor dysphonia.

Blitzer, Brin, Stewart, Aviv, and Fahn (1992) reported on 32 patients with abductor spasmodic dysphonia. Most patients required bilateral posterior cricoarytenoid muscle injection and improved to an average of 70% normal function, less than that observed in patients treated for adductor dysphonia. Ten patients also received cricothyroid muscle injection and/or Type 1 thyroplasty resulting in further improvement.

Woodson and Murry (1993) have treated eight patients with abductor spasmodic dysphonia. All have required frequent, bilateral injection with the duration of the benefit lasting only 4–8 weeks. The presence of breathy voice breaks, diaphragmatic spasms, and low vocal volume have been observed in these patients following botulinum toxin injection. In general, abductor SD appears to be a more complex syndrome, with frequent involvement of respiratory muscles, and intermittent or sustained failure of activation of adductor muscles during phonation. This may explain the less consistent improvement of patients treated with BOTOX® for abductor SD.

Speech Pathology

In the early stages of spasmodic dysphonia, voice therapy is often recommended. It may serve to reduce the severity of the spasms under controlled speaking conditions. It may also serve diagnostically to indicate the severity of the problem beyond the information obtained from objective data. Voice therapy for adductor spasmodic dysphonia relies on techniques that reduce the tightness in the laryngeal area. By reducing the tightness, and consequently increasing the breath flow rate, the pitch breaks and spasms may be reduced. Other techniques suggested include the use of a whisper voice (probably impractical for most speaking situations although it works well in the therapy environment), speaking on inhalation, establishing easy voice onset, and speaking with an overall higher pitch (Freeman, Cannito, & Finitizo-Hieber, 1985).

Few objective data suggest that therapy techniques are carried over outside of the clinic. The use of biofeedback instruments as well as listening to one's own samples of clear voice may also help; nonetheless, most patients report little lasting success with voice therapy. In general, patients who feel that treatment was helpful were in therapy for a long time with a dedicated clinician. A further complication to voice therapy is the need to be ever vigilant in controlling the speech output. This often leads to frustration in the long term despite some short-term benefits. Patients even report an unwillingness to use a different pitch level, altered prosody or rate to overcome the spasms because these changes are perceived by the patient as "not my voice." A recent report of 17 patients by Murry and Woodson (1995) suggests that patients with adductor SD significantly lengthen their time between injections when as few as five voice therapy sessions are given after the first injection. They found a mean increase of 12.5 weeks between injections for patients undergoing a voice therapy program based on symptom reduction of hyperfunctional, supraglottic phonation. In addition, they reported evidence of carryover to later injections compared to a group that received only BOTOX® with no voice therapy.

For abductor spasmodic dysphonia, there is even less information regarding voice therapy. The goal of voice therapy is to increase the consistency of adduction. This can be accomplished by practicing materials devoid of voiceless consonants. By gradually inserting voiceless consonants into the practice material, the patient may learn to abduct and adduct the vocal folds consistent with the voiceless and voiced intervals of the speech material.

There are occasional anecdotal reports describing improvement of spasmodic dysphonia after voice therapy; however, there is little evidence that voice therapy alone has a long-term benefit for adductor or abductor spasmodic dysphonia. Lack of success and frustration in therapy experienced by both patients and clinicians has prompted the search for other methods of treating this problem.

SUMMARY

Although the use of botulinum toxin has given patients with spasmodic dysphonia functional voice use for extended periods of time and has enhanced our knowledge of the disorder, the key to understanding this disorder is to understand the pathophysiology of spasmodic dysphonia and the pathophysiology of spasmodic movement disorders. The success of implantable laryngeal nerve stimulators (Freedman et al., 1988) along with the combined approaches of laryngeal surgery and/or voice therapy as treatment methods for spasmodic dysphonia remains to be explored as treatment tools. In the course of these increased treatment options, a more thorough knowledge of the disorder within the framework of other focal dystonias may be developed.

Research in spasmodic dysphonia should include efforts to determine its etiology and pathophysiology and to search for associated defects which, if corrected, could improve function in these patients. Such research may involve extensive imaging, electrophysiologic, and biochemical studies.

REFERENCES

Aminoff, M. J., Dedo, H. H., & Izdebski, K. (1978). Clinical aspects of spasmodic dysphonia. *Journal of Neurology, Neurosurgery and Psychiatry, 41,* 361–365.

Arnold, G. E., (1959). Spastic dysphonia I: Changing interpretations of a persistent affliction. *Logos, 2,* 3–14.

Aronson, A. (1977). *Psychogenic voice disorders.* Philadelphia: W. B. Saunders.

Aronson, A. (1980). *Clinical voice disorders: An interdisciplinary approach.* New York: Thieme.

Aronson, A. E. (1979). Spastic dysphonia: Retrospective study of one hundred patients. Unpublished manuscript.

Aronson, A. E., Brown, J. R., Litin, E. M., & Pearson, J. S. (1968). Spastic dysphonia II: Comparison with essential (voice) tremor and other neurologic and psychogenic dysphonias. *Journal of Speech and Hearing Disorders, 33,* 219–231.

Aronson, A., & DeSanto, L. W. (1983). Adductor spastic dysphonia: three years after recurrent laryngeal nerve resection. *Laryngoscope, 93,* 1–8.

Aronson, A. E., & Hartman, D. E. (1981). Adductor spastic dysphonia as a sign of essential (voice) tremor. *Journal of Speech and Hearing Disorders, 46,* 52–58.

Aronson, A. E. (1985). *Clinical voice disorders* (2nd ed.). New York: Thieme.

Basmajian, J. V., & DeLuca, C., (1985). *Muscles alive: Their function revealed by electromyography* (5th ed.). Baltimore: Williams & Wilkins.

Blitzer, A., Lovelace, R. E., Brin, M., Fahn, S., & Fink, M. (1985). Electromyographic findings in focal laryngeal dystonias (spastic dysphonia). *Annals of Otology, Rhinology and Laryngology, 94,* 591–594.

Blitzer, A., Brin, M. F., Fahn, S., & Lovelace, R. E. (1988a). Clinical and laboratory characteristics of focal laryngeal dystonias: Study of 110 cases. *Laryngoscope, 98,* 636–640.

Blitzer, A., Brin, M., Fahn, S., & Lovelace, R. E. (1988b). Localized injections of botulinum toxin for the treatment of focal laryngeal dystonia (spastic dysphonia). *Laryngoscope, 96,* 193–197.

Blitzer, A., Brin, M. F., Stewart, C., Aviv, J., & Fahn, S. (1992). Adductor laryngeal dystonia: A series treated with botulinum toxin. *Laryngoscope, 102,* 163–167.

Boone, D. (1971). *The voice and voice therapy.* Englewood Cliffs, NJ: Prentice.

Brodnitz, F. S. (1976). Spastic dysphonia. *Annals of Otology, Rhinology and Laryngology, 85,* 210–214.

Burton, K., Farrell, K., Li, D., & Calne, D. B. (1984). Lesions of the putamen and dystonia: CT and magnetic resonance imaging. *Neurology, 34,* 962–965.

Cannito, M., & Johnson, J. (1981). Spastic dysphonia: A continuum disorder. *Journal of Communicative Disorders, 14,* 216–223.

Critchley, M. (1939). Spastic dysphonia in inspiratory speech. *Brain, 62,* 96–103.

Crumley, R. (1990). Regeneration of the recurrent laryngeal nerve. *Otolaryngology—Head and Neck Surgery, 90,* 442–447.

Dedo, H. H. (1976). Recurrent laryngeal nerve section for spastic dysphonia. *Annals of Otology, Rhinology and Laryngology, 85,* 451–459.

Dedo, H. H., & Izdebski, K. (1984). Evaluation and treatment of recurrent spasticity after recurrent laryngeal nerve section: A preliminary report. *Annals of Otology, Rhinology and Laryngology, 93,* 343–345.

Dordain, M., & Dordain, G. (1972). L'epreuve du "a" tenu au cours des tremblements de le voix (tremblement idiopathique et dyskinesie volitionnelle, leurs rapports avec la dysphonie spasmodique). *Revue, Laryngologie, Otologie, Rhinologie, 93,* 167–182.

Feldman, M., Nixon, J. V., Finitzo-Hieber, T., & Freeman, F. J. (1984). Abnormal parasympathetic vagal function in patients with spasmodic dysphonia. *Annals of Internal Medicine, 100*(4), 491–495.

Finitzo, T., & Freeman, F. (1989). Spasmodic dysphonia, whether and where: Results of seven years of research. *Journal of Speech and Hearing Research, 32,* 541–555.

Ford, C. N., Bless, D. M., & Lowery, J. D. (1989). Treatment of spasmodic dysphonia with visually directed minimal injections of botulinum toxin. *Otolaryngology—Head and Neck Surgery, 101,* 161.

Freedman, M., Toriumi, D. M., Grybaukus, V. T., et al., (1988). Implantation of a recurrent laryngeal nerve stimulator for treatment of spasmodic dysphonia. *Annals of Otology, Rhinology and Laryngology, 98,* 193–197.

Freeman, F. J., Cannito, M. P., & Finitizo-Hieber, T. (1984). Classification of spasmodic dysphonia by perceptual-acoustic-visual means. In G. A. Gates (Ed.), *Spasmodic dysphonia: State of the art 1984* (pp. 5–13). New York: The Voice Foundation.

Freeman, F., Cannito, M. P., & Finitizo-Hieber, T. (1985). Getting to know spasmodic dysphonia patients. *Texas Journal of Audiology and Speech Pathology, 10,* 14–19.

Heaver, L. (1959). Spastic dysphonia II. Psychiatric considerations. *Logos, 2,* 16–24.

Hornykiewicz, O., Kish, S. J., Becker, L. E., Farley, I., Shannon, K. (1986). Brain neurotransmitters in dystonia musculorum deformans. *New England Journal of Medicine, 316,* 347–353.

Jankovic, J., & Patel, S. C. (1983). Blepharospasm associated with brain stem lesions. *Neurology, 33,* 1237–1240.

Jankovic, J., Svendson, C. N., & Bird, E. D. (1988). Brain neurotransmitters in dystonia. *New England Journal of Medicine, 316,* 278–279.

Levine, H., Wood, B. G., Batza, E., Rusnov, M., & Tucker, H. (1979). Recurrent laryngeal nerve section for spasmodic dysphonia. *Annals of Otology, Rhinology, and Laryngology, 88,* 527–530.

Ludlow, C., & Conner, N. (1987). Dynamic aspects of phonatory control in spasmodic dysphonia. *Journal of Speech and Hearing Research, 30*(2), 197-206.

Ludlow, C. L., Baker, M., Naughton, R. P., Hallett, M. (1987). Intrinsic laryngeal muscle activation in spasmodic dysphonia. In R. Benecke, B. Conrad, & C. D. Marsden (Eds.), *Motor disturbances* (pp. 119–130). New York: Academic Press.

Ludlow, C. L., Naughton, R. F., Sedory, S. E., Schulz, G. M., & Hallett, M. (1988). Effects of botulinum toxin injections on speech in adductor spasmodic dysphonia. *Neurology, 38,* 1220–1225.

Ludlow, C. F., Hallett, M., Sedory, S. E., Fujita, M., & Naughton, R. F. (1990). The pathophysiology of spasmodic dysphonia and its modification by botulinum toxin. In A. Berardelli & R. Benecke (Eds.), *Motor disturbances II* (pp. 274–288). London: Academic Press.

McCall, G. N., Skolnick, M. D., & Brewer, D. W. (1971). A preliminary report on some atypical movement patterns in the tongue, palate, hypopharynx, and larynx of patients with spasmodic dysphonia. *Journal of Speech and Hearing Disorders, 36,* 446–470.

Miller, R. H., & Woodson, G. E. (1991). Treatment options in spasmodic dysphonia. In J. A. Kaufman & G. Issacson (Eds.), *Otolaryngology Clinics of North America: Voice Disorders, 24*(5), 1227–1237. Philadelphia: W. B. Saunders.

Miller, R. H., Woodson, G .E., & Jancovic, J. (1989). Botulinum toxin injection of the vocal fold for spasmodic dysphonia: A preliminary report. *Archives of Otolaryngology—Head and Neck Surgery, 113,* 603–605.

Murry, T., Zwirner, P., & Woodson, G. E., (1991). *Unilateral v. bilateral botulinum toxin treatment.* Presented at the Pacific Voice Conference, San Francisco, CA.

Murry, T., Cannito, M., & Woodson, G. E. (1994). Spasmodic dysphonia's emotional status and botulinum toxin treatment. *Archives of Otolaryngology—Head and Neck Surgery, 120,* 310–316.

Murry, T., Woodson, & G. E. (1995). Combined-modality treatment of adductor spasmodic dysphonia with Botulinum toxin and voice therapy. *Journal of Voice, 9,* 460–465.

Nygaard, T. G. (1989). Dopa-responsive dystonia: 20 years into the L-dopa era. In N. P. Quinn & P. G. Jenner (Eds.), *Disorders of movement: Clinical and physiological aspects* (pp. 323–337). London: Academic Press.

Ozelius, L., Kramer, P. L., & Moskowitz, C. B. (1989). Human gene to torsion dystonia located on chromosome 9q32-34. *Neuron, 2,* 1427–1434.

Parnes, S. M., Lavarato, A. B., & Myers, E. N. (1978). Study of spastic dysphonia using video fiberoptic laryngoscope. *Annals of Otology, Rhinology, and Laryngology, 87,* 322–326.

Rabuzzi, D., & McCall, G. (1972). Spasmodic dysphonia. *Transactions of the American Academy of Opthalmology and Otolaryngology, 76,* 724–728.

Reich, A., & Till, J. (1983). Phonatory and manual reaction times of women with idiopathic spasmodic dysphonia. *Journal of Speech and Hearing Research, 26,* 10–18.

Robe, E., Brumlik, J., & Moore, P., (1960). A study of spastic dysphonia. *Laryngoscope, 93,* 1183–1202.

Rosenfield, D. B., Donovan,D. T., Suleck, M., Viswanath, N. S., Inbody, G. P., & Nudelman, H. B. (1991). Neurologic aspects of spasmodic dysphonia. *Journal of Otolaryngology, 19*, 231–236.

Sanders, D. B., Massey, E. W., & Buckley, E. R. (1985). Botulinum toxin for blepharospasm, single fiber EMG studies. *Neurology, 35*, 271–272.

Schaffer, S. D. (1983). Neuropathology of spasmodic dysphonia. *Laryngoscope, 93*, 1183–1204.

Sharbrough, F. W., Stockard, J. J., & Aronson, A. E. (1978). Brain stem auditory evoked responses in spastic dysphonia. *TransAmerican Neurology Association, 103*, 198–201.

Shipp. T., Izdebski, K., Reed, C., & Morrissey, P. (1985). Intrinsic laryngeal muscle activity in a spastic dysphonia patient. In R. Benecke, B. Conrad, & C. D. Marsden (Eds.), *Motor disturbances I* (pp. 119–130). New York: Academic Press.

Swenson, M., Zwirner, P., Murry, T., & Woodson, G. E. (1992). Medical evaluation of patients with spasmodic dysphonia. *Journal of Voice, 6*, 320–324.

Traube, L. (1871). Spastische Form de nervosen Heiserkeit. *Gesammelte Beitrage, Pathology and Physiology* (Berlin), *2*, 677.

Watson, B. D., Schaffer, S. D., Freeman, F. J., Kondraske, G. V., Dembowski, J. D., & Roark, R. M. (1991). Laryngeal electromyographic activity in abductor and adductor spasmodic dysphonia. *Journal of Speech and Hearing Research, 34*, 473–482.

Watson, B. E., MacIntire, D., Roark, R. M., & Schaffer, S. P. (1992). *Statistical modelling of electromyographic activity in spasmodic dysphonia and normal control subjects.* Paper presented at the American Speech-Language-Hearing Association, San Antonio, TX.

Woodson, G. E., & Murry, T. (1993) A review of 155 cases of spasmodic dysphonia. Unpublished manuscript.

Woodson, G. E., Zwirner, P., Murry, T., & Swenson, M. (1991). Use of flexible laryngoscopy to classify patients with spasmodic dysphonia. *Journal of Voice, 5*, 85–91.

Zwirner, P., Murry, T., Swenson, M., & Woodson, G. E. (1991). Acoustic changes in spasmodic dysphonia after botulinum toxin injection. *Journal of Voice, 5*, 78–84.

Zwirner, P., Murry, T., Swenson, M., & Woodson, G. E. (1992). Effects of botulinum toxin therapy in patients with adductor spasmodic dysphonia: Acoustic, aerodynamic and videoendoscopic findings. *Laryngoscope, 102*(4), 400–406.

Zwirner, P., Murry, T., & Woodson, G. E., (1993a). Perceptual-acoustic relationships in spasmodic dysphonia. *Journal of Voice, 7*(2), 165–171.

Zwirner, P., Murry, T., & Woodson, G. E. (1993b). A comparison of bilateral and unilateral botulinum toxin treatments for spasmodic dysphonia. *European Archives of Oto-Rhino-Laryngology, 250*, 271–276.

Index